NURSING ADMINISTRATION

NURSING ADMINISTRATION

Theory for practice with a systems approach

CLARA ARNDT, R.N., M.S.

Lecturer in Nursing Service Administration,
University of California,
Los Angeles, California

LOUCINE M. DADERIAN HUCKABAY, R.N., B.S., M.S., Ph.D.

Assistant Professor, School of Nursing,
University of California,
Los Angeles, California

Illustrated

The C. V. Mosby Company

Saint Louis   1975

Library of Congress Cataloging in Publication Data

Arndt, Clara, 1905-
  Nursing administration.

  Bibliography: p.
  Includes index.
  1. Nursing service administration. I. Huckabay,
Loucine M. Daderian, 1939-   joint author.
II. Title. [DNLM: 1. Nursing, Supervisory.
2. Organization and administration. WY105 A747n]
RT89.A76   658′.91′61073   75-4893
ISBN 0-8016-0312-9

CB/CB/B 9 8 7 6 5 4 3 2 1

FOREWORD

This book was developed during a time of unprecedented challenge for nurses who are engaged in coordinating, directing, and evaluating nursing services and education. Sweeping social changes are involving every segment of the health professions and the organizations designed to meet health needs. The external forces for change—consumer demands, scientific knowledge explosion, and rapid technical advances—coupled with the processes involved in creating a humanistic environment that fosters growth for every member of the nursing staff, mandate that a new and different approach be utilized for those in positions of leadership. The administrator cannot rely on a "bag of tricks," but must be well grounded in all aspects of the role. This book provides the theoretical background for effective administrative practice.

Within this volume the authors have identified and analyzed the major components of administration, utilizing a systems approach as their unifying theme.

They have drawn from several accepted major schools of thought and have used research findings as a basis for suggested action. Of, perhaps, most importance of all, they have provided viable alternatives for thought and action for both the novice and seasoned administrator.

Ms. Arndt and Dr. Huckabay have provided the profession of nursing with a unique profile of the knowledge base, skills, and personal attributes needed by each nurse administrator who desires to create and maintain a nursing care system for the delivery of optimum and individualized care to patients, as well as a system of nursing education designed to prepare creative, independent nurse practitioners for today and tomorrow.

Rheba de Tornyay, R.N., Ed.D.

Dean and Professor,
School of Nursing,
University of California,
Los Angeles

v

PREFACE

This book is based on the premise that administrative theory improves administrative action.

The significant expectation of an administrative theory, and for that matter of research, is that it will establish criteria for competence in administrative work and will also attract nurses of ability to whom the accountability for needed health care organizational success can be entrusted.

Administrative theory, well understood, is a basis for improving administrative action of all practicing nursing administrators. Knowledge of the functions of an administrator and of the concepts involved in planning, organizing, directing, and controlling is an essential prerequisite for the modern practicing nursing service administrator.

The ability to reflect all decisions against a background of knowledge of administrative theory is a powerful aid to an administrator in today's complex world of health care administration. The knowledge that administrators in other fields of work face the same problems gives all administrators the strength and depth of perception necessary to make them better administrators than those who ignore the lessons to be learned.

That is not to say that experience is always the best teacher and that lessons learned can be applied blindly. A student of administration knows that experience per se can be the poorest teacher if experience in one situation is applied to another without careful examination of all the conditions prevailing in each situation to ascertain that they are precisely the same.

The ability to test alternatives in a body of knowledge lends strength to the direction to be taken. When facts can be substituted for opinion, they certainly can prevail.

To the practicing nursing service administrators, theory forms the skeleton on which to build a body of knowledge; and when based on research, theory adds substance to that knowledge. In the human body the muscles provide the forces for action; likewise, in the administrator's body of knowledge the actions are energized by the forces of leadership, commitment, and competition. In the human body, the brain and the nerves provide the sensitivity and precision of action; similarly, in the administrator's body of knowledge the policies of integrity provide the sensitivity and acuity of observation necessary to direct the body of knowledge down the road to success.

Administrative theory and research are invaluable to the practicing administrator and to the student of administration, provided they are motivated by it. If the student is stimulated, this book has accomplished its mission.

This book, then, addresses itself to two audiences: practicing nurse administrators and nursing students interested in the field. This book is also very useful to the nursing practitioner in the clinical area and to supervisors and administrators of other health related agencies. Because the majority of persons filling the role of nursing service administrator are women, the pronoun she has been used in referring to this position. We intend no slight to the men who have entered this field in recent years.

Our purpose is to provide the practicing nursing service administrator and the student of nursing administration with a unique theoretical framework to use as a map or guide to action. Working with this model and operationalizing the different concepts will enable them to add to their own body of nursing knowledge. We have set forth a comprehensive but simple framework for the administrator of any health care system, an eclectic theory of administration that is general enough to apply to any administrative situation. This book is based on scientific research conducted by behavioral and management scientists, as well as by ourselves. Certain components of the administrative theory and the conceptual model that are presented in this book are original. Other aspects are synthesized in a manner to enable the nursing service administrator to put the theory to work.

We have taken into consideration the recommendations of Claude S. George, Jr., who pointed out in *The History of Management Thought* that a new theory is not needed but that there is a need for an evolving all-encompassing and eclectic theory of administration general enough to apply to any administrative situation and based on the following four schools of administrative thought: the scientific management school, the administrative process school, the behavioral science school, and the management science, or quantitative, school. In taking these recommendations into consideration, we found that three broad objectives for this book evolved: (1) to think of the administrative process as a complex of simultaneously variable factors rather than as a set of specific techniques,

(2) to incorporate knowledge of the several disciplines, and (3) to provide for economical ways of ordering practice.

Following the objectives, we find that theory is the constant but unseen companion of administration. No administrator can function long without it, yet few are aware that they use it. Fewer still can state what their theories are.

Much of the work of the nursing service administrator is problem solving. For the solution of most important nursing service problems, four things are required: models, concepts, analytical process, and data. The first three are intimately associated with the theories of administration.

Chapters 1 and 2 of this book are concerned with theory and model building. Whenever a nursing service administrator undertakes to solve a problem, she does so with some idea of the relationships involved. This idea of relationships constitutes a model. Our specific objectives for these two chapters were (1) to provide the administrator with a sound administrative theory, one on which to build a new organization, revitalize an already existing organization, solve problems, and make needed change; (2) to see the organization as an open system, as a whole, with all its parts related and interconnected; (3) to provide the administrator with needed tools for evaluation, her own work, her personnel, and the output, or patient care; and (4) to give consideration to the ever present constraints and provide for feedback.

Chapters 3 to 7 of this book are concerned with concepts. No nursing service administrator can manage without a large number of concepts, which are essentially abstractions and generalizations she derives from the particulars of her experience. As is true with models, concepts are employed by many nursing service administrators unconsciously. They use such words as planning, accountability, expense control, and management development. Each of these stands for a concept that embraces a great many individual events, such as discussions and operating decisions. Specific objectives for these chapters include the administrative functions of (1) setting objectives, both organizational and individual; (2) building an environment for their achievement; (3) measuring results; (4) using the functional processes of administration, planning, organizing, directing, and controlling; and (5) seeing health care organizations as dynamic systems.

Chapters 8 to 10 are concerned with analytical process and data. When a nursing service administrator is confronted with a problem, she needs not only some concepts and some ideas of relationships but also an analytical process with which to attack the problem. Specific objectives for these chapters concern (1) analyzing problems with a systems approach and utilizing the administrative processes (composite process) as a diagnostic tool, giving considerations to restraining forces; and (2) making a nursing service diagnosis, classifying the problem to determine the technique, or techniques, to be used in the resolution of the problem.

Chapters 11 to 13 are concerned with education, leadership, and the future. They focus on a rationale for curriculum development and a presentation to help give direction for decisions concerning how to teach. In any health care facility the situation is so complex that the administrator no longer directs a nursing service program but must give leadership. Consideration is given to possible kinds of leadership, depending on the situation. Specific objectives for these chapters are to (1) develop the critical characteristics needed in the nursing administrator, (2) develop the abilities of the nursing service administrator and make a success of the department of nursing, (3) prepare the nursing administrator educationally and experimentally to function at a quality leadership level, (4) develop a stated philosophy and goals, and (5) prepare a needed curriculum for the preparation of the nursing administrator.

The future for nursing service administration looks bright; the nursing profession has the needed knowledge, skills, and attitudes. The problem still is, to a certain extent, and has been for a long time, with the implementation of that knowledge.

The planning of this book was a cooperative venture from its inception. Each author contributed suggestions and materials to chapters written by the other.

We consider the administrative theory presented in this book to be sound and hope that nurses will use it to better advantage than our own writing may suggest and if possible in a science-practice relationship. Many nurses talk about theory, few write about it, and even fewer practice it.

We appreciate permission to use the "Synthesis of Administrative Theories" developed by Claude S. George, Jr., in 1972, as a basis for our administrative nursing service model and to use the environmental constraint model developed by Farmer-Richman and published by Business Publications, Inc., in 1971. We are also indebted to the Institute for Development of Education Activities, Inc., an affiliate of the Charles F. Kettering Foundation, for giving us permission to quote from their 1968 monograph, *An Idea,* and to Eliah E. Porter, who in 1972 assisted with the development of the "Systems Frame of Reference." We are grateful to the architects of "Conceptual Framework for Hospital Planning," J. J. Souder, W. E. Clark, J. I. Elkind, and M. B. Brown, for allowing us to quote from their work; to the many students who have contributed their ideas; and to the participants of the workshop sponsored by the Western Interstate Commission on Higher Education in Nursing, who contributed much to the isolation of the nursing service problems.

It is impossible to thank and to name individually the many people who contributed to our book, either directly or indirectly, through their writing of books and articles and who have helped us maintain focus on our ideas of nursing service administration.

Last, but by no means least, we are especially thankful to Dean Rheba de Tornyay, University of California, School of Nursing, Los Angeles, for the reading of the entire manuscript and to Teresa Joseph for working with us on the rough draft of this book.

Clara Arndt
Loucine M. Daderian Huckabay

CONTENTS

4 ADMINISTRATIVE COMPOSITE PROCESS: CONCEPTUAL AND PHYSICAL ACTS, 61

5 ENVIRONMENT, 108

6 EVALUATION AND MEASUREMENT, 136

NURSING ADMINISTRATION

Chapter 1

A BRIEF HISTORY OF ADMINISTRATIVE THEORY AS APPLIED TO NURSING SERVICES

In the century and a quarter that marks the history of the formal study of administration a good many distinct "thoughts" have emerged. Often these thoughts have developed into so-called schools of thought. Administrative ideas polarized at various times around such subjects as division of labor; work simplification and measurement; separation of physical work from the intellectual work of planning; the behavior of people in organizations and their goals and objectives; and finally, quantitative analysis, operations research, and systems.

These polarization periods reflected the problems of the times in which they were popular and they succeeded in promoting interest in and studies of the administrative process as it was then understood.

It is notable that in the third quarter of the twentieth century the pace of thought and ideas quickened and that the contributors included a different group of people. Newcomers such as engineers, mathematicians, economists, physicians, nurses, psychologists, sociologists, and philosophers turned their attention to studies of the administrative process. Many contributions to administrative literature came from the minds of such men and women who introduced new knowledge and new scientific insights and demonstrated their applicability to the administrative process. A number of the new thoughts and ideas have

survived and continue to influence contemporary administrative thought.

Many nursing service administrators who have taken a critical look at their own activities might feel overwhelmed at their findings. If the student or practitioner of nursing service administration feels that the subject is complicated, each is justified. Nursing service administration is indeed many faceted and multidimensional. But like any subject within the context of nursing, it can be, and has been, studied from many points of view.

After a brief look at some attempts at this, we shall be prepared to study the growth and development of administrative theory. Earlier study of theory can be regarded as attempts to identify, isolate, and study the components of administration and to define the requirements of what constitutes adequate administration. Trends and patterns can be seen to emerge.

Among these emerging elements are integration and innovation as functions of sound nursing service administration. Indeed, integration is one of the keys to the smooth working of any health care organization. Without it no agency can properly use its resources such as personnel, other disciplines, funds, materials, and services. And again, the agency must be integrated in some way with the needs and activities of the community it serves. Integration implies knowing, appraising, and interacting

1

with all the subcomponents of the total agency or system. The administration must also have a dynamic response to present and future needs of people. It must be innovative to future challenges.

Today, such statements almost seem axiomatic. But it has not always been so. Administration like economics, physics, and sociology had to pass through several stages of development. Administrative science as we know it today is in some respects a twentieth-century concept. It has attained its position, however, through the efforts of a host of scholars and practitioners working in its behalf over the centuries. The nursing service administrator must realize the need to draw from and utilize concepts from the various theories of administration or periods of thought. Administrators also must have a historical perspective concerning their growth to use the theories rationally. These various administrative theories have been brought together into an understandable and meaningful whole by Claude George (1972). His concepts form the core of our administrative model within the systems framework.

Administration contains a body of traditional or classically derived theory, which provides both a conceptual framework and terminology, as is true in most fields of study. This traditional system is mainly deductive, and there is a danger that it will be judged on the basis of its logical consistency or theoretical elegance rather than on its ability to predict or explain phenomena in the real world. Another use for such a system is as a means of classifying knowledge.

The nursing service administrator and student might justifiably ponder why such a theory has been so long in developing, why many of the ideas seem so self-evident today. Indeed, the administrator and student might well ask why there is such a profusion of ideas and doctrines. A brief look at the problems of the nineteenth century and some sampling of today's problems might bring clarification. We stress that nursing service administration must be built on sound theory and practice. Indeed, if nursing is to meet its share in furnishing the knowledge, skills, attitudes, and the leadership in health care delivery, nursing service administration must be based on a sound and flexible core of theory. Innovative solutions to present and future problems will not be forthcoming otherwise.

A BRIEF REVIEW OF ADMINISTRATIVE THEORIES

The development of administrative theory may be broadly classified into three periods. The first one, the classical period, was concerned essentially with the management of work. It dates from about 1895 on. Its major contributors were F. W. Taylor, the Gilbreths, and H. L. Gantt. Various management pioneers saw their ideas evolve through time into one or more aspects of management theory, culminating in what became known as the scientific management school by about 1910 to 1915.

The scientific management school evolved from the systematic observation of the methods of production—research and analysis of shop operation. Although concerned with specific techniques, all centering on efficiency and production, it is nevertheless firmly grounded in theory. As the first body of management concepts, it has served managers well and has provided a foundation on which scholars can build and improve.

Between the classical and neoclassical periods occurred the administrative process school, which developed from classical theory by about 1929. The focus was on administrative theory. Major contributions were made by Henri Fayol and James D. Mooney. This school built a theory of administration around the process involved in managing. It was concerned with the establishment of a conceptual framework and the identification of the principles underlying it. Because administration is viewed as a process, this school approaches the analysis of the process by investigating the manager's functions of planning, organizing, staffing, directing, and controlling.

The second period, known as the neoclassical, dates from about 1925. It was concerned with human relations and behavioral science foundations. The focus of this period was on human relations theory, motivation, work groups in organizations, and leadership. Its major earlier contributors were Gantt and Munsterberg. The behavioral science school, which dates back to about 1930, grew out of the leaders' recognition that the individual is central to any cooperative endeavor. They reasoned that inasmuch as managers get things done through people, the study of management must be centered on the workers and their interpersonal relations. The behaviorists concentrate on items such as motivations, group dynamics, individual drives, and group relations. The school is eclectic and incorporates most social sciences, including psychology, sociology, social psychology, and anthropology. It ranges in scope from how to influence individual behavior to a detailed analysis of sociopsychological relationships.

The modern period began about 1940. The focus of this period was on organization theory and systems analysis. The distinctive qualities of this theory are its conceptual-analytical base, its reliance on empirical research data, and its integrating nature. These qualities are framed in a philosophy that accepts the premise that the only meaningful way to study organization is to study it as a system. Again, as in previous periods, management pioneers saw their ideas evolve through time into one or more aspects of administration theory. Modern organization concepts evolved into the quantitative school of thought by about 1946. Its most obvious characteristic is the use of mixed teams of scientists from several disciplines working together and sharing their knowledge on the study and effective solution of a

problem. The work is variously labeled operations research, operational research, and management science; the work group may consist of a mathematician, a physical scientist, an economist, an engineer, and a statistician. By analyzing the problem from an operations research, or management science, point of view, one should obtain a better solution than could otherwise be achieved. It is a scientific method utilizing all pertinent scientific tools for providing a quantitative basis for managerial decisions. It grew out of the recognition by leading managers that closely integrated research teams were needed to fathom the diverse ramifications of various alternative paths of action.

Before the advent of mathematical models and the electronic computer, administrators were faced with the problem of planning and controlling their organization's operations. They would still have to perform these functions if the field of management science did not exist today. The point is that management science is not management. Mathematical models are useful only insofar as they are an aid to the administrator or manager as she performs the functions of planning and controlling. One of the goals of management science is to enable the manager to be a better planner or controller or both. The dates given represent the time of widespread attention and acceptance rather than of first introduction. Actually the genesis of these theories can be traced to much earlier times (George 1972). Because each school is associated with a particular contribution or research effort, our discussion is focused on certain authors. Although it is difficult to place sharp boundaries around divisions within history, certain thought patterns or schools into which various writings fit can be distinguished.

Later this functional classification will be used as a basis for formulation of theoretical constructs. In this chapter, historical and comparative frames of reference will be used with a strong eclectic effort. The emphasis will be pragmatic. The central processes of administration must consider all viewpoints. In this way the practitioners of nursing service administration and the student will be able to relate their thoughts to those from their practices, studies, and readings.

It was probably inevitable that the oldest administrative theories should focus only on productivity, inevitable because of the social-Darwinian doctrines of moral utility, which equated ultimate good with ultimate economic return to society. The Industrial Revolution had turned the socio-economic structure inside out, and such drastic changes and concomitant influences, although not always for the good of society, were justified according to this nineteenth-century philosophy. The pioneering administrative theorists, even if they were geniuses, were not immune from such influences.

Productivity was conceived of as having two dimensions: (1) effectiveness equals *results* (total treatments given or medications passed) and (2) *efficiency* (ratio of treatments given or medications passed to labor cost); more commonly efficiency was the ratio of output to an arbitrary standard of performance.

Scientific management school

The originator of the first great classical theory of scientific management was Frederick W. Taylor (1856–1917). His scientific management school was of fundamental and germinal importance in shaping thought and is still influential today. Although modified and expanded somewhat by Henry L. Gantt, Frank B. and Lillian M. Gilbreth, and others, Taylor's views were based directly on his own engineering and labor background. He rose from laborer to chief engineer at the Midvale Steel Works, was later at Bethlehem Steel Works, and still later became a consultant. His views, first published in 1895 and expanded in 1903

and again in 1911 (Taylor 1911), were based on four main principles:

1. The development of an ideal or best method. This included the analysis of each job to determine the "one best way" of doing it. The proper method was recorded on a job card, and the employee was paid on an incentive basis, given a higher rate for work beyond the standard.
2. The selection and development of the person. This involved selecting the right person to do a particular job and educating that person in the proper method.
3. The bringing together of the method and the selected, educated person. This, Taylor felt, would cause a mental revolution on the part of management. Workers would show little resistance to the improved methods, he felt, because of the greater earnings they would receive.
4. The close cooperation of managers and employees. This principle involved primarily the division of labor between managers and workers, with managers given the responsibility for the planning and "preparation" of work.

Taylor and his associates advocated knowing what work had to be done and getting it done in the most effective and efficient manner. They were concerned with division and specialization of work, the measurement of work and effort, and the efficient and human expenditure of effort. The practice and emphasis were on the physiological rather than on the psychological and sociological aspects of behavior in the work situation. The writings of the pioneers for scientific management do, however, indicate interest in the broader aspects of the well-being of people at work. Attention to standardized methods at the operative level is different from a focus at the administrative level of an organization.

Contemporary to the scientific management school was the era of the Industrial Revolution. At the time when modern nursing was taking shape the western world was suffering all the evils of the Industrial Revolution. The shift from muscle and water power to steam power had not released society from drudgery.

Life was an inexpensive commodity and death was common. Social, health, and sanitary practices intensified contagion. Slums, malnutrition, and abuses of labor had grown as factories replaced the home as the primary place of production.

Although scientific medicine was in its infancy, the physical sciences that had fostered the technical advances of the Industrial Revolution were well established. But, as the laboratory sciences and medical practice began to work together a foundation was laid for immunology, pasteurization, aseptic surgery, anesthesia, and most of public health. Thus the mortality and morbidity trends began to reverse by the turn of the century. By this time also the hospital, with its evermore specialized services, could begin to offer reassurance of safer care. A rationale, both protective and defensive, was adopted for the promotion of health and safety. A dramatic improvement in statistics tended to support the health care criteria chosen. But to quote Wooden (1961:91-104):

> Yet, it must be recognized that it was in combating the threats of the past that these defensive efforts served as effective weapons. In the context of today's greater progress . . . our index of performance can no longer be the death rate. Many of the routinized and proceduralized defenses have become merely outmoded controls, altogether devoid of their original meaning.
>
> The broad and seemingly blind obedience to these patterns today can only be explained by the enormous degree of security which, through actual experience, has understandably become attached to them, and which accounts for much of the ritualism associated with them and thus for the reluctance to relinquish them.

This evolution has been and is being influenced by the early and present development of industrial administration practices. The doctrine of moral utility is and was applied to most hospitals in a more humanitarian way, but here was an overlap of interests. Both institutions existed to contribute to society—industry through economics and the hospital as a guardian of worker's health or the custodian of the

nonproductive. The philosophy of the Industrial Revolution was used to rationalize social activities.

With a shift again in power sources, this time from coal to petroleum, new prototypes of administration came forth, as has been sketched above. In this second phase of the Industrial Revolution, emphasis was placed on organizational efficiency, such as was found in the central nursery and fixed feeding schedules. Perhaps the hospital had caught a "disease" or at least a "symptom" from industry. But with the advent of specialization as early as the 1900s, the hospital ward was being viewed as a machine—dispensing care. A patient-centered machine perhaps, but still a machine. Taylor's influence was felt in such ideas as matching the personnel to the machine for optimum output, in this case a declining death rate.

The roots of today's more ritualized, but less individualized, approach can be seen in this attitude. Such early mechanistic and organizational emphasis would have tended to reinforce Victorian ritualistic behavior. It must not be forgotten that these approaches and behaviors did have a very large measure of success. On the other hand, we must not be bound by convention. If the nurses are forced to function not as therapeutic agents but rather as other resources by which the status quo of the system is imposed on their patients, something is wrong. If the environment of care is rigid and inflexible, if standards of expectations are imposed, and if necessary relationships become a barrier between the nurses and their patients, neither will prosper.

In the formulation of administrative prototypes the early use of job standards and written instructions was a signal advance. Surely eccentricity should not be encouraged to the point of becoming a disruptive influence. Yet inflexible administration and overroutinized nursing procedures can block the nurse in professional growth, destroy the patient's therapeutic potential, and adversely affect the social milieu of nursing. All organizational services or production, including health, have their dilemmas. These are usually due not so much to personal shortcomings as to the nature of the organizational environment. In spite of recent writings by scholars and research findings, most health care organizations do not concentrate on individual differences, neither in their staffs nor in their patients.

Administrative process school

The next great development, the administrative process school of thought, began as a separate area of attention about 1930. This school of thought differed from the scientific management school by tending to be deductive rather than inductive; it focused on the organization as a whole rather than upon a single process such as production or service alone. Its suggestions for an ideal organizational design were based on such ideas as scalar levels, span of control, line and staff, and departmentation. The administrative process school built a theory of administration around the process involved in administration, the establishment of a conceptual framework for it, and the identification of the underlying principles.

A fundamental tenet is that administration is universal both in theory and practice whenever it is operative, such as in hospitals, clinics, private practice, or public agencies. Because administration is viewed as a process, this school approaches the analysis of the process by investigating the administrator's functions of planning, organizing, directing, and controlling. Inasmuch as these functions deal with the individuals involved, this school is somewhat eclectic in that pertinent aspects of the social sciences are recognized. Up to this point, however, these aspects have not been actively incorporated in the administrative process school.

Henri Fayol (1841–1925) fathered this stream of administrative thought. His original and perceptive listing of the functions of administration still reads like a current book, and his classical analysis has stood the test of time. Like many classics, it was not appreciated at first and did not become widely known until after a second English translation in 1949 (see Fayol 1949). It was "discovered" in the United States during the 1950s.

Behavioral science school

The behavioral science school grew out of the early efforts of leaders such as Gantt and Hugo Munsterberg to recognize and cope with the problems of the individual in organization. Cooperation is a central doctrine of this school. If administrators get things done through people, the early leaders reasoned, the focus must be on the workers and their interpersonal relations. There is concentration on such items as motivation, group dynamics, and individual drives. This school is eclectic in that it borrows from most social sciences, such as psychology, sociology, and anthropology. Its scope ranges from studying an individual nurse's behavior in detail to the complexities of a hospital considered as a anthropological subculture. The human element is central in any work situation.

Mayo (1933) and his colleagues made a landmark study of factors affecting worker activity, productivity, and efficiency at Western Electric's Hawthorne Chicago plant. The results were surprising to say the least. For no matter how the controlled variables were manipulated, production increased. The researchers were forced to the conclusion that human factors in the work situation were more important than the physical factors.

This behavioral science school borrowed from the psychological doctrine current at the time and also yielded much data and many concepts that were soon incorporated into the general body of psychology. Some ideas were truly revolutionary, as they affected selection and placement of personnel, recruitment, job analysis, and incentives; personnel departments began to appear with the outward change of careful selection and placement of personnel. As one would expect, these early personnel departments did little other than help make transfers between departments and help start recreational activities. But with the spread of the new concepts about personnel relations, these early departments began to perform duties that administrators recognized as of general importance. The depression of the 1930s, however, served momentarily to stop their progress. Others were not so new; indeed, it was Lillian Gilbreth, generally considered a Taylorist, who wrote the first book on industrial psychology (Gilbreth 1914). The recognition that organizations, including hospitals, were complex social systems and that the questions arising from this social nature could be handled by the research methods of psychologists has had a profound impact to this day. Now, of course, the viewpoint of the industrial behavior science student is based more on studying the organization as a whole, and the organizational psychologist must consider the systems characteristics of the whole organization. In this respect the behavioral science school tends to overlap the thought-provoking quantitative school.

Quantitative school

The quantitative school is the most recent to appear and has impinged on society and the general public more than all the other schools combined. It is based on a collection of diverse techniques generally using logic and a rationalistic model to analyze the operation of an organization. The knowledge of various disciplines is brought to bear on the problem under consideration. A typical case might involve a social scientist, a physicist, an engineer, and an anthropologist. Subspecialities often encountered include operations research, linear programming, critical-path-method, program evaluation and review technique (PERT), systems theory, econ-

ometrics, model theory, queuing theory, strategy and game theory, simulation, Markov chains, information theory, and cost effectiveness. Other names sometimes used for this school include management science, operations research, and decision theory.

If a single characteristic can be isolated as making this school unique, it is the approach, which involves scientific method and the belief that a phenomenon is not understood until it is quantified. There is much reliance on symbolic communication and interdisciplinary teamwork.

The quantitative school has shown fruitful results in many areas of administration, especially in providing tools for a quantitative basis for decision making. Steps in this process usually consist of the following:

1. Formulating the problem
2. Building a mathematical model to represent the system under study
3. Deriving a solution from the model
4. Testing the model and the solution
5. Establishing controls over the solution
6. Putting the solution to work, implementation

These steps have diverse ramifications in choosing between alternate decisions. Considerable mathematics may be involved; statistics and probabilities may be the only way to deal with fluctuations in variables. Electronic data processing and giant computers may be needed to reduce the theoretical models to manageable, practical aids. Indeed it is the high-speed computers with their vast data handling and computational abilities that have brought the quantitative school out of a purely academic setting and into the administrator's daily practice.

Of course, no one claims that the computer is the whole answer to the problems of society, health care organizations, or nursing. Indeed, it is the mystique of the computer, possibly more than anything else, that has shown the need not to neglect the human problems as expounded by the studies of the behavioral science school.

Many times the transition to a computerized or automated system within any organization, including health, has caused more turmoil than was first imagined by the proponents of the new ideas and devices. This does not mean that the innovations were without value. Most of them have by now proven themselves to be more than a good investment by reducing costs, saving time for the nurse to serve the patient more, and thus improving care of the patient.

Again, proper functioning of the computer is dependent on proper motivation and education of those people to gain an understanding of why these devices or improvements are introduced. When people understand, then change is accepted on an easier basis. The computer is complex but not nearly so complex as people.

Computer systems can now free a nurse from much of the time-consuming tasks such as writing nursing care plans, copying physicians' orders, transcribing patients' drug prescriptions, assigning staff, and determining rotation patterns. But if nurses are not willing to accept electronic devices as helpful, they are not much further along than their sisters and brothers of three generations ago.

Other classifications of administrative thought

We have presented four periods of polarized thought or schools of administrative ideas with a more important purpose in mind, namely to synthesize the ideas, in accordance with the thinking of Claude George (1972). It is interesting to see how some other writers taken at random, with various other purposes, have classified administrative thought.

Mary Arnold (1968) classifies four different approaches to administrative theory: structural, process, decision-making, and systems. Ernest Dale (1965) divides the thinking into four schools: scientific management, school efficiency, human relations, and administrative. Kast and Rosen-zweig (1966) divide the theory into behavioral science, operations research, and continuations of earlier classical and neo-classical theory. Levey and Loomba (1973) break theirs into five categories: scientific management, administrative management, human relations school, behavioral school, and management science. Newman, Summer, and Warren (1967) list four approaches: productitivity, behavioral, rationalistic-model, and institutional concepts. And finally, Paul Gordon (1966) labels his categories traditional, behavioral, decisional, and ecological.

Advantages and limitations of each school of thought

Practitioners may not have applied theory as intended by authors, but there are limitations in each school as listed in the following tabulation.

Advantages	Disadvantages
I. Scientific management school	
Emphasis on	
1. Clear-cut goals and objectives	1. Tends to neglect consideration of human and social values
2. Improved performance and efficiency	2. Usually omits co-ordination of diverse functions
3. Reduced cost and the scientific method	3. Usually does not apply to whole organization
4. Technical expertise	4. Tends to be prescriptive rather than situational
5. Work level and technical aspects of production	5. Seems to contain paradoxes in the decision-making process
6. Philosophy based on effective operation	6. Building an organization without people
II. Administrative process school	
Emphasis on	
1. Administrative functions and their study	1. Tends to view administration as distinct from organization
2. Administration as a subject separate from its application	2. Results are difficult to measure
3. Administrative principles	3. Lack of individual involvement

4. Administrative mission

4. Coordination seen as a function rather than as a result of administrative processes

III. Behavioral science school

1. Recognizes human and social needs
2. Stresses cooperation
3. Stresses teaching and supervision
4. Emphasis on recognition of informal organization

1. Can lead to fragmentation
2. Individual can lose sight of total organization
3. Building people without organization
4. Lack of integration of human facets of behavior

IV. Quantitative school

1. Aids rational decision making
2. Adaptable to almost any problem
3. Stresses models and mathematics
4. Emphasis on interdisciplinary scientific teamwork
5. Emphasis is on output

1. Can be complicated
2. Can be initially costly
3. May require outside experts
4. Building organizations without people

Viewed in terms of systems concept, either one of the four schools of thought can make for a closed system or an open system, or a partly closed and a partly open system.

A closed system is one in which the final state is determined by initial conditions. An open system is one in which the same final state can be reached from different initial conditions and by different paths. A closed system has negative feedback. In open systems there is more than one way to achieve a cause and effect relationship.

Table 1 presents the open and closed system concepts in a diagrammatical form.

CONTRIBUTION OF DIFFERENT SCHOOLS OF THOUGHT TO NURSING SERVICE ADMINISTRATION

This introductory account shows that principles of general administrative theory, as practiced in business and industry, are applicable to health care organizations.

Table 1. Blending of the four schools of thought in terms of systems concepts

Scientific management	Open or closed system or both	Administrative process	Open or closed system or both	Behavioral	Open or closed system or both	Management science—quantitative	Open or closed system or both
Planning	o/c	Planning	o/c	Motivation	o/c	Decisions	c
Organizing	o/c	Organizing	o/c	Group norms	o/c	theory	
Controlling	o/c	Controlling	o/c	Flatter organization	o	Linear programming	c
Directing	o/c	Directing	o/c	T-Groups	o	Inventory control	c
Unity of command	c	Line-staff	o/c	Management by objective	o	Break-even points	c
Specialization	c	Specialization	c	Job enrichment	o	PERT	c
		Span-of-control	c	Situational Leadership	o	Business gaming	o
				Decentralization	o		

Symbols: o = open; c = closed; o/c = open and closed.
Characteristics of open and closed systems:
  o = Open system → leads to increased creativity, decreased routinization.
  c = Closed system → leads to decreased creativity, increased routinization.
  o/c = Open and closed systems → lead to either increase or decrease in creativity and routinization.
  A partly open and partly closed system may lead in some areas of administration to creativity and in other areas to routinization.

For example, hospital and industry show complex organization, both have formal and informal groups and subgroups, both have mutual interactions with a community and a larger environment, both are related to the total society, both utilize power or authority, both have a product, and both use specialized services.

Areas of difference may be found: the product is different, that of the hospital is people; the preparation for leadership is not necessarily the same; hospitals tend to use normative authority; industry is more decentralized than hospitals. An illustration of a problem common in industry and health organizations can be drawn from the increasing dependence upon specialized services.

The economist Galbraith, as cited in Deliége (1974), states that the real authority in commercial organizations belongs to the experts who form what he calls the technostructure. Galbraith's analysis concerns Western commercial companies whose purposes are purely economical; this is not the case with health care organizations, which have a set of functions. Furthermore, in the commerical companies, experts have a career that is well integrated with the very objective of the organization; the common purpose is growth and profit making. On the other hand, the medical and nursing experts of Western health care facilities are often involved in an individualistic career and are more concerned about the care patients receive than about economical efficiency or effectiveness. Not only do medical and nursing experts often advise the administration, but they constantly make crucial and vital decisions; they bear

alone the whole responsibility for their actions. We conclude that the medical and nursing technostructure is not identical with that of industry. Nurses may have more knowledge than their supervisors.

These and other areas have been studied and some results presented graphically in research publications. Schurr (1969) shows how both types of organizations are under pressure.

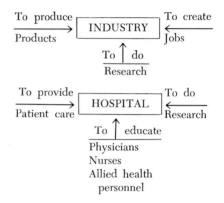

Note that there is not the pressure on the hospital to create jobs; on the contrary, it supplies employees for a special labor market.

Social scientists at the Tavistock Institute have encompassed the social and cultural values and demands of people such as hospital employees and patients in a study to show how external factors influence a sociotechnical system; they used the analogy of material being imported, converted, and finally exported (Trist and Rice 1963).

Thus, many external factors become internal factors because hospital workers, like patients, do not shed their culture when they cross the threshhold of a hos-

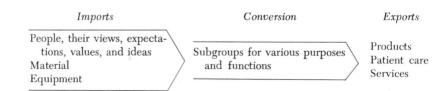

pital. The Tavistock researchers found this true of industrial workers also.

Through a detailed analysis of basic variables, Etzioni (1961) separates hospitals from business and industry. He has three main categories of organization based on the type of authority used and kind of member involvement.

Category I	Category II	Category III
		Normative authority use of membership, status, and intrinsic value rewards
	Predominantly utilitarian use of economic	
Pure coercive power	nomic rewards	
Concentration camps	Business and industry	Religious organizations
Prisons	Business	Hospitals
Custodial institutions	unions	Colleges and institutions
Coercive unions	Peacetime military organizations	Voluntary associations
		Professional associations

We have seen how in the late nineteenth century and first years of the twentieth century the modern hospital started to take shape. As it grew and changed so did nursing services and their administration. Many of the early top officials were nurses, the "wardens" or "superintendents of nurses." Supervision of patient care and the teaching of student nurses were the main responsibilities. The model for authority was largely based on holdover ideas harking back to the religious and military hospitals of the past (Bullough and Bullough 1969).

Other administrative functions were handled by various members of the board of trustees; therefore, responsibility was divided and fragmented. Any coordination achieved was due to board meetings, each member speaking for a particular specialty, for example, finance, maintenance, or personnel. In these early days, nursing service administration went largely unrecognized as an essential component of hospital operation.

About the time of World War I the situation began to change in the hospitals, as it did in industry. The growth of industry and its shift from private, single proprietorship to larger and more complex structures have been alluded to at the beginning of this chapter. One result of this was the development of the earliest administrative theory, the scientific management school. So too, changes occurred in the administration of the increasingly complex and larger hospitals. Many things happened almost simultaneously; new knowledge in science and medicine, new procedures, new laboratories, x-ray tests, an ever increasing number of nursing schools, and many more educated nurses were just some of the developments requiring coordination and direction.

The scientific management school tended for the most part to regard all facilities, including personnel, as resources to be administered. The proper function of administration was considered to be to increase efficiency and improve production, that is, patient care. No qualitative change had occurred in the nature of administrative thinking from the days of the single owner. Fundamental changes had occurred in ways of carrying out the primary function of organizations, that is, making profits or caring for patients. The workers' or nurses' roles changed but administration as an art did not alter its basic nature until the advent of the administrative process school.

Stewart (1934:15) observed that the emphasis on efficiency and standardization in business and industry before World War I had a considerable effect on nursing; as a result, nursing education moved in the direction of inflexibility, with nurses expected to follow a set pattern and with spontaneity discouraged.

Along with problems stemming from the technical and other innovations were economic and financial problems. Hospitals had grown too big and complicated for the trustees to administer completely.

Johnson (1966) identified five stages of

administrative authority in the transition from late nineteenth-century to mid-twentieth-century health care. Hospitals were administered in turn by a superintendent of nurses, stage 1; a business manager and board of trustees, stage 2; a hospital superintendent and trustees, stage 3; an administrator, stage 4; and finally an executive vice-president, stage 5. All stages coexist in the United States today.

Between 1915 and 1930 the position of business manager gradually evolved. During the 1920s the active administrative role of trustees declined considerably. Concerned at first with finance, the business manager was subordinate to the trustees as was the superintendent of nurses. The two positions needed some coordination and liaison, which was supplied by the trustees.

The role of the business manager grew. Other functions soon fell on this person's shoulders, such as responsibility for service departments, purchasing, payroll, billing, and many daily affairs of the hospital. Some functions were transferred from the trustees and some from the superintendent of nursing. As the business manager demonstrated competence and filled a real need, the position was accepted more widely. Business managers or chief executive officers were recruited from trustees, physicians, nurses, or religious members in religious hospitals.

This pattern lasted less than 20 years; the acceleration of change of the thirties and forties forced still further administrative reorganization. Again concern was felt for the impact of science, financial questions, and the growth of specialties. Administration began to be concerned with the problem of recruiting full-time people.

Change was felt on all fronts. The behavioral sciences, which indirectly came about from scientific management studies, research, and experiments, ushered in an interest in the human aspects of nursing operations. Scientific management had emphasized technical matters, but nursing service administrators were soon to accept the need to consider other factors. Administrative studies expanded to include such areas as human relations, morale, and group dynamics. Nurses had always dealt with people, but now there was an emphasis on skill in dealing with people. Administrators, it was felt, must not only be familiar with industrial engineering but with human engineering as well.

To meet the need for nursing service administrators, especially the ones with this new orientation, academic education programs were established at the graduate level in universities. People choosing this new career were well accepted. Although the title *superintendent* still exists in a few places, its meaning and definitive term is *administrator. Executive director* and

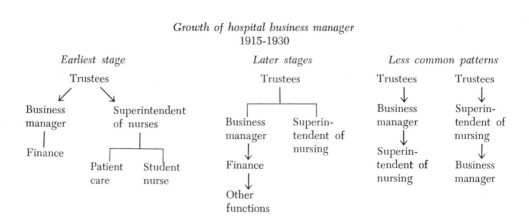

Growth of hospital business manager
1915-1930

| *Earliest stage* | *Later stages* | *Less common patterns* |

executive vice-president are growing in popularity as titles and as concepts.

Administration is still evolving at an accelerating pace. Boards of trustees of health care organizations are becoming more like boards of directors of industry. The executive director and the nursing administrator have greater responsibility, including community relations. They are on the threshhold of even greater responsibilities, including those relating to shifting patterns of bureaucracy and the new medical staff relationships (Levey and Loomba 1973).

Change is a dominant theme of our time. By now it should be obvious that we feel change has impinged and will continue to impinge on nursing from all quarters.

During the late twenties and thirties there was great concern about nursing education. According to Russell (1958): "Some of the strongest programs of nursing education came into existence during this period." A new voice was heard throughout education. The democratic philosophy of John Dewey gave a new direction to nursing education. Its aim was the "development of the individual and the progressive enrichment of his life experience, on the one hand, and the construction and improvement of society on the other" (Stewart 1947).

The W. K. Kellogg Foundation gave new direction to nursing service administration through the financing of research in this important area and by assisting again through funds in establishing university programs in nursing service administration in 16 schools throughout the nation (Mullane 1959; Finer 1961).

NATURE OF THEORY

We now draw the reader's attention to the nature of and criteria for evaluating theory to review the most commonly used empirical research methods and to suggest some basic considerations involved in assessing the validity of research findings.

Nursing service administrators and students in the field of administration have witnessed heated controversy over the proper approaches to nursing service administration and management as an academic discipline because of the different schools of administrative thought and recent developments in research methodology.

This discussion presents criteria for evaluating theory and empirical research methods and suggests some basic considerations for assessing the validity of research findings and theory. Also discussed and advanced are guides for integrating theory and research findings in solving problems in nursing service administration. A clear understanding of these concepts and their relationship to the day-to-day practice of administering can be of great value to practicing administrators as well as to students of nursing service administration. The most commonly held belief regarding theories of administration and particularly of nursing service administration is that it is a set of "ought to's," that is, a set of rules that tells one how to administer.

Filley and House (1969) describe a theory as the frame of reference that students and practitioners of administration use for thinking and for making decisions. A theory is not something apart from practice; it is the basis for application of practice. The real world is complex and must be put to order in a systematic fashion; theoretical formulation is the ordering process.

Theory serves two functions; it functions as a tool and as a goal. Marx (1963) states that as a tool, theory serves to direct empirical research by generalizing new predictions not otherwise likely to occur. As a goal, theory integrates and applies empirical findings. Theories are an economical and efficient means for abstracting, codifying, summarizing, integrating, and storing information.

Components of theory

The important components of theory are concepts, propositions, and laws. A *concept* is a term to which a particular meaning has been attached. Concepts are class names that may refer to objects, events, properties of objects, events, and to relationships between them. A *proposition* is a provisional statement that makes predictions about empirical data. Predictions are often derived from theoretical propositions; they indicate what the researcher expects to find. *Laws* are statements of regular, predictable relationships among empirical variables. They also mean a strongly established theoretical or abstract set of principles.

A theory is described by Griffiths (1964:100) as "a deductively connected set of laws. Certain laws are the axioms or postulates of the theory and are usually called assumptions. Their truth is not so much self-evident as it is taken for granted, so that the truth of other empirical assertions called theorems can be determined."

Types of theory construction

There are four types of theory construction: theoretical model, inductive, deductive, and functional. Their differentiation is based on the way in which they relate to empirical data.

Marx (1963) and Filley and House (1969) describe a *theoretical model* as a conceptual analogue used to suggest a framework for empirical research. It affects a researcher's approach to empirical data, but it is not changed by the data. The major difference between the model and other forms of theory is its insensitivity to the data.

An *inductive* theory is a form that summarizes empirical relationships and avoids the elaboration of deductive logic. It is the data that develops the theory. Researchers begin with a set of observations, and based on observations, they develop or induce a generalization or principle to predict or explain the pattern of relationships they have observed. The flow of logic is from data to abstraction. A *deductive* theory emphasizes its conceptual structure and the substantive validity of its laws. It is constructed from empirical data, is used to view empirical research, and is modified as new or different relationships appear. Stress is placed on the logical internal consistency of its propositions. The flow of logic here is from abstraction to data.

A *functional* theory is viewed as a provisional means for collecting and analyzing data. Premature elaboration of a sophisticated logical system is a void. A functional theory is more tentative and less formal than deductive theory.

The classical scientific administrative and management theories are largely functional, although many of the recent theories have been inductive in nature. They are based mostly on an accumulation of experience in dealing with work groups and emerge in descriptions of standardized jobs, in separate planning units, and in special selection procedures.

Characteristics and criteria of theory

How can a researcher or a nursing service administrator decide which theory to accept and which to reject? Filley and House (1969) have suggested five criteria for acceptability of a theory. First, a theory must be internally consistent; that is, its propositions should be free from contradiction. It should allow the theorist to make "if-then" propositions and to test them. The second characteristic of a sound theory is its external consistency, which means that a theory must be consistent with observations and measures of real life. This criterion of a theory is commonly referred to as the test of empirical reference. Third, a theory must have the possibility to prove its predictions wrong, and its predictions should also be verifiable. The fourth characteristic of a theory is its generality. Finally, a practical theory must have the attribute of scientific parsimony. That is, if two theories, both accurately predicting events, are supported by evidence, then the less complex of the two should be selected.

Theories also have seven descriptive dimensions. The first descriptive dimension is a method of development in which the flow of logic is either from abstraction to data or from data to abstraction, and the second, exposition, which means that a theory may be expressed verbally or quantitatively. The third dimension is purpose; a theory is said to be prescriptive if it prescribes what should take place; for example, "every one in an organization should understand the responsibility and authority of his job" (Filley and House 1969:32). A descriptive theory explains what is rather than what should be. The fourth dimension is scope; a theory may be either microscopic or macroscopic. Microscopic theory starts with a small unit of analysis, for example, a single person or small group, and builds the whole theory; macroscopic theory starts with the entire environment of the phenomenon and then moves to smaller units within it. The fifth dimension of a theory is the orientation. A theory may be discipline oriented if it is originated by experts in a specific area of knowledge; for example, we may find theories of hospital administration, business management, and experts in each of these disciplines. Problem-oriented theory focuses on the question at hand and draws knowledge from any appropriate source.

Mutual dependence of parts is the sixth dimension of a theory. It focuses on the extent to which the various parts of the theory are interrelated. At one extreme is static theory. Its rules are said to be fixed and unchanging, and the relationship between the factors of the theory is simple. Dynamic theory has more complex relationships and more interdependencies. For example, consider a worker's willingness or lack of willingness to participate in the organization and meet its goals. The dynamic model of March and Simon (1958) suggests that the less the job satisfaction of workers, the higher is their search for alternative sources of satisfaction. This may include either leaving the organization, staying and producing, or staying and not producing. March and Simon also indicate that worker search behavior is stimulated by the expected value of rewards, that is, the greater the expected value of reward, the greater the search and the higher the level of job satisfaction and aspiration. Increasing aspiration levels also decrease satisfaction, though. Therefore, a worker's decision to participate and the specific performance level are determined by a balance between positive and negative forces. This example illustrates how the dynamic theory explains an employee's decision to participate in a complex manner but more realistically than static theory (see Filley and House 1969).

Another characteristic of a theory is its applicability. Bennis, Benne, and Chin (1962) have proposed a set of criteria for valid practical application of social science theory that also applies for practical application of administrative theory. Such a theory should be able to take into consideration the behavior of people operating within specific institutional environments and should be able to account for interrelated levels within the social change context. A theory should include variables the practitioner can understand, manipulate, and evaluate. It should select from among variables those that are most appropriate to a specific local situation in terms of its values, ethics, and morality. It should also accept the premise that organizations and groups, as units, are as liable to empirical research and analytic treatment as the individual. Finally, a theory should take into account the external social processes of change as well as the interpersonal aspects of the collaborative processes (see Filley and House 1969).

Therefore, a theory that has practical value provides the nursing administrator with a description of her environment. It serves to broaden her range of knowledge, for by deriving predictions from theory, she is able to relate specific facts to broader explanations. She uses theory to guide her search for finding variables that relate to her practical problems and in her effort to formulate optimum solutions. According to Filley and House (1969), a scientist attempts to describe and predict behavior without attempting to guide it, but the practitioner attempts to predict and control behavior in ways that are judged to be desirable. The practitioner derives guides from theory that are useful for analysis of problems, prediction of events, and control of variables. In reality, knowledge of theory enables the practitioner to better solve problems that arise in her own specific environment.

Because much of today's theory in the field of administration has been developed from the practical experiences of administrators or on the basis of uncontrolled observations, it has provided some significant and useful information for the development of prescriptions, guides, and principles to guide action. The actual empirical tests of these principles, however, are rare. Therefore, it is of extreme importance that instead of the administrator confining herself exclusively to observing applications and violations of a principle in actual practice before she can evaluate its validity, she can turn to other academic disciplines for previously conducted studies based on analogous hypotheses, from which valid inferences may be drawn. An example of analogous research would be the study by Gulick (1937) on the principle of unity of command. Gulick states that "no individual should receive orders or directions from more than one person" (see Filley and House 1969:35). The rationality for this principle being that as a person receives orders from too many people in an organization, the chances are that the orders will conflict and create uncertainty in the employee in deciding which order carries the

highest priority. Therefore, the employee may develop feelings of frustration and anxiety and may delay in the decision-making process. Since the principle of unity of command is based on the expectation of conflict, we can draw useful inferences from the behavioral sciences of psychology and sociology about role conflict, which state that conflicts arise when incompatible role demands or expectations are made of a person as an employee or citizen.

Summary

Nursing service administration in health care organizations has had a slow beginning but a steady rise toward a theoretical foundation. From the beginning of scientific management, nursing service administration learned to look at the tasks to be performed and to consider the most effective and efficient ways for their accomplishments. The process period taught the planning, organizing, directing, and controlling functions as the administrative duties but different from the work at the "bench" so to speak, and essential to the survival of the organization. The behavioral sciences with their emphasis on individual differences pointed to people as the most important variable to accomplish the purpose of the organization. Administration was considered the science of managing people. With the rapid advent of the quantitative science period we begin to think of the organization as a whole; we are beginning to use the scientific method and are now able to measure our inputs and outputs.

We have taken the administrative theories representing the best of the four schools of administrative thought and have placed them within a systems framework constructing a model or cognitive image as a guide for practicing nursing service administrators and students to consider the concepts, expand their use, and add new knowledge (see Fig. 2-7). Administrative history puts present-day administration on the shoulder of past learning, making it unnecessary for every administrator to find the way anew from the labyrinth of administrative theory.

Possessing a variety of theoretical frameworks is like possessing a reservoir of potential energy stored within the cognitive repertoire of the individual; this potential energy is ready to be transformed into kinetic energy whenever the nursing service administrator is called on to take action. In short, a theory is a guide to action.

REFERENCES

Arnold, M. F.: Professionalism and changing concepts of administration, J. Nurs. Educ. **7**(1): 5-50, 1968.

Bennis, W. G., Benne, K. D., and Chin, R.: The planning of change: readings in the applied behavioral sciences, New York, 1962, Holt, Rinehart & Winston, Inc.

Bullough, V., and Bullough, B.: The emergence of modern nursing, ed. 2, New York, 1969, Macmillan Pub. Co., Inc.

Dale, E.: Management theory and practice, New York, 1965, McGraw-Hill Book Co.

Deliége, D.: The sociological framework surrounding patients, Int. Nurs. Rev. **21**(1):16-20, 1974.

Etzioni, A. A.: Comparative analysis of complex organizations, Glencoe, Ill., 1961, The Free Press.

Fayol, H.: General and industrial administration, London, 1949, Sir Isaac Pitman & Sons, Ltd.

Filley, A. C., and House, R. J.: Managerial process and organizational behavior, New York, 1969, Scott, Foresman & Co.

Finer, H., Administration and nursing services, New York, 1961, Macmillan Pub. Co., Inc.

George, C. S., Jr.: The history of management thought, ed. 2, Englewood Cliffs, N. J., 1972, Prentice-Hall, Inc.

Gilbreth, L. M.: The psychology of management, New York, 1914, Sturgis & Walton Co.

Gordon, P. J.: Transcend the current debate on administrative theory, Hosp. Admin. **11**(2): 6-23, 1966.

Griffiths, D. E.: The nature and meaning of theory in behavioral science and educational administration. In Griffiths, D. E., editor: The 63rd yearbook of the national society for the study of education, Chicago, 1964, University of Chicago Press, pp. 95-119.

Gulick, L.: Notes on the theory of organization. In Gulick, L., and Urwick, L.: Papers in the science of administration, New York, 1937, Institute of Public Administration.

Johnson, E. A.: The continuing evolution of the hospital administration, Hosp. Admin., **11**(2): 47-59, 1966.

Kast, F. E., and Rosenzweig, J. E.: Hospital administration and systems concepts, Hosp. Admin. **11**(4):17-33, 1966.

Levey, S., and Loomba, P. N.: Health care administration: a managerial perspective, Philadelphia, 1973, J. B. Lippincott Co.

March, J. G., and Simon, H. A.: Organizations, New York, 1958, John Wiley & Sons, Inc.

Marx, M. H.: Theories in contemporary psychology, New York, 1963, Macmillan Pub. Co., Inc.

Mayo, G. E.: The human problems of an industrial civilization, New York, 1933, The Viking Press, Inc.

Mullane, M. K.: Education for nursing service administration, Battle Creek, Mich., 1959, The W. K. Kellogg Foundation.

Newman, W. H., Summer, C. E., and Warren, E. K.: The process of management, ed. 2, Englewood Cliffs, N. J., 1967, Prentice-Hall, Inc.

Russell, James E.: National policies for education, health and social services, Garden City, N. Y., 1955, Doubleday & Co., Inc.

Schurr, M. C.: A comparative study of leadership in industry and the nursing profession. II. Int. J. Nurs. **16**(2):115-132, 1969.

Stewart, I.: The educational program of the school of nursing, Geneva, 1934, International Council of Nurses, p. 15.

Taylor, F. W.: Principles of scientific management, New York, 1911, Harper & Brothers.

Trist, E. J., and Rice, A. K.: The enterprise and its environment, London, 1963, Tavistock Publications, Ltd.

Wooden, H. E.: Impact of the industrial revolution on hospital maternity care, Nurs. Forum **1**:91-104, Winter 1961.

ADDITIONAL READINGS

Roethlisberger, F. J., and Dickson, W. J.: Management and the worker, Cambridge, Mass., 1939, Harvard University Press.

Stull, R. J.: Management of the American Hospital. In Hague, J. E., editor: The American hospital system, Pensacola, Fla., 1961, Pensacola Hospital Research and Development Institute, Inc.

Chapter 2

ADMINISTRATIVE THEORY WITHIN SYSTEMS FRAME OF REFERENCE

Modern science and technology have influenced the conversion of health care institutions into increasingly more complex, diversified organizations. Increase in knowledge has subsequently increased specialization. This factor has made co-ordination of patient care difficult.

Nursing service administrators, long educated in the art of doing and immersed in the day-to-day operation of an organization, seldom can take time to examine ways in which the theory of administration can be of help to them in solving the pressing problems of a modern health care institution. Yet there are concepts that can serve as maps for the harassed administrator as she journeys through the labyrinth of interrelationships and complexities of her organization.

One of these concepts, the processes of administration, is presented in this chapter and, for that matter, throughout the book. We urge that nursing service administrators check their thinking against these four essential ingredients of this process: planning, organizing, directing, and controlling. We urge that nursing service administrators not treat such matters as the fragmentation of health delivery services or the conflict between public, voluntary, and proprietary sectors of medical care as though they were only medical problems and that they not view the inability of existing health organizations to respond adequately to changing community health needs and the startling increase in health

care cost as if they were unrelated to the health care organization as a whole. Using this approach, we formulated a model or cognitive map that will carry the nursing administrator step-by-step through the job of examining the four basic functions of nursing service administration in terms of the system as a whole.

For decades the nursing service administrator's functions have been defined as planning, organizing, directing, and controlling. How have these functions changed? The truth is that the functions themselves have not changed, but how we employ them has. The point of view can make a big difference in the way an administrator observes and relates the facts of a situation. Much depends on the administrative ability to establish an orderly relationship among factors in the social and economic environment, on the institution's purpose and standing within the community, and on the operation of the nursing service organization. The nursing service administrator must be aware of the totality of the institution, but this is an abstract ideal unless the thinking of organizational activities is in terms of the objective, the plans for attaining the objectives, the organizational system created to do the job, and of the controls required to adjust to an evolving situation.

An environment conducive to the attainment of organizational and individual goals lies at the end of a long chain of interrelated activities. No single link in the

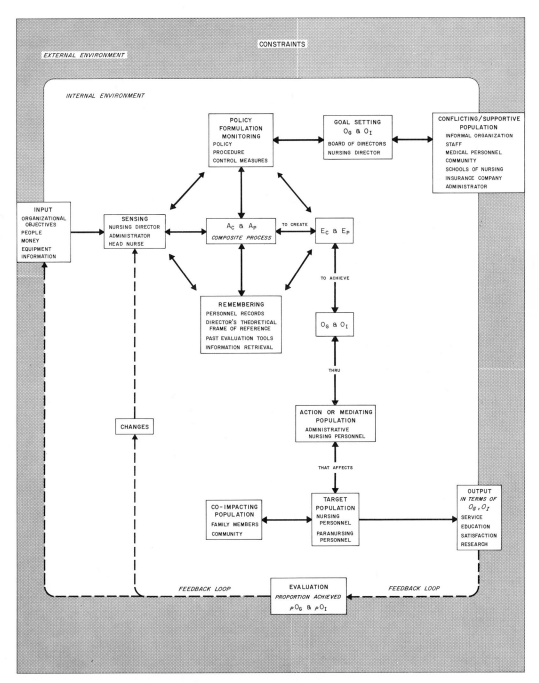

Fig. 2-1. Administrative model within systems frame of reference.

chain seems less important than another, although a good many theoretical discussions of service maximization seem to focus primarily on such items as cost control, optimum levels of output, and the equating of marginal resources and marginal costs. Although these factors are certainly important and deserve careful attention, they need to be put in perspective by the administrator responsible for the total organization. Far more of what the institution wants to stand for concerning quality service to people, education of health care personnel, research in the control and prevention of disease, and cost control is possible when the focus is placed on the basic design of the overall institution, notably on the direction in which it is going, its scheme of operations, and the interconnections of its parts. The key to success lies in the process of administration.

The task facing the nursing profession is to evolve a general theory for nursing service administration that incorporates the appropriate aspects of past theories and disciplines. In short, what is needed is not a new theory but a synthesis embracing the totality. To better illustrate our concept of administrative theory for nursing service, we have constructed a model or concise formula, a conceptual analogy used to suggest a framework for action (Fig. 2-1 and Table 2).

The ingredients that went into the making of the model were (1) the functions of the nursing service administrator, (2) the nursing service organization as an open system, (3) influence of external environment, constraints, (4) the nursing service organization as a dynamic entity not restricted to itself or to interrelationships of internal subsystems, (5) organizational goals and individual goals as measurable entities via the feedback loops, (6) change considered a constant in modern health care organizations, and (7) the concepts grouped as interdependent, interrelated, and interactive.

By separating the administrative func-

Table 2. Explanation of symbols

Notation	Term
A	Achievement
Ac	Conceptual acts
Ad	Administration
AdA	Administrative achievement
Ap	Physical acts
C	Controlling
D	Directing
Ec	Conceptual environment
Ep	Physical environment
f	"A function of"
O	Organizing
Og	Organizational objectives
Oi	Individual objectives
P	Planning
p or %	Percentage
>	Greater than

tions or processes from the environment in which they actually occur, we have a model that appears to be a useful means for evaluating the administration.

Our approach to building the model was to define nursing service administration and the nursing service administrator today. Nursing service administration is the process of setting and achieving objectives by influencing human behavior within a suitable environment. The nursing service administrator, on the other hand, creates the environment that is conducive to the performance of acts by other individuals—acts that will accomplish the institution's objectives, or goals, as well as achieve the objectives or goals of the participating individuals. Determining the collective objectives of a nursing service organization and generating an environment for their achievement, therefore, is the total function of a nursing service administrator. A nursing service organization may be defined, therefore, as a social organization within which people have achieved stable relations among themselves to facilitate obtaining a set of objectives or goals.

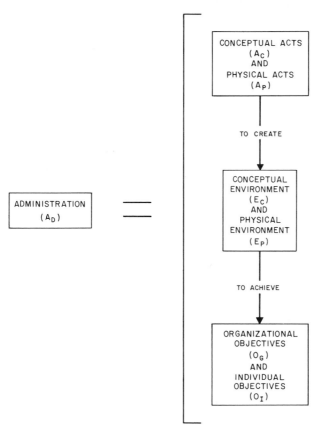

Fig. 2-2. Administrative theory.

CORE COMPONENTS OF THE ADMINISTRATIVE THEORY MODEL
Administrative theory

The heart of our model or cognitive map is the administrative theory (Fig. 2-2). The act of administration *(Ad)* is conceptual *(Ac)* and physical *(Ap)*, which combine to create a conceptual and physical environment *(Ec* and *Ep)* in terms of individual *(Oi)* and organizational *(Og)* objectives. Conceptual acts are concerned with thinking, ideation, philosophizing, putting ideas together, and making decisions. Physical acts are concerned with communication, teaching, self-actualization, and the implementation of the planned and organized program or translated knowledge into doing. The conceptual acts are realized through the intellectual pro-

cesses of planning and organizing, whereas the physical acts are realized through the doing process of directing and controlling.

The administrative process is not a series of separate functions of planning, organizing, directing, and controlling that can be performed independently. Instead, administration is a composite process made up of these individual components. None of these functions can be performed without involving the others, but by utilizing all four as a composite process, the nursing service administrator carries out the duty of generating a physical and conceptual environment conducive to the coordinated participation of team members or participants. In this sense the nursing service administrator becomes a composite process specialist.

The work environment with which administrators are concerned involves two parts: conceptual and physical. The conceptual environment *(Ec)* is concerned with the mental facet of the interpersonal relationship that affects a nurse's attitude toward work and the place of work. The conceptual or mental interpersonal–relationships environment that administrators generate is aimed at creating for each person a positive attitude or frame of mind that will have a salutary effect on the employee's willingness to participate in the health care enterprise. This environment aims at creating a frame of mind that will enable each person to understand why it is to one's advantage to expend efforts to achieve the objectives of the institution, it being "to the person's advantage" only when one is enabled directly or indirectly to reach one's personal goal or goals.

The second part of the environment with which nursing service administrators are concerned is physical *(Ep)* in nature, and this environment includes all the physical aspects of which it is composed. The esthetic qualities of the health care facilities of the institution and the architectural planning of life-space constitute a significant principle of the philosophy underlying the patient and personnel centered approach, since these aspects deal solely with human qualities. In particular, many of the purely biophysical and biochemical tensions imposed on personnel and medical staff, which are inevitably transmitted to the patient, can to a marked degree be prevented through hospital planning and design. Furthermore, time and space impressions bear direct relation to human interaction and, thus, to stress reduction or stress production.

An administrator's prime task, therefore, is the creation of a healthy physical and mental, interpersonal relationship, work climate that will induce others to willingly contribute their efforts to achieve the objectives of the institution. Without this proper physical-conceptual environment or work climate, the participant's efforts may be ineffective or even lacking.

The administrative theory has been strengthened through the systems frame of reference. Exposure to the widening dissemination of the systems theory and its increasing applications to so many fields, including health, provided the point of entry. The systems frame of reference, as applied to the field, can best be understood as a complex set of related, interacting social factors and institutional mechanisms responding to a subset of societal needs and demands, that is, those related to their health. A systems approach forces us to pinpoint and describe the successive states of the system and to assess each of them in terms of its contribution to meeting the purpose of the system. It demands further that we accurately examine and describe the environment within which the system functions and that we gauge the impact that environment has on the system—how it provides inputs to it and absorbs its outputs and what kinds of constraints it places on the system as it seeks to fulfill its purpose.

We need to identify and describe the boundaries of the health system, as we would do for any system under study. This requires us to make distinctions between the health care system and other socially relevant systems with which it relates (interfaces), such as education, employment, and housing. Agreed that these boundary definitions may be arbitrary, but this is one way we can set limits to one field and subject it to careful inquiry, analysis, and evaluation. In the broadest sense we are forced to identify and, through systems analysis, describe all those transactions taking place within the system if we are ever to be in a position to assess or evaluate its effectiveness.

External environment: the nursing service organization as an open system

The second part of the model emphasizes the external environment (Fig. 2-3). A health care organization does not exist in a vacuum. It exists in association with

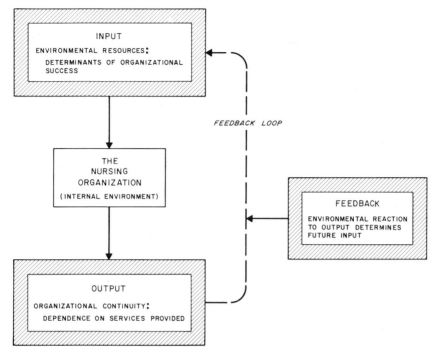

Fig. 2-3. External environment: elements of the environment include people, physical resources, climate, economic conditions, attitudes, and laws.

its environment, which provides resources and limitations. If the organization is to remain socially useful and economically stable, it must continually adapt to its environment, which is constantly changing. Failure to adequately adapt to the environment is a major cause of organization failure.

A nursing service organization and its environment are interdependent; the organization depends on its environment for the resources and opportunities necessary for its existence (Fig. 2-3, input). Too, the environment determines the limits of the organization's activities. The environment will contribute valuable resources to the organization only if the organization provides desired services to the environment (Fig. 2-3, output). The activities of the organization when doing so must be acceptable to the environment. For example, nurses must serve people and assume responsibility for services rendered without excessively delegating direct people services to nonprofessional staffs. Through

feedback the environment reacts to the services rendered by and the activities of the nursing service organization (Fig. 2-3, feedback). The environment evaluates the services and determines the future resources that it will contribute and the restrictions that it will place on the organization.

Constraints: external environment

The nursing service organization is influenced by the external environment. Its constraints may be divided into four classes: educational, sociological-cultural, legal-political, and economic (Fig. 2-4).

1. Educational constraints include such things as personnel lacking in knowledge, the availability of specialized professional and technical education, the prevailing attitude toward education, and the extent to which education matches requirements for skills and abilities. The educational factors may support or limit effective nursing service administration.
2. Sociological-cultural constraints include a great number of factors. Some of the most

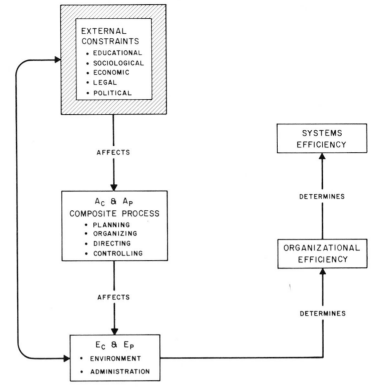

Fig. 2-4. Constraints. (From Donnelly, J., Gibson, J., and Ivancevich, J.: Fundamentals of management, Dallas, Tex., 1971, Business Publications, Inc., p. 400.)

important are the general attitude of colleagues and society toward nursing administrators; the dominant views of authority and subordinates; the extent of cooperation from professional organizations, unions, and administration; and the prevailing view in the country toward health and the significance of its cost.

3. Legal-political constraints include such things as political stability and the flexibility of law and legal changes regarding health.

4. Economic constraints include such factors as the basic economic status in the country, whether within the health care industry private or public ownership prevails, whether it is a competitive economy based on sound money, and the extent to which the government controls economic and health care activities.

By analyzing the external environmental constraints, it was found that these constraints definitely influence practice in specific instances. Separating them from the administrative processes narrowed the concept of administration to administra-

tive functions and in so doing became a useful means for evaluating the administrator and for presenting what may make effective administration differ between varying environments. An additional advantage of this approach is that it can be a useful practical aid for nursing service organizations in different environments. By specifying the areas of external constraints that may exist and by identifying the elements within each area, this approach provides nursing administration with an orderly framework within which to perform the composite process in varying environments.

Information and energy flow: sensor, decision-making mechanism, and environment processor

The fourth part of the model (Fig. 2-5) emphasizes flows of information, material resources, and energy through the organi-

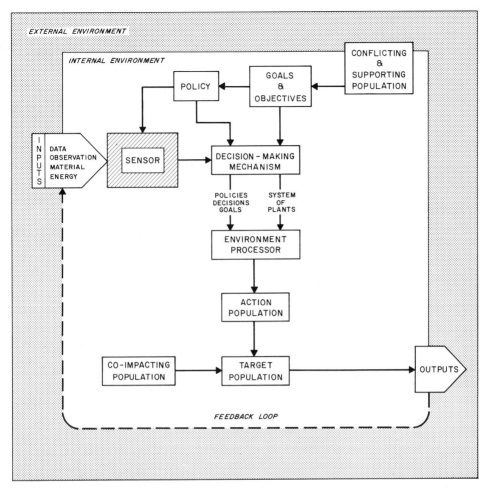

Fig. 2-5. Information and energy flow: sensor, decision-making mechanism, and environment processor.

zation (inputs), which is itself composed of three entities—a sensor, a decision-making mechanism, and an environment processor. The sensors, nursing administrator and associates, receive information from stimuli (data and observations) extracted from the internal nursing service organization and from the external environment. Information flows not only to points of decision but also throughout the health care organization in a network of communications. The decision-making mechanism uses information as the basis for deciding what should be done and for ordering the environment processor to do it. Material flow is a primary concern of the environment processor. Material flow ranges from the acquisition of equipment and supplies to the distribution of services to patients. The decision-making mechanism plans the activities of the processor-*environment*. The energy flow consists of human and nonhuman forms. An example of a nonhuman form is electronic energy. The various forms of energy are combined with materials and information by the processor as the plans made by the decision-making mechanism are executed.

The processor-environment consists of all the administrative and operational functions relating to nursing administrative decisions. Specifically, the processor-environment includes not only the physical acquisition, conversion, and distribution activities, but also the administrative functions of planning, organizing, directing, and controlling. Also implied are all the informal, face-to-face, interpersonal relationships required in executing the decisions.

Systems reference is useful for conceptualizing important facets of organizations that may be omitted from nonsystems approaches. For instance, the systems approach emphasizes the significance of the decision-making–decision-execution feedback loop, which operates via the environment. In addition, it shows that the systems view of organizations does not restrict itself to interrelationships of internal subsystems. For example, the supervisor, a processor, performs all those activities associated with the operation and control of the services, personnel, and research development. This position is not distinct from that of the administrator, or sensor mechanism, in that it may be the instrument for carrying actions, such as reorganization. Thus, the supervisor completes the feedback loop by creating the information, material, and energy flows back to the environment.

Measurements: action population

The primary fundamentals of health organization deal with those phases of administration that include policy formulation and organization structure. The operating fundamentals deal almost entirely with the operating phase of administration. The primary fundamentals of organization may be stated as (1) regard for the aim and objectives of the institution, (2) the establishment of definite lines of administration with the organization structure, (3) the placing of fixed responsibility among the various persons and departments within the organization, and (4) regard for the personal equation.

The operating fundamentals may be stated as (1) the development of an ade-

quate system, (2) the establishment of adequate records to implement the system and to use as a basis of control, (3) the laying down of proper operating rules and regulations within the established organization in keeping with the established policies, and (4) the exercise of effective leadership.

Fig. 2-6 is the fifth component of the model and measures goal accomplishment. Using the formula devised by George (1972), we can measure whether we have accomplished our objectives.

Inasmuch as the physical and conceptual acts $(Ac$ and $Ap)$ of administration (Ad) may be expressed as a compound of planning (P), organization (O), directing (D), and controlling (C) with varying percentages whose total is unity, then

$$(Ac + Ap) = \%_1 P + \%_2 O + \%_3 D + \%_4 C$$

Where

$$\sum_{i=1} \%_i = 1$$

and

$$\%_i > O$$

Therefore

$$Ad = [(\%_1 P + \%_2 O + \%_3 D + \%_4 C) \rightarrow (EC + Ep)] f(Oi, Og)$$

It may well be that an organization's goal is 90% achieved, whereas the individual's goals are 20% realized. Under these conditions employee resistance may well result. This resistance, in turn, would cause a change in administrative actions to effect a greater achievement of individual goals. If, however, the organization's goal is only 10% achieved, then some change will be made by the administrator in her actions to effect a greater than 10% achievement of the organization's goal. A good or effective administrator, therefore, is one who promotes high achievement in individual as well as in organizational goals.

Given the preceding, one may express

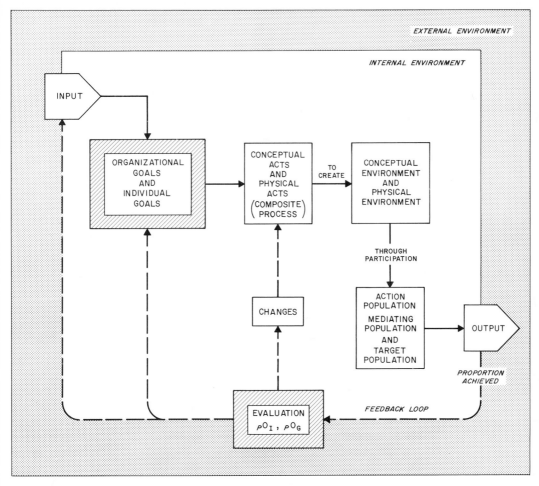

Fig. 2-6. Measurement: action population.

administrative achievement *(AdA)* as the percentage *(p)* that the goals of the organization and the employee are realized.

$$AdA = p \, (Oi + Og)$$

Likewise, if we recognize that administrative acts *(Aad)* are a function of the percentage of $Oi + Og$, then

$$Aad = f(pOi + pOg)$$

If Og is known, Oi is a function of it. Thus

$$Oi = f(Og)$$

and

$$Og = f(Oi)$$

If we recognize that administrative acts are functions of goals and that the effectiveness of these acts is expressed in a percent relation to goal achievement, then we see that the percentage of achievement changes an administrator's conceptual and physical acts, which yield the conceptual and physical environment $[(Ac + Ap) \rightarrow (Ec + Ep)]$, a function of the goals.

Change

The administration of change implies a systematic process. The part of our model concerned with the change process is presented in Fig. 2-7. It consists of five subprocesses that are linked in a logical sequence. To undertake a change program, an administrator considers each of them,

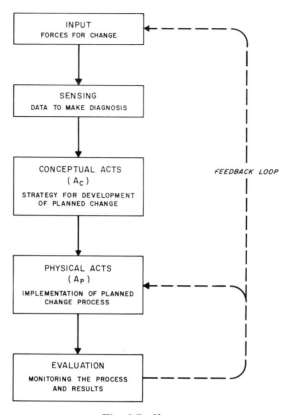

Fig. 2-7. Change.

either explicitly or implicitly. The prospects for initiating successful change is enhanced when an administrator explicitly and formally goes through each successive step.

The change process presumes that inputs in terms of forces for change, externally and internally, are continually acting on the institution; this assumption reflects the dynamic character of the modern world. At the same time it is the administrator's, or sensor's, responsibility to analyze and sort the information that is received from the organization's control system and other sources in the form of measurement of objectives, which reflect the magnitude of change (Og and Oi) forces. The information is the basis for recognizing the need for change; it is equally desirable to recognize when change is not needed. But once the nursing service administrator recognizes that some-

thing is not functioning, a diagnosis of the problem must be made and relevant alternative change techniques identified. The change technique selected must be appropriate to the problem, as constrained by limiting conditions. One example of a limiting condition is the prevailing character of group norms. The nursing groups may support some of the change techniques but disapprove of others. Further limiting conditions may include leadership behavior and the formal organization.

The fact that a change program can be undermined underscores the fact that the choice of change strategy is as important as the change technique itself. One well-documented behavioral phenomenon is that people tend to resist change or at least to be reluctant to undergo change. An appropriate strategy for implementing change is one that, according to Kurt Lewin (1947), seeks to minimize resistance or the restraining forces and to maximize employee commitment. Finally, the nursing service administrator, in cooperation with the coimpacting and target population, implements the change and monitors the change process. The model includes feedback to the implementation phase and to the input, or forces-for-change, phase. The feedback loops suggest that the change process itself must be monitored and evaluated. Moreover, the feedback loop to the initial step recognizes that no change is final. The framework suggests no final solution, rather, it emphasizes that the modern nursing service administrator works in a dynamic setting wherein the only certainty is change itself.

Systems frame of reference

Fig. 2-1 brings together into a single entity all of the separately discussed parts. It emphasizes the mutual interrelatedness and interdependency among the parts as well as the need for integration.

What does administrative theory within a systems frame of reference have to offer? In the first place, any theory seeks to provide a verifiable systematic explanation of the world about us and to suggest other lines of inquiry to test, enrich, or even invalidate it. For the nursing service administrators, if any theory is to be really serviceable, it must enable them to understand the problems of a here-and-now situation and must provide assistance when a course of action is needed. In addition, it must be flexible enough to be employed in the variety of situations that a nursing service administrator encounters. The model (Fig. 2-1) makes operative the processes of administration and the open systems concept by providing a framework that satisfies the conditions mentioned above. Specific situations that this model serves may be listed as (1) the designing of a new nursing service organization, (2) the diagnosing of nursing service problems, and (3) the changing of an already existing organization from low accomplishments to new heights of accomplishments.

The core of the model is the administrative theory based on a synthesis of knowledge derived from four schools of scientific thought (scientific management, process, and behavioral and management science).

New thinking has been introduced, first, by separating the functions of administration (planning, organizing, directing, and controlling) from the environment in which administration actually occurs. By so doing, the administrative process has been accepted as a means of more effectively meeting objectives. Second, the administrative process has become a tool for diagnosing problems by asking pertinent questions concerning the setting of objectives, by planning to meet the objectives, by organizing for the accomplishment of the plan, by directing and implementing the designed plan, and by establishing controlling mechanisms. Third, constraints stemming from the external environment have an effect on the administrative process. By separating the administrative functions from its consideration of the external environmental factors that can influence actual practice in specific instances, the administrative process appears to be a useful means for evaluating administration and for presenting what may make effective administration differ between different environs. By specifying the areas of external constraints that may exist and by identifying the elements within each area, the administrative process provides administration with an orderly framework within which to perform the administrative functions in varying environments.

Conceptual thinking is instituted by the model shown in Fig. 2-1, as the organization is looked on as an open system. An open system means that it influences and is being influenced by the external environment through the process of "influence reciprocity," which results in a dynamic (changing) equilibrium. A health care organization provides an excellent example of the process of influence reciprocity and, therefore, of an open system.

Goals and objectives are received as inputs from the environment. How well the objectives are accomplished, however, depends on the means employed, namely, the administrative process. Output is determined by how well the objectives (quality of service in nursing) are accomplished. Through feedback, further input is received or withheld by the environment, depending on the quality of output.

The systems frame of reference brings into sharp focus the external environmental forces. The administrator, in the role of the sensor (Fig. 2-5), receives stimuli, data, and observations from the environment. The information is analyzed, and decisions are made and communicated to the processes of administration in the form of goals, objectives, policies, and systems of plans. But, while the sensor is analyzing data, other energy—human and material—flows directly from the environment into the system; conversion takes place in the internal environment and is transported in the form of output service to the external environment. The point is made that the system never rests and is in a dynamic state of equilibrium.

The goals of organizations are growth, stability, and interaction. If the output of the system is unsatisfactory to the external environment, this information will be received via feedback at the input level, at which point resources will be restricted or withheld depending on the extent of the dissatisfaction with the service. The nursing service administrator is made aware of needed changes through sensing the input and through new thinking about the administrative process, a tool to make an adequate nursing diagnosis.

In summary, the model describes the following two concepts:

1. The administrative process. By separating the administrative process from the actual environment in which administration takes place, the administrative process has become (a) a means to accomplish objectives and a tool for designing a new or renovating an old organization, (b) a tool for diagnosing organizational problems, (c) a tool for bringing about change through feedback, and (d) an evaluation tool for administration.

2. The systems frame of reference, or open system. The concept focuses on the environment (a) input, (b) transformation, (c) output, and (d) feedback.

The administrative process, as a system, shares characteristics with all other systems; it is illuminated by present knowledge about systems and is also shadowed by the limitations of present knowledge about the nature and workings of systems. To see administration as a system is to view the process from a broad perspective; to understand more comprehensively its nature, its structure, and its process; to be able to deal with the interrelationships that characterize the operation as the whole; and to be able to serve as the designer and engineer of the system by means of which any whole is administered.

Whereas previously it was enough to view the administrative process as relating to a job at the place of work, the techniques of planning, the relations of employees to one another, the qualities of leadership, the nature of decision making, and other aspects of activities in organizations, we have recently become conscious of the need to deal in a conceptual way with the entire process. We have discovered synergy, learned that the whole is greater than the sum of its parts, and come to realize that there is a clear need for building ideas of wholeness, on the framework of which a more adequate conceptual image of administration can be built.

The need is now apparent for integrating knowledge about the complete process and discovering how much we know about the concept of administration in its entirety. The knowledge that helps us to look at the whole, as distinct from the parts, is the knowledge that in the future will be the most substantive and valuable in the field of administration.

In the past, organizations were looked upon essentially as people, structures, and organizations in which the principal characteristic is the structural relationship that exists between and among the human participants. Since the concept of structure has been put in better perspective, the process of organization has come into clearer view and has come to be recognized as being of no less importance than its structure. With systems insights we are able to visualize process, to work with it, to model it, to simulate it, and to reckon with it as a vital aspect of reality. The more one deals with process, and reflects on its relationship with structure, the more one sees that systems are indivisible; "structure" and "process" are only names that we as individuals have given to aspects of the system to which we have confined our observations.

In theory, then, the new organization is a whole—a system. It is neither structure nor process; it is both.

CORRELATION OF COMPONENT PARTS OF ADMINISTRATIVE THEORY MODEL

The second part of this chapter covers three areas: (1) the explanation of the nature of the systems approach, its rationale, the component parts, and characteristic that are specific to a systems approach; (2) the application of the administrative theory within the systems frame of reference and its operationalization; and (3) illustration of the subsystems of a health care organization as an open sociotechnical system.

Description of the systems approach

Systems are made up of sets of components or parts that work together for the achievement of the objectives of the enterprise. It is a way of looking at a social and technical organization as a whole. A system is a complex of elements in mutual interaction.

Systems can be considered in one of two ways: closed or open. A closed system is used mostly by the physical sciences and is applicable to mechanistic systems. The physical sciences view the system as self-contained. Traditional organization theories and still earlier concepts in the social sciences were a closed system. Traditional administrative theories concentrated only on the internal operation of the organization and tried to utilize the highly rationalistic approaches taken from physical science models. The physical science models considered the organization to be sufficiently independent to the extent that its problems could be analyzed in terms of internal structures, tasks, and formal relationships without reference to the external environment. A characteristic of a closed system is its tendency toward entropy and a static equilibrium. Entropy is a measure of ignorance, disorder, disorganization, randomness, or chaos. During this chaotic state a closed system has no further potential for energy transformation or work. A closed system tends to increase in entropy over time and moves toward greater randomness and disorder.

An open system, on the other hand, is in continuous interaction with its environment and achieves a steady state or dynamic equilibrium while retaining its capacity for work and energy transformation. A steady state refers to the maintenance of a constant ratio among the components of the system, given a continues input. Open systems exchange energy and information with their environment, that is, inputs and outputs. A nursing service organization is such a system.

It is not possible for a system to survive without continuous input, transformation, and output. A general model of a social organization as an open system is illustrated in Fig. 2-8.

A system needs to receive enough input of resources to maintain its operations

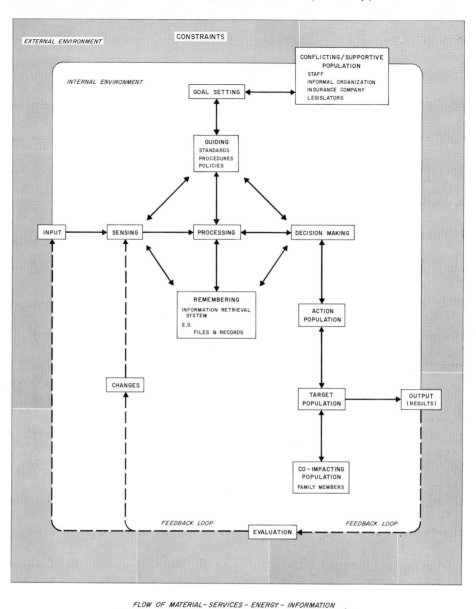

Fig. 2-8. General model of a social organization as an open system. Arrows indicate relationships, communication, and direction of flow information, material, services, and energy.

and to export its transformed product into the environment in sufficient quantity to survive and to continue its cycle.

Let us put the above systems model into operation and apply it to the health care organization. The hospital as an open sociotechnical system receives two types of input: work input (patients, food, ma-terials such as equipment and machinery, and information such as community's needs for patient care services and the expectations of the community) and sus-taining input (people, for example, physi-cians, nurses, technicians, and experts in other related fields; funds; and knowledge) (see Fig. 2-1). Inputs into the organization come from the external environment and from within the organization; for example, in the evaluation of outputs, feedback is provided as an input to the organization for improvement and changes.

The inputs (people, funds, equipment) undergo *sensing* by assigned people in their departments. For example, if the input is a patient entering the system, the admission office handles the processing; if it is money, the cashier takes care of that part; if it is a nurse seeking employment, either the nursing administrator or the personnel officer does the sensing. Assigned people who are performing the sensing duties in their departments are guided by hospital policies, procedures, and standards and may resort to other types of information—*remembering*, which is an information retrieval system, for example, patient records, files, and performance records.

The planning and implementation phase of the transformational process is called *processing*. The person who is dealing with this phase is also guided by the policies and procedures of the hospital and may need more information, in which case the person will resort to remembering. For example, if the nursing administrator is faced with a sudden influx of patients owing to a disaster, the processing will include such activities as the planning, organization, directing, and controlling for safe delivery of patient care services. The decision making in this situation deals with achieving the goals of safe delivery of care; for example, the nursing administrator will resort to a preplanned program for the management of a disaster, which may entail opening a new clinical unit and recruiting extra nurses. The personnel through which the decisions that were made are being implemented, for example, assistant nurse administrators, coordinators, charge nurses, and team leaders, are called the *action population* or *processor-environment*. The staff members, for example, nursing and paranursing personnel

and ultimately the beneficiaries, patients, are called the *target population*. The families of staff members and patients are called the *coimpacting population*. Service in the form of safe delivery of care, patient satisfaction, employee satisfaction, research, and education form the *output*.

Outputs of social organizations can be classified in two major categories: (1) objective, such as quantity and quality of production and service, absenteeism, turnover, and profits and (2) subjective or attitudinal, such as the satisfactions that the staff members and administrators derive from participation in the organization. Job satisfaction is the sum of several satisfactions. For example, it may include intrinsic job satisfaction, satisfaction with the superiors, with programs of the organization, with personal achievements, with one's peers and co-workers, or with one's advancements (Triandis 1968; Dabas 1958; Roach 1957; Twery, Schmid, and Wrigley 1958). Employee morale is also one of the most frequently cited concerns in the literature of organization theory. Morale is the concept specifying the congruence of individual and group goals. It deals with the "persistence of individuals in reaching the group goals and the absorption of the individual in activities leading to reaching these goals" (Triandis 1968:68).

These outputs then undergo evaluation by the organization or the community or both, which are the consumers of health care delivery systems. Results from these evaluations in the form of information, criticism, or comments, on areas that need improvement and change, or funds return to the organization through the feedback loop as inputs. The cycle then repeats itself.

The goals and values of the department, more specifically, the organizational objectives and individual objectives, are termed *goal setting*. These objectives guide the whole functioning of the system. Goal setting is commonly referred to as *man-*

agement by objectives. The outputs are measured in terms of these objectives and the degree to which these objectives are achieved.

Those people who are either within the organization or outside the organization and who may enhance or deter the functioning of the organization as a system to meet its goals are the *conflicting and supportive population.* The same people may act in either role. For example, when the informal organization within a department is antagonized by the formal organization, the people will work against the goals of that department or act as an obstacle to the achievement of the organization's goals by not cooperating. If, however, the formal organization cooperates with the informal organization, the informal organization can be a positive force that facilitates the achievement of the goals of the organization. Other conflicting or supportive populations for a health care organization can be the legislators, staff members, schools of nursing, professional organizations and associations, labor unions, and insurance companies.

The concept of *constraints* that affect the whole system can be such variables as tradition, fiscal budget, physical structure and size of the institution, religious beliefs, and other implications. Constraints affect the accomplishment of the goals and objectives of the institution.

The advantages of using the systems frame of reference in illustrating the functioning of an organization or a department within an organization are as follows. First, the systems frame of reference makes visible who does what. Visibility in the system determines areas of accountability. It avoids overlap of responsibility and accountability. Second, errors and problems tend to become more easily detected. Third, intervention is more specific because personnel can identify the phase within which errors have occurred. Fourth, the systems frame of reference provides for economy of time and energy.

OTHER CHARACTERISTICS OF OPEN SOCIOTECHNICAL SYSTEMS

1. The view of an organization as an open sociotechnical system suggests that there are boundaries that separate it from the environment. Closed systems have rigid inpenetrable boundaries. Open systems have more permeable boundaries among themselves and a broader supersystem. The concept of boundary helps specify what is inside or outside the system. According to Chin (1969), the boundary of a system may exist physically, for example, the skin of a person or the number of people in a group. Also, the boundary of a system may be viewed in a less tangible way by placing boundaries according to what variables are being focused upon or by determining the steps in a process. A system can be viewed in terms of multiple roles of a person or varied roles among members in a small work group or in a family. The components or variables used are roles, acts, expectations, communication, influence, and power relationship. The concept of *boundary* is operationally defined by Chin (1969: 300) as "the line forming a closed circle around selected variables, where there is less interchange of energy (or communication, etc.) *across* the line of the circle than within the delimiting circle."

One of the key functions within any organization is that of boundary regulations between systems. Likert (1961) points out that one of the primary roles or functions of management is to serve as a linking pin or boundary agent between the various subsystems to ensure integration and cooperation. The research findings of Arndt and Laeger (1970a and b) point out that the nurse administrator is a focal person who occupies a position within a diversified role set. Kast and Rosenzweig (1970) further stress an additional managerial function, that of serving as boundary agent between the organization and its environment. For example, nursing service administrators possess such a critical role. They can serve as a link between the institutional level (hospital administrator or the board of trustees) and the technical core (nursing department). They can also function as a boundary agent or link between the community (environment of the system) and the nursing department.

2. The concept of *interface* refers to the area of contact between one system and another; for example, the hospital has interfaces with many other systems that are outside the organization, such as professional associations, the local community, suppliers of materials, prospective employees, unions, and state, local, and federal governmental agencies. There are many transactional processes across systems boundaries at the interface involving transfer of people, funds, material, energy, and information. Within the internal environment of the hospital organization an interface is the area of contact between one subsystem and another where the output of one step becomes input for another, for example, between sensing and processing and between processing and guiding.

3. A characteristic of all systems, whether physical, biological, or social, is that they can be considered in a hierarchical sense. A system is composed of subsystems and at the same time is part of a supersystem. Large organizations are generally hierarchical in structure. For example, people are organized into groups, groups are a part of departments, departments are organized into divisions, and divisions into companies (Kast and Rosenzweig 1970). According to Simon (1960), hierarchical subdivisions are not unique to human organizations but are characteristic of almost all complex systems. He states that "the reasons for hierarchy go far beyond the need for unity of command or other considerations relating to authority" (Simon 1960:40-42). Hierarchical structure is based on the need for a combination of subsystems progressing into a broader system to coordinate activities and processes.

There are two types of hierarchy within complex organizations, hierarchy of processes and of structures.

4. Open systems display *progressive segregation*. This process occurs when the system divides into a hierarchical order of subordinate systems that gain some degree of independence of each other.

5. Open systems are *self-regulating*. Central to the success of open systems is the concept of organization equilibrium. According to Chin (1969), a system is assumed to have a tendency to achieve a balance among the various forces operating within and on it. The term *equilibrium* is used to denote when the balance of a system is thought of as a fixed point or level, for example, body temperature at 98.6° F. Steady state, on the other hand, refers to the balanced relationship of parts that is not dependent on a fixed equilibrium point or level, for example, the functional relationship among clinical units in a hospital, regardless of the level of service. In most cases, however, the term equilibrium is used to cover both types of balances.

Equilibrium may be static or dynamic. In a condition of static equilibrium a system responds to a stimulus or a change in its environment by a reaction or adjustment that tends to restore the system to its original state. We rarely find such instances in human relationships because of the variability of individuals. In a condition of dynamic equilibrium the system responds to a stimulus or a change in its environment by a shift to a new balance or by a modification of its goals (Lonsdale 1964; Chin 1969).

A system in equilibrium responds to disturbances from the outside in three ways: (1) by resisting or disregarding the disturbances or by protecting and defending itself against the intrusion, for example, a small group (nursing team) refuses to talk or discuss a problem of unequal patient load or of unequal power distribution raised by a member, (2) by using homeostatic forces to restore the former balance, for example, the small group talks about the problem that was brought up by a member or convinces the member that it is not "really" a problem, or (3) by accommodating to these disturbances or by achieving a new equilibrium, for example, talking about the problem may result in an equalization in patient load distribution or a shift in power relationships among members of the group. Team leaders or administrators should assist the group or the organization in responding to the third of these three ways.

6. Open systems maintain their steady equilibrium in part through the dynamic interplay of subsystems operating as functional processes; that is, the different parts of the systems operate without persistent conflicts that can be neither resolved nor regulated (Griffiths 1964).

Because the components within systems are different from each other or are not well integrated, either changing or reacting to change, or because disturbances and intrusions from the outside occur, we need ways of dealing with these differences. These differences lead to varying degrees of tension within a system. The internal tensions that arise out of the structural arrangements of the system are referred to as stresses or strains of the system. But when tensions conglomerate and become sharply opposed along the lines of two or more components, they are referred to as *conflicts* (Chin 1969).

Systems have both adaptive and maintenance mechanisms. To maintain an equilibrium, maintenance mechanisms ensure that the various subsystems are in balance and that the total system is in accord with its environment. The forces of maintenance mechanism help to prevent the system from changing too rapidly and also tend to prevent the various subsystems and the total system from getting out of balance. The adaptive mechanisms are necessary to keep the system in dynamic equilibrium, one that is changing over time. Thus, the adaptive mechanisms help the sys-

tem to respond to changing internal and external requirements. Some forces within the social organization are geared toward maintenance of the systems; some are geared toward adaptation. Often these two forces will cause tension, strain, and conflict, natural manifestations that should not be considered unhealthy. Chin states that the presence of tension and conflict within a system is viewed as shameful and to be done away with, but "tension reduction, relief of stress and strain, or conflict resolution become the working goals of practitioners but some times at the price of overlooking the possibility of increasing tensions and conflict to facilitate creativity, innovation and social change" (Chin 1969:301).

The identification and analysis of how tension operates in a system and the utility of systems analysis for the practitioners of change are of great importance. These tensions lead to two kinds of activities, those that do not affect the structure of the system (dynamics) and those that alter the structure itself (system).

7. Another characteristic of an open system is its *feedback* mechanism. Open systems maintain their steady state, in part, through feedback. Feedback is that portion of the output of a system that is fed back in a loop to the input and affects succeeding outputs by adjusting the way the system responds to inputs and to the properties of being able to adjust future conduct by past performance. Through feedback the system continually receives information from its environment, which helps in its adjustment. The feedback input is used to steer the operation of the system. The *sensory organ* of the organization functioning to process the information feedback is the individuals or groups within the administrative hierarchy assigned the role of assessing the information and then sending the right signal with new information and perhaps instructions back to the action points, so they may continue or modify action and behavior, as necessary. One of the problems to watch for, if

the feedback loop is to work properly, is sensitizing the sensory organ of the organization so as to decrease any blockage and increase receptivity. Programs in sensitivity education for administrators attempt to increase and unblock the feedback process of persons (Tannenbaum, Weschler, and Massarek 1961; Lonsdale 1964; Chin 1969).

8. Open systems display *equifinality;* that is, identical results can be obtained from different initial conditions. In physical systems (closed systems) there is direct cause and effect relationship between the initial conditions and the final state. However, biological and social systems (open systems) operate differently and display equifinality. This view suggests that the social organization can accomplish its objectives with varying inputs and with varying internal activities. Thus a social system is not restrained by the simple cause and effect relationship of the closed system. The concept of equifinality of an open system is of great importance for the administration of complex organizations. As opposed to the cause and effect relationship of the closed system, which suggests that there is only one best way to meet an objective, the equifinality of the open system suggests to the administrator that varying bundles of inputs into the organization can be utilized and that they can transform these in different ways and can achieve satisfactory output. An important implication of this view is that the administrative function is not necessarily one of seeking a rigid and best optimal solution to a problem, but rather one of having available a variety of satisfactory alternatives and solutions to problems of decision.

Making the administrative model of an organization operational
A SYSTEMS FRAME OF REFERENCE

In this discussion administrative theory is applied to the administration of nursing services within health care institutions. This theoretical framework can be utilized for the administration of any type of sociotechnical organization, and the major concepts apply to the administration of departments, units, or teams within any organization that deals with people and technology.

The example used to make the administrative theory operational is at the level of the nursing service administrator, who is responsible for operating the department of nursing within the health care institution. Fig. 2-1 illustrates the sequential functioning of the system at this level.

The inputs into the system are people (personnel and patients), funds, equipment, information in the form of new knowledge, and feedback information from the output. Therefore, the quality of output is an essential variable that affects the input. Some aspects of organizational objectives that are set forth by the community also act as input into the system.

Next comes the sensing process, that of analyzing, sorting, allocating, and channeling of information and resources to proper destinations. Sensing is done by nursing administrators or assistant administrators, also known as the sensors. As the different inputs are communicated the administrator sensors them according to the charter, philosophy, policies, procedures, goals, and objectives of the institution. Sensing is a conceptual process that precedes planning. For example, if the nursing administrator is appointed to open a new nursing service department, the administrator utilizes this framework to organize the nursing department. In this situation the items that need sensing are (1) patients, to ensure proper care, (2) nurses with different professional preparation to staff clinical units or outpatient clinics, (3) available funds to plan the budget, (4) equipment and machinery to ensure proper functioning, and (5) pertinent information, such as new knowledge and environmental needs to help plan the nursing division of the health care institution. While sensing the inputs the nursing service administrator may need to resort to remembering, to retrieve pertinent information to do efficient and effective sensing. The administrator also relies heavily on the learned and acquired theoretical and practical knowledge base in planning the new nursing department.

The third phase of administrative activity is the composite process, which is separated into *conceptual acts* and *physical acts*. Conceptual acts are cognitive in nature and deal with the planning and organizing aspects of administration. Physical acts are more functional and technical in nature. They are the doing part of the administrative act. They deal with directing and controlling. The planning function deals with setting specific organizational and individual goals and objectives. The *conceptual environment* is concerned with the work of building a milieu that is conducive to the practice of professional nursing in which patients receive optimal care. The conceptual environment deals with such things as employee morale and employee satisfaction from work. It is concerned with relationships among people working together, human relationships, relationships between the formal and informal organizations, and people having a voice in their work situation.

The *physical environment* encompasses the architectural design of the institution, which accommodates or fits the patient care design. For example, an interdisciplinary health team approach to patient care requires that the different members of the health team have a place that is sufficiently comfortable physically to meet and discuss patient care problems. Equipment and supplies are part of the physical environment. The organizational structure (people structure), vertical and horizontal with communication channels, is part of the physical environment of the organization. The physical and conceptual environments are very much interrelated and must be in balance to achieve the goals, values, and objectives of both the organization and the individuals within the organization.

Another phase of administrative activity is setting organizational and individual objectives. This takes place at the same time that planning is initiated. The overall *organizational objectives* are set forth by the board of trustees, the hospital administrator, and the nursing service administrator. Those objectives that specifically deal with the nursing department and the delivery of patient care are set forth by the nursing administrators and their associates, utilizing the organization's framework of thinking. They receive inputs from the policies and standards of the institution. Their past experience and their learned theoretical frame of reference also guide them in establishing organizational objectives for the department of nursing.

The *individual objectives* are set forth by the individual employee in consultation with the immediate superior. Inputs into the establishment of individual objectives are the employee's expectations, capabilities, educational preparation, and the specific job description, which is prepared by the organization.

The nursing service administrator creates the environment to achieve the goals through the *action, mediating,* or *processor population,* for example, the administrative nursing personnel, such as the assistant nurse administrator, nursing coordinators, or head nurses. The nursing service administrator cannot do everything and, therefore, delegates certain tasks to others with due delegation of authority, responsibility, and accountability to perform the task; this constitutes the sixth phase of the administrative activity. The decisions that are made by the nurse administrator are implemented by these action people, who in turn affect the *target population*. In this case the target population is the nursing and paranursing personnel, who are concerned with direct patient care, and ultimately the benefactors of care, the patients. They are the consumers of the total administrative process. They are either the benefactors or the victims of the administrative process. The target population, in turn, is influenced by the *coimpacting population,* meaning their family members or members in the community who influence the nurses, either positively or negatively. For example, a family member can press on the target person (nurse) to ask for more money (raise) or better working hours. Or, the family member may affect the target person, positively by asking the nurse to keep the job and suggesting that the remuneration is adequate and the working hours excellent.

The results and the consequences of the functioning of the whole administrative system is exported to the environment as outputs in terms of organizational and individual objectives, for example, the patient care service, contribution to community, research, education, and employee satisfaction.

These outputs are then evaluated in terms of organizational and individual objectives, and the proportion achieved in each case is determined. This evaluation is done by the organization itself (nurse administrator and heads of other departments) and by the community, and the deficiencies and recommendations for changes are then fed back as inputs into the system through the feedback loop. In this way the cycle continues.

In addition to the administrative cycle there are two factors that influence the functioning of the system: a *conflicting* and *supporting* population and the *constraints.*

A conflicting and supporting population is inherent in any organization. It influences either positively or negatively the operation of the system. For example, if the nursing administrator does not have the backing of the staff or other departments, the programs of the nurse administrator may fail. However, if there is full support, then a better environment can be created to achieve the goals of the organization.

Every institution has constraints that affect the operation of the organization. An example of constraint is tradition. If the leadership within the organization is tradition oriented, they may discourage the testing and implementation of innovative ideas. Another example of constraint is the economy and the financial status of the nation as a whole. For example, inflation or depression affect adversely the budget of the organization.

Subsystems of a health care organization as an open sociotechnical system

The health care organization can also be viewed as a structural sociotechnical system with five primary subsystems or components: goals and values, administrative composite process consisting of conceptual acts and physical acts, conceptual environment, the physical environment, and technology. One way of viewing the organization as a sociotechnical system is shown in Fig. 2-9. These subsystems are integral parts of the overall organization.

The sociotechnical view of an organization was originally set forth by Trist and his associates at the Tavistock Institute. His concept of a sociotechnical system arose from the consideration that any production system requires a technical organization, for example, equipment, machinery, and process layout, and a work organization that deals with people who carry out the necessary tasks. A work organization has psychological and sociological properties of its own that are different and independent of technology.

Therefore, an organization is not simply a technical or a social system, but it deals with the integration of human activities around different technologies. The technical aspects of an organization affect the types of inputs and outputs of the organization. However, the conceptual environment with its social system determines the effectiveness and efficiency of the utilization of the technology.

Before an organization is created its originators have certain purposes in mind.

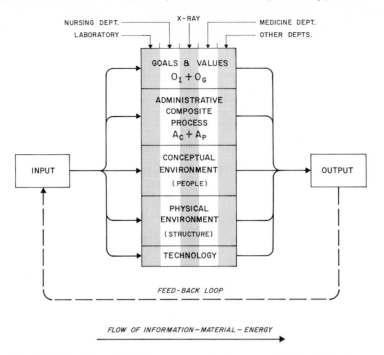

Fig. 2-9. Subsystems of health care organizations as sociotechnical systems.

The originators commonly ask themselves about the aims, purposes, *goals,* and *objectives* of the organization, for example, what do they want to accomplish and why and how should they go about planning and making sure that when these plans are put to reality that they will obtain the desired outcome and accomplish the goal. Churchman (1968:31) states the management scientist's test of objectives of a system: "the determination of whether the system will knowingly sacrifice other goals to attain the objective." Precise and specific objectives of an organization can be tested in terms of measures of performance of the overall system. This measure may be a score that tells us the degree or the proportion to which the organizational and individual objectives have been accomplished. The higher the score, the better the performance.

In the determination of a measure of performance, the nursing service administrators will seek to find as many relevant consequences of the system's activities as possible. Admittedly, the nursing service administrators too will make errors and will have to revise their plans and strategies as they get feedback and in the light of further evidence.

An example of the types of goals and values that the nursing department within the sociotechnical organization of a hospital sets forth might well be (1) quantity and quality patient care services, for example, 6.6 hours of care per patient per 24 hours and according to standards set, (2) advancement of nursing research, measured in terms of numbers and quality of research produced per year, (3) professional growth of personnel in terms of provision for the practice of clinical specialization, utilization of employees' full potential in terms of their educational preparation and interests, and (4) financial balance. These objectives are measurable. Such a set of objectives can be adopted by the nursing service department.

The second subsystem of an organization is *technology.* The technical aspect of the organization is formed by the task requirements of the organization, which vary widely. It is shaped by the specialization of skills and knowledge required, the types of machinery and equipment, assessment of tools involved, and the layout of facilities. Furthermore, it is the technology that determines the type of human resources and input required. For example, an aerospace industry is a technology that requires the employment of scientists, engineers, craftsmen, and other highly educated and trained people. Hospitals require the employment of medical scientists, physicians with different specializations, nurse specialists, technicians, personnel managers, and other skilled workers. Similarly, the nursing department within the health care institution may require the employment of nurse administrators, clinical nurse specialists, staff nurses with different educational preparation, and other skilled paranursing personnel. Technology is an important factor in determining the structure of the organization, relationships between jobs, and behaviors expected of personnel.

The third component of an organization is its *physical environment*. It deals mainly with architectural structure, people structure, physical layout of facilities, and utilities.

The structure of the human organization deals with the ways in which the tasks of the organization are divided into functional or operating units and with the coordination of units. In a formal sense, structures can be viewed as set forth by the organization in the form of a vertical versus horizontal chart, by positions according to authority, task and job description, and rules and procedures. Structure is also concerned with patterns of authority and influence and patterns of communication and work flow. Organizational structure formalizes the relationship between the technical subsystem and the conceptual environment. However, there are many interactions and relationships that occur between these two subsystems and bypass the formal structure, for example, the informal organization.

The fourth component of every social organization is its *conceptual environment*. It deals with the human element, people and their psychosocial needs. It consists of interactions, expectations, aspirations, sentiments, and values of participants. The conceptual environment and the technical subsystems are interdependent. Because change in any one subsystem will have repercussions on the others, they cannot be looked at separately but must be considered in the context of the total organization.

The *administrative composite process (ACP)* is the final subsystem of the organization. Its main trust or concern is the overall administration of the total organization. Others refer to this component as a managerial subsystem (Kast and Rosenzweig 1970; Parsons 1960). There are three managerial levels in the hierarchical structure of complex organizations: the technical level, the organizational level, and the institutional or the community level (Parsons 1960) (Fig. 2-10).

The technical level is involved with the actual task performance in the organization. It deals with the nursing department and is concerned with the delivery of direct and indirect patient care. The technical system is not only involved with the physical skill utilizing little knowledge, but it also includes technical activities utilizing great scientific knowledge and skill, for example, research and development and services control. The scientist performs technical tasks in a research laboratory; the physician and the nurse perform technical tasks in health care institutions. The people that work at this technical level within the nursing department are the action population and the target population. In complex organizations, many technical tasks are performed by highly educated and professional people as well as by skilled and unskilled people.

The function of the organizational level

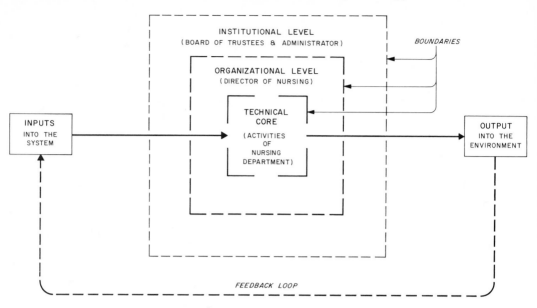

Fig. 2-10. Administrative levels of an organization.

is coordination or integration of the task performance of the technical core, for example, the nursing department and the integration into the technical core of the inputs (funds, information, and energy). The position of nursing service administrators is at the organizational level. Her administrative functions are the coordination and integration of the patient care services provided by the nursing staff. In addition, the administrator integrates appropriate input into the technical core. The organizational level is mainly concerned with the intraorganizational interactions.

The institutional level is involved in relating the activities of the organization to its external environment. The organization needs to receive continuous inputs from the community so that it can carry on its transformational activities. For example, in a hospital situation the board of trustees, the administrator, and more recently the nursing service administrator, in addition to her work at the organizational level, work at this institutional level.

Therefore, the subsystems of the administrative composite process cover the entire organization by directing the technology, by organizing personnel according to position description and assigning tasks according to activities, by integrating other resources, and by relating the organization to its environment. It should be pointed out that the orientation at each level is different; for example, the technical level deals primarily with technical and economic rationality. The boundaries at the technical level are less permeable to inputs from the environment than are the boundaries on the organizational and institutional levels. The boundaries at the institutional level are permeable to intrusions and inputs from the environment, over which it has little control. Therefore, the administrator at this level should have an open system view and concentrate on adaptive and innovative strategies. The nursing service administrator at the organizational level operates between the institutional level and the technical core and mediates and coordinates the two. For example, the nursing service administrator who operates at this level helps to transform the uncertainties of the environment into the economic technical rationality necessary for input into the technical core (Fig. 2-10).

Therefore, the ACP subsystem in the organization involves three levels: the technical core activities, the intraorganizational activities, and interinstitutional relationships. Theoretically these roles are separated in many organizations, but the distinctions are not always clear.

With regard to these three levels, Parsons (1960) has observed that there is relative independence among the three levels of organization and that it is not realistic to talk about a "line authority" extending from the institutional level to the organizational and down to technical level. He indicates, however, that there is a break in line authority between these levels. For example, a hospital administrator cannot exert absolute authority over the professional person, because the hospital administrator's knowledge is limited in a specific area. The administrator must rely on the professional person's specialized expertise. The administrator can veto a recommendation submitted by the specialists but cannot propose alternatives. Therefore, it is necessary that appropriate means of articulation and adjustment at the boundaries be made. It does not mean that these levels can operate independently. They are interdependent. For example, personnel at the institutional level need to perform effectively so that the organization can receive the necessary inputs from the environment for the technical level to perform properly. Conversely, the technical level must produce outputs in the form of services or products efficiently and effectively to make sure that the organization receives environmental support.

In reviewing the historical evolution of organization, we find that the traditional, classical management theory emphasized the structural aspect of the physical environment and of the administrative subsystems and that its main concern was developing principles. The process school originated by Fayol stressed the administrative process of planning, organizing, directing, and controlling and made the distinction between physical and conceptual activity. The human relationists and the behavioral scientists have emphasized the psychosocial aspects of human needs. Their main focus has been on motivation, group dynamics, and individual drives. The management scientists or the quantitative school of thought have emphasized the economictechnical aspects of the physical environment and are more concerned with decision making and control processes. Thus, we can see that each of these approaches to organization and management has emphasized only one primary subsystem and has mostly ignored the importance of the others. The administrative theory that is presented in this book within the systems frame of reference is a synthesis of the four schools of thought, views the organization as a structured sociotechnical system, and takes into consideration each of the primary subsystems and their mutual interaction and interdependence.

REFERENCES

Arndt, C., and Laeger, E.: Role strain in a diversified role set: the director of nursing service. I. Nurs. Res. **19**(3):253-259, 1970*a*.

Arndt, C., and Laeger, E.: Role strain in a diversified role set: the director of nursing service. II. Sources of stress, Nurs. Res. **19**(3):495-501, 1970*b*.

Chin, Robert: The utility of system models and developmental models for practitioners. In Bennis, W. G., Benne, K. D., and Chin, R., editors: The planning of change, New York, 1969, Holt, Rinehart and Winston, Inc., pp. 297-312.

Churchman, C. W.: The systems approach, New York, 1968, Dell Pub. Co., Inc.

Dabas, Z. S.: The dimensions of morale: an item factorization of the SRA employees inventory, Personnel Psychol. **11**:217-234, 1958.

George, C. S., Jr.: The history of management thought, Englewood Cliffs, N. J., 1972, Prentice-Hall, Inc.

Griffiths, D. E.: Administrative theory, New York, 1959, Appleton-Century-Crofts, chapter 4.

Griffiths, D. E.: The nature and meaning of theory. In Griffiths, D. E., editor: Behavioral science and educational administration, the 63rd

Yearbook of National Society for the Study of Education, Chicago, 1964, University of Chicago Press, pp. 95-119.

Kast, F. E., and Rosenzweig, J. E.: Organization and management: a systems approach, New York, 1970, McGraw-Hill Book Co.

Lewin, K.: Group discussion and social change. In Newcomb, I. and Hartley, E., editors: Readings in social psychology, New York, 1947, Holt, Rinehart & Winston, Inc.

Likert, R.: New patterns of management, New York, 1961, McGraw-Hill Book Co.

Lonsdale, R. C.: Maintaining the organization in dynamic equilibrium. In Griffiths, D. E., editor: Behavioral science and educational administration, the 63rd Yearbook of National Society for the Study of Education, Chicago, 1964, University of Chicago Press, pp. 142-177.

Parsons, T.: Structure and process in modern societies, New York, 1960, The Free Press of Glencoe, pp. 60-96.

Roach, D. E.: Dimensions of employee morale, Am. Psychol. **12**:443, 1957.

Simon, H. A.: The new science of management decision, New York, 1960, Harper & Row, Pubs.

Tannenbaum, R., Weschler, I. R., and Massarek, F.: Leaders and organization: a behavioral science approach. II. New York, 1961, McGraw-Hill Book Co.

Triandis, H. C.: Notes on the design of organization. In Thompson, J., and Vroom, V. H., editors: Organizational design on research, Pittsburgh, 1968, University of Pittsburgh Press, pp. 57-102.

Twery, R., Schmid, J., and Wrigley, C.: Some factors in job satisfaction: a comparison of three methods of analysis, Educational and Psychological Measurement, **28**:189-201, 1958.

ADDITIONAL READINGS

Cleland, D. I., and King, W. R.: Management: a systems approach, New York, 1972, McGraw-Hill Book Co.

Donnelly, J., Gibson, J., and Ivancevich, J.: Fundamentals of management, Dallas, Tex., 1971, Business Publications, Inc.

Etzioni, A.: Modern organizations, Englewood Cliffs, New Jersey, 1964, Prentice-Hall, Inc.

Filley, A. C., and House, R. J.: Managerial process and organizational behavior, Glenview, Ill., 1970, Scott, Foresman & Co.

Getzels, J. W.: Administration as a social process. In Halpin, A. W., editor: Administrative theory in education, Chicago, 1958, Midwest Administration Center, University of Chicago Press, pp. 150-165.

Guyton, A. C.: Textbook of medical physiology, ed. 4, Philadelphia, 1971, W. B. Saunders Co.

Hicks, H. G.: The management of organizations: a systems and human resources approach, ed. 2, New York, 1972, McGraw-Hill Book Co.

Johnson, R. A., Kast, F. E., and Rosenzweig, J. E.: The theory and management of systems, ed. 2, New York, 1967, McGraw-Hill Book Co.

Kahn, A.: The study of society: a unified approach, Homewood, Ill., 1963, Richard D. Irwin, Inc.

MacEachern, M. T.: Hospital organization and management, ed 3, Chicago, 1957, Physicians Record Co.

March, J. G., and Simon, H. A.: Organization, New York, 1958, John Wiley & Sons, Inc.

Marx, M. H.: Theories in contemporary psychology, New York, 1963, Macmillan Pub. Co., Inc.

Maslow, A. H.: Motivation and personality, New York, 1955, Harper & Row, Pubs.

Mussallem, Helen K.: The nurse's role in policy making and planning, Int. Nurs. Rev. **20**(1):9, 1973.

Newport, G. M.: The tools of management, Reading, Mass., 1972, Addison-Wesley Pub. Co., Inc.

Petit, T. A.: A behavioral theory of management, Academy of Managerial Journal **2**:346, December 1967.

Sayles, L.: Managerial behavior, New York, 1964, McGraw-Hill Book Co.

Smith, L.: Two lines of authority: the hospital's dilemma, Mod. Hosp. **84**(3):12, 1955.

Thompson, J. D.: Organization in action, New York, 1964, McGraw-Hill Book Co.

Trist, E. J., and Rice, A. K.: The enterprise and its environment, London, 1963, Tavistock Publications Ltd.

Chapter 3

GOALS AND OBJECTIVES: ORGANIZATIONAL AND INDIVIDUAL

Any consideration of the essential conditions of a good department of nursing must begin with a statement of its philosophy; this gives the rationale for whatever actions are taken. Oftentimes a statement of philosophy appears to be a vague statement about beliefs, so abstract that we perhaps read it once, understand very little, and tuck it away in one of the policy books. It is used only when dignitaries visit the health care institution and for accreditation purposes. It will be the concern of this chapter to examine a concrete philosophy of nursing service administration, discuss the mission of nursing that arises from the philosophy, and finally discuss both organizational and individual goals and objectives and see how they can be utilized by the nursing service administration.

Basic philosophy of nursing service administration

A philosophy of nursing service may be described as an intentionally chosen set of values, primary ends, which serve as criteria for a choice of means to accomplish the end goal. These criteria also indicate the limitation on the choice of means and intermediate ends. These primary ends are prescriptive in that they select one form of action over another and that they direct behavior toward the alternative chosen. Implicit in these choices is the knowledge or judgment of what is desirable or undesirable. This is in contrast to the scientific findings and theories that we have discussed so far, which are descriptive. These scientific findings describe and accurately predict consequences, and of course, the nursing service administrator must know the consequences of a decision to reach certain primary ends.

It is also true that an individual's philosophy is created in the mind—a conceptual act. A philosophy gives one the ability to understand oneself, others, and the world around. The same holds true on the organizational level.

A basic philosophy of nursing service administration gives us a sense of our mission, an understanding of interrelationships between the system and its subsystems, and a complete understanding of our overall objectives and values. This basic philosophy should serve as a directive on how to achieve our given purpose. It shall also contain a statement of premises governing the organization. A viable philosophy such as this will encourage contributions from people at all levels, resulting in its further development and eventual adoption.

Put in another way, the philosophy underlying administration of nursing services, or any other health institution, is based on the following important points. These criteria are also in agreement with recommendations of the World Health Organization (Goddard 1958).

1. Achieving the individual and organizational goals (O_i and O_g) requires expenditure of effort. The quality, quantity, timing, and

45

cost of this effort are all interrelated and must be given constant attention.

2. Decisions must be based on verifiable facts. This applies at all levels and in all phases of planning, execution, and control of work plans.

3. The successful nursing service administrator uses appropriate delegation. To avoid wasting time, it is necessary to give pertinent authority and responsibility at the lowest possible organizational level, consistent with written job descriptions and agency policy.

4. The major thrust of nursing service administration is to achieve both O_i and O_g by applying conceptual acts (A_c) and physical acts (A_p) to create a conceptual environment (E_c) and a physical environment (E_p). Success is definitely related to the part of the conceptual environment that is affected by financial as well as other factors.

5. Effective communication is needed in all interrelated and interdependent components of a system. The nursing service administrator can maintain equilibrium only if communication flows properly in all networks, both vertically, that is, from the top down and from the bottom up, and laterally.

6. Administration of nursing services must stay flexible enough to meet and adapt to the changing needs of the organization, individuals, community, and society in general.

Factors influencing the nature and the mission of nursing services in health care institutions

One of the most important factors influencing the nature and mission of nursing services is the health care institution itself, whether it be a hospital, a clinic, or any other health care agency. Another important factor is whether or not the mission is to provide episodic or distributive care to members of the community.

Other influencing factors are the rapid development of medical and nursing skills and knowledge, recent advances, and the proliferation of technological and pharmaceutical aids to medical and nursing practice. All of these changes cause a tremendous amount of additional input into the system of nursing services, which will cause disequilibrium among the subsystems of the organization unless there is change and adaptation. If the influx of input increases too much and/or too fast, some of the resultant problems may be ones of structure, technology, or behavior. For example, new machinery such as complex EKG equipment or kidney machines require the hiring, training, and educating of additional nursing and paranursing personnel with new status and positions that effect the nursing organization and the physical structure housing the equipment. Technological problems may erupt stemming from inadequate currency (inefficient training and education of technical nurse specialists) to function in these new areas of health care. Behavioral problems may result when the nomothetic (organizational) role required of these new positions is incongruent with the personality characteristic of the person filling these roles.

Other factors influencing the mission of nursing services are the geographic mobility of population, the effectiveness of preventive medical and nursing care, and the increased life span. Enlargement and extension of health services to our population has added another influx of inputs into the nursing service system, in terms of increased numbers of older patients who, in the main, require restorative type of care. Most of these patients need to be taken care of at home and in extended health care facilities. These factors also cause problems of structure and technology.

The traditional triad of physician, nurse, and patient has been complicated by the interworkings of different kinds of people with different professions, the health team. For example, we now have a health team composed of the medical social worker, family therapist, occupational therapist, physiotherapist, physicians, nurses, and many others. Within the nursing profession itself there is confusion among the different kinds of registered nurses. There are those who are diploma graduates, associate degree graduates, B.S. degree graduates, M.A. degree graduates, and even doctoral degree graduates. Delineation of roles and responsibilities overlap, often resulting in problems of accountability, responsibility, and role conflict.

The fact that health care has become the predominant social force in our society makes it interrelated with economical and political aspects of our culture; its functioning requires a complicated social structure. Since nursing personnel constitute the largest single group within the health care delivery system, all these variables—economic, political, and cultural—affect the functioning and the social structure of the nursing department the most.

SETTING OF GOALS AND OBJECTIVES

Now that we have clarified our philosophy and mission it is time to address ourselves to the main concern of this chapter —goals and objectives, both corporate and individual.

As touched on earlier, one of the basic strategies of planning is the setting of goals and objectives. Strategy is defined as the union of plans, goals, objectives, and major policies needed to bring the organization from its present state of affairs to a desired position at a specific future point in time.

The strategic plan of an organization is at the peak of all contributing plans. A strategic plan is important because it delineates the goals of the organization, becomes the model for guiding the direction of the subsidiary plans of the organization, determines the compatibility of the overall plan with other plans, and finally directs the organization in decisions involving the actual delivery of the product, in this case the delivery of health care services in the present and in the future.

Goals are broad statements of direction; they are plans in the guise of results-to-be-achieved and include such items as purposes, objectives, missions, deadlines, standards, and targets. The goal structure sets the stage for the relationship between an organization and its environment. By no means do we want to oversimplify, because

the process of establishing goals is complex, involving whole sets of objectives put on the organization by the external environment and by the individuals making up the organization. Goals are the ultimate targets in planning and represent the end point toward which organizing, directing, and controlling are aimed.

Objectives are specific, desired accomplishments that are to be effected in a specified time period. Achieving objectives makes possible the achievement of overall goals.

Objectives are more specialized than goals; therefore, their development requires greater technical expertise. The following are basic questions to be asked:

1. What output indicators are appropriate to what we wish to accomplish?
2. What success criteria are to be applied?
3. What are the givens? That is, under what conditions and time limitations does the expected behavior, or outcome, have to occur?
4. Who is the target person (persons, groups, or departments) responsible for accomplishing the stated objective?

Of course the resolution of these questions involves discussion, negotiation, and concensus, as does the process of establishing goals. The process here, especially in setting goals and objectives in nursing service departments, is more specialized, parochial, since those primary involved will be the nursing administrator, personnel advisor, and clinical nurse specialists who will first develop objectives and then report back to the clientele group, such as consumers of patient care, employees, professional organizations, and special interest groups, for their evaluation of how well the objectives suit the goal.

The combination of internal organizational expertise and clientele evaluation is very critical because (1) it encourages clientele involvement beyond the goal-setting stage and (2) it enables and forces the technician and specialists to explain clearly and operationalize their objectives to the clientele group, which is mostly made up of nontechnicians.

Value of objectives

Clearly defined and integrated organizational objectives have several primary values. First, all members are encouraged to work toward a common goal. Objectives make behavior in organizations become more rational, coordinated, and thus, more effective. When objectives are used, people know what they should be trying to accomplish. Secondly, the use of specific and concise objectives provides a kind of idealized standard by which actual performance can be measured. Thirdly, clear-cut objectives serve as motivators because the individual can see and relate personal objectives to the work of the organization. The individual can see that achievement of personal objectives are dependent on the organizational objective and will then direct personal effort and behavior toward the achievement of the objectives of the organization. Fourth, the objectives of the organization tell the community something about the relative importance the organization places on the interests of the various components of the community and something about how the organization plans to use its activities to pursue those interests.

Inputs into the development of objectives in nursing service administration

Inputs to the development of an organization's goals and objectives come from several sources: (1) the sociocultural values and norms in which the health care institution is located, (2) the organization's various clientele groups and consumers of health care facilities, such as patients, employees, physicians, and shareholders, and (3) values and goals of the board of trustees or top managment, both personal and collective.

All of these inputs affect the formulation of the organization's goals and objectives. Since the nursing division is one of the major departments of the organization, these inputs will also affect the formulation of the nursing department's goals and objectives. So, in addition to the above inputs, the organization's overall goals and objectives serve as inputs to the development of the nursing service department's goals and objectives

SOCIOCULTURAL VALUES AND NORMS AS INPUTS

The health care institution and its different departments have many diverse objectives. The hospital and its nursing service are affected by the impact of sociocultural values and norms. We borrowed a definition from Cleland and King (1972: 230) by using *value* to mean assessments of worth of objects and states by individuals. The very development of the hospital or the health care institution as a private, voluntary, nonprofit institution is a reflection of the community's value system. Emphasis on patient care and treatment and prevention of disease permeates the value system and objectives of the health care institution even though there are constraints of technology, economics, and organizational abilities (Georgopoulos and Mann 1962).

Oftentimes nurses experience role conflict when their administrative functions interfere with their perceived role of providing direct care to the patient. An example of this is the increasing tendency of nurses in administrative jobs to want to return to the bedside (Georgopoulos and Mann 1962).

Something else that determines the value system of health care organizations and their nursing services is the emphasis on patient welfare. The educational process and the standards of conduct that are prescribed by specific professional groups reinforce this value system. Examples of this are the pledge of Florence Nightingale for nurses and the Hippocratic oath for physicians. This common goal of *patient welfare* enables the individual participants to perform their highly specialized and professionalized skills toward a common goal, which helps provide the voluntary coordination of activities.

INPUTS FROM ORGANIZATION'S VARIOUS CLIENTELE GROUPS

Before setting the objectives of the organization, people in top management, such as the board of trustees, administrators, and department heads, must answer some basic questions, Who are the claimants of the health care institution? Are they the consumers of patient care, or is it the community? Is it a group of doctors or a single individual such as an administrator? If it is a profit-making organization, are the claimants the shareholders? What is the nature of the service or business the organization is involved in? The answers to these questions determine the goals of the enterprise and help define the scope of its activities. Determination of the nature of business is equivalent to determining the kinds of services rendered or the type of product produced. So by answering these basic questions, an organization determines exactly what business it is in—questions such as What is the nature of the organization, what can it do or offer, what is it capable of doing, what are its potentialities, and what might it have an opportunity to do?

Goal development may also require the actual involvement of the various clientele group. For example, the goals of a school district must be developed and agreed on through involvement of various community leaders and groups. Planning-study groups are set up to draft a statement of goals, which are reviewed and revised as necessary. The important point is involvement. Similarly, the development of goals and objectives of the health care organization may require the involvement of various community leaders, special interest groups who are financially contributing to the development of the organization, and other community groups and professional nursing organizations on local, state, and national levels.

VALUES AND GOALS OF THE BOARD OF TRUSTEES OR TOP MANAGEMENT

Establishment of organizational goals is basically a function of implementing the values of the people at top level management, for example, the trustees, administrators, and department heads. Values are personalistic concepts. There is no formal structure or agreement that tells the director which values are right, which are wrong, or which have priority over the other. Each of us has personal values, and these values are all different.

When top management determines the goals and objectives of the organization its values are set implicitly. In so doing, personal values play an important role. Furthermore, the two additional aspects of *group values* and *multiple value systems* also contribute to the complexity of the problem of objective setting.

Generally speaking, most organizational objectives are set by a group of individuals, each individual having a different value system. The problem of determining a collective value for the group is a difficult one. There simply is not a way to take the individual values and develop from them the group values. Some organizations get around this by using any of the following three decision-making arrangements: the participant-determining, the parliamentarian, or the democratic-centralist. In the participant-determining and the parliamentarian arrangement, each group member can theoretically exert the same amount of influence on a decision. The difference between the two is that the participant-determining group demands consensus, whereas the parliamentarian demands a plurality vote. The democratic-centralist group places authority in one person, and that person's decision is binding. In addition, everyone has two value systems, those emanating from personal preferences and those emanating from the organization. Both systems play important roles in making decisions and in setting organizational objectives. Most of us are motivated by the possible effect of our organization on our own future interests and promotions, as well as its influence on the purely organizational outcome. Therefore, every decision made by the nurse administrator and people in top management must reflect, to some extent, their personal and organization value systems. Just knowing this should prove helpful to the nursing service administrator.

Criteria for setting goals and objectives

At this point it will be useful to review the criteria for setting goals and objectives; there will be a detailed discussion of these goals and objectives later.

An organization's objectives are criteria by which materials, personnel, and specialists are selected; content and area of performance are outlined; instructional procedures are developed; and evaluative measures are prepared. All aspects of an organization's program are means by which the purpose of the organization is accomplished. Therefore, if we want to study the organizational program systematically, we first must know the direction toward which the organizational objectives are aimed.

A statement of objectives should meet the following criteria: specific, operational, and flexible. The expected terminal behavior must be stated in observable or measureable terms. The criteria of acceptable performance also must be specified.

MAKING OBJECTIVES OPERATIONAL AND SPECIFIC

First making an objective operational means to describe the terminal behavior in terms of expected outcomes. In terms of observable behavior this is the behavior the employee will be exhibiting to show that the objective has been achieved. For example, at the completion of a program of instruction or orientation, or both, on team nursing, the staff nurse will be able to identify in writing or discuss orally the major concepts and principles of team nursing. Secondly, a statement of objectives should define a desired terminal behavior by describing the important conditions under which the behavior is expected to occur. For example, given a team composed of one registered nurse (RN), one licensed vocational nurse (LVN), one nurse's aid, and 12 patients, the team leader will be able to (1) delegate responsibility of patient care to appropriate nursing personnel, that is, make assignments, and (2) conduct a team conference once during the eight-hour work shift. Thirdly, a statement of objectives should specify the criteria of acceptable performance by a description of how the student or employee must enact the terminal behavior to be acceptable. Also, if the time element of the objective is crucial, then the date for achievement of the objective is important and should be established. For example, with 12 patients and a team of three members (one RN, one LVN, and one NA), each patient will receive 3.3 hours of direct patient care during an eight-hour work shift.

Some behavioral scientists call this aspect of writing objectives *quantification* (Kast and Rosenzweig 1970). In other words, when objectives are quantified, they can then be translated into explicit plans, such as numbers of patients treated, budget, and number of incident reports reduced. This provides a relatively clear-cut framework around which activities can be organized and performance measured. Developing explicit quantitative goals enhances clarity and makes objectives operational.

Two of the reasons administrators fail to explain the objectives of the organization to their employees are the lack of specificity of objectives and the failure of administrators to make these objectives operational.

When objectives are made specific for each position in the organization, they become operational. This is commonly called *management-by-objectives* and is usually defined in accordance with the degree to which personnel participate in the setting of the objectives.

Management-by-objectives is a technique of work planning, review and performance appraisal; it is not concerned with rating of the individual on dimensions such as initiative, honesty, and aggressiveness. The purpose of management-by-objectives is to develop and use job-related criteria that are observable, measurable, or verifiable as the basis of evaluation. With the use of measurable objectives that have been agreed on by the superior and the staff members, behavior becomes predictable, the soundness of decisions can be assessed while they are being made, work performance can be evaluated, and the individuals can analyze their own experiences and determine the improvement of their own performance.

Making objectives flexible

In the midst of all the clamor for clarity in organizational goals and objectives, it is wise to consider the possible virtues of vagueness for flexibility. In an environment of multiple objectives it is extremely difficult to focus on more than a few at any one time. Short-term goals and contributing objectives may be stated explicitly, whereas medium- and long-term goals and central objectives can be stated in a more flexible and general way.

Kast and Rosenzweig (1970) emphasize the need for flexibility in writing goals and objectives. If goals are stated in general terms, there is room for organizational participants to fill in details according to their own perception and experience and to possibly modify the pattern more to their own liking. Ultraprecision can destroy flexibility, making it ever more difficult for individuals and organizations to adapt to changing conditions. Keeping the goals general also provides for the possibility of achieving them by various means. The concept of equifinality, achieving the same end via different means, is an important concept in viable systems. Provision for flexibility also fosters serendipity, which in this case means the achievement of a specific worthwhile goal by accident. When objectives are stated in such a way as to give the individual more flexibility in electing different means of achieving them, these kinds of results become much more common.

At the organizational level, mediation and compromise are essential ingredients in coordinating activity and integrating long-term and short-term goals.

We are not advocating this approach explicitly. We still feel the best approach is to strive for clarity as a means to make goal setting operational, but one should also realize that the inability to do so may not necessarily be catastrophic.

ORGANIZATIONAL AND INDIVIDUAL OBJECTIVES

There is a good deal of controversy today with regard to the nature of both organizational and individual objectives. Some writers in recent management literature are arguing that the primary objective of an organization is profit. Still others say that it should be service to the consumer or to society. Some writers claim that individual behavior is motivated by increased financial reward, shorter working hours, and adequate security. Others believe that individual behavior is directed toward performance of interesting and meaningful jobs and opportunity to progress in the organization and to develop skills, and professional capabilities (Filley and House 1969).

Organizational objectives

Historically, the classical organization theorists viewed organizational objectives as rational goals that added up to more than the sum of the individual goals of its members. The workers are bound together because they share a common goal; thus, they come to value the organization itself as a means of doing things. So, the individual identifies with the organization and its objectives, and the organization takes on a specific identity that makes it more than a nominal grouping of individuals.

Classical theorists classify organizational objectives into three categories: primary, secondary, and social.

The *primary objectives* of an organization, or a department within the organization, are defined by those the organization serves. Primary objectives are achieved by providing services or product for the consumers of the organization. For example, in the case of hospital nursing service the consumers are the patients, the nursing staff, and the community. The primary objective of nursing service within any health care institution is to provide quality patient care service, creating an environment that is conducive to the delivery of optimum patient care and staff satisfaction. Thus, one can trace primary objectives down to the level of an individual's job assignment.

Secondary objectives are used to reach primary objectives and are usually met through the staff who perform supportive tasks such as coordination, interpretation, facilitation, and analysis. Secondary objectives are also directed toward providing economy and efficiency in the performance of the organization itself. For example, the personnel department does not contribute directly to patient care. It contributes indirectly by hiring employees (nursing and paranursing personnel), who in turn provide direct patient care. The personnel director contributes directly to the achievement of secondary organizational objectives, which in turn facilitate the attainment of the primary objective (patient care in this case).

Social objectives deal with the organization's contribution to society. The community imposes certain conditions such as health, safety, and labor practices. The or-

ganization must set up social objectives to meet these conditions. The health care organization may contribute to the social, educational, and physical betterment of the community in the form of provision of better health care facilities and to economic betterment by means of providing employment of health care workers.

As mentioned, objectives can also be classified in terms of time because time is an important variable and very closely related to organizational objectives. Relative to time, then, organizational objectives can be classified in three categories: long-term or visionary objectives, medium-term or attainable objectives, and short-term or immediate objectives.

Visionary objectives are the ultimate, the "dream" objectives of the organization. This could be a goal to be achieved in 25 years with the advances of technology. Setting up a time table for these kinds of goals is obviously extremely difficult. Medium-term objectives are much more attainable, as sound estimates of time and expenditures can be made.

The third category obviously refers to the kinds of objectives that can be achieved at the present moment without additional technological development. For example, staffing the four-bed coronary care unit with four qualified nurse specialists and utilizing computer facilities in planning the staffing patterns of clinical units or processing personnel records are the kinds of immediate objectives found at lower levels of complex organizations. Higher levels of organizations are more concerned with the visionary objectives. It is the administrator's responsibility to see that all these objectives on the different levels are realized.

When organizational and individual objectives are achieved together, it is called mutual reinforcement. For example, health care institutions benefit when they help the individuals reach their objectives. Both are interdependent. The concept of mutual reinforcement of objectives is based on *Law of Effect* by Thorndike (1911):

Of the several responses made to the same situations, those which are accompanied or closely followed by satisfaction to the animal or human will, other things being equal, be more firmly connected with the situation so that when it recurs, they will be more likely to recur; those which are accompanied or closely followed by discomfort to the human or animal will, other things being equal, have their connections with that situation weakened, so that when it recurs, they will be less likely to recur. The greater the satisfaction or discomfort, the greater the strengthening or weakening of the bond.

Overwhelming evidence supports Thorndike's law. The main generalizations to be drawn from this law are that rewarded responses tend to be repeated in given situations and unrewarded responses tend to be discontinued (Thorndike 1911; DeCecco 1968).

When individual and organizational objectives reinforce one another, the organization prospers and so do its members. It is, of course, necessary that the two kinds of objectives be compatible but not necessarily identical. This point will be explained in more detail when we discuss relationships between organizational and individual objectives.

In conclusion, organizational objectives deal with several dimensions, which should be kept in mind when one is actually writing and implementing them. Organizational objectives should (1) indicate the level of the organization to which the objective applies, (2) indicate the time when the objective is expected to be accomplished, (3) indicate the criteria of acceptable performance, and (4) indicate or write in specific, behavioral, and measurable language the kind of performance, task, product, or service that is to be accomplished.

Individual objectives

Since a health care institution is a sociotechnical system, the individual constitutes its essential component. Historically, classical theorists (Taylor 1919) view individual objectives in terms of task and economic perspective. For them, the individual attains an objective by subordinating it to the objectives of the organization. The behavioral theorists (Argyris 1957a; Davis 1951; Mayo 1945) view individual objectives from a psychosocial point of view. They suggest that if organizations integrate the individual objectives into their systems and realistically foster the achievement of them, then the organization may better achieve its own objectives. The classical approach states that employees will work harder with material rewards (Taylor 1919). Chester Barnard (1938) was one of the first writers to acknowledge motivating factors other than those of financial reward.

As we have seen, an individual's objectives are based on individual needs. Murray and co-workers (1938:54) described a need as "a hypothetical process the occurrence of which is imagined in order to account for certain objective and subjective facts." He also defined need more fully as "a force which organizes perception, apperceptions, intellection, conation and action in such a way as to transform in a certain direction as existing, unsatisfying situation" (Murray and co-workers 1938: 124).

There are three essential factors that influence the behavior of individuals in response to a need:

1. The nature of the need and how intense it is. An intense hunger or thirst need may require immediate satisfaction by eating or drinking.
2. The physical and mental disposition or the make-up of the individual. For example, the individual's physical strength, sensory organs, and sensitivity of his nervous system all affect behavior in perceiving needs and the means of satisfying them.
3. The physical and social environment of the individual.

These three factors interact with one another in varying degrees of strength. It can be seen that no two people will react to a given situation in the same way, nor will an individual necessarily react the same way at different times. Thus, an important key to an effective organization is the nurse administrator's recognition that each nurse under supervision has many constantly changing needs that affect and direct the nurse's behavior.

Relationship between individual and organizational objectives

The complete scope of the relationship between organizational and individual objectives can range from totally opposing, in which achievement of one is just the opposite of the other and obvious conflict exists between the two, to partially opposing, in which there is some agreement between the two objectives, to neutral, in which there is indifference in the sense that they don't hurt each other. Obviously, the compatible relationship is one in which individual and organizational objectives are in harmony and the achievement of one fulfills the achievement of the other. The individuals keep their separate identities and, at the same time, respect the organization's need for cooperation. The success of the majority of organizations is due to compatible individual and organizational objectives. At the other end of the spectrum the individual and organizational objectives are the same. Individuals may completely subordinate themselves to the organization's objectives and allow themselves to be controlled by it. This is not a desirable situation, but unfortunately there are firms that would like nothing better than this situation.

Our suggestion is that instead of seeking to make organizational and individual objectives identical, organizations should try to bring individual and organizational objectives into a working relationship that will contribute to the success of both. This relationship aims for compatability, not conformity.

Argyris (1957a and b) states that there is an inherent conflict between the objectives of the organization and those of the individual because the formal organization creates situations in which individuals become dependent, subordinate, and passive and are kept from using all of their potentialities. If the organization promotes an atmosphere in which self-fulfillment and organizational fulfillment are given equal time, the conflicts can be circumvented.

Lonsdale (1964) also pointed out that, to satisfy the needs of its employees, an organization offers certain inducements or incentives, hoping that the employees will then be motivated to carry out their roles with sufficient effectiveness. The resulting job satisfaction and productivity constitutes morale.

When the interests of both the individual and the organization are integrated, Davis (1951) calls it morale building. This process fosters the individual's interdependency between personal objectives and those of the organization. One way to attain this integration is by increasing the participation of staff members in seting objectives. This gives the employee a feeling of worthwhileness or belonging.

Like Davis, Drucker (1954) and many others suggest a participative approach to establishing objectives. Drucker states that managers' goals must be defined by the contributions they have to make to the success of whatever company or department of which they are a part. Both these management writers state that individuals should subordinate their objectives to those of their organization.

McGregor (1960) suggests that this integration is a reflection of the way individuals perceive their organization's objectives as a way of achieving personal objectives. The closer they see the relationship between these objectives and their own, the greater will be their commitment to the organization. Furthermore, McGregor suggests that the integration of Oi and Og depends on this perception and this commitment.

Integration probably starts with orientation and is enhanced by job enlargement, employee-centered leadership, democratic leadership, formation of groups based on employee needs, and participative decision making. Appropriate delegation, as noted in our discussion of philosophy, is also very important.

Obviously, if an organization knows and appreciates individual objectives, it is in the possession of an effective administrative tool. Any organization exists by offering rewards in exchange for contributions and by structuring itself so that it provides the individual with the opportunity to move toward personal objectives in a manner that contributes to major organizational objectives.

Most nurses will state that they became nurses to "get involved," "to help people," or some related motivation. Such intangibles must be considered in planning organizational structures. Objectives are seen not only as bases on which to design the organization but also as tools for eliciting motivation and teamwork (Filley and House 1969).

Filley and House drew up the following four propositions that summarize what classical and modern organizational theory have to say about objectives:

1. Client or customer satisfaction is necessary if the organization is to survive, grow, and function as a profitable operation. Failure to provide such a value will result in the opposite effect, an unprofitable operation. The work of Dent (1959) and Healey (1956) supports this proposition. Dent's survey revealed that management of large, successful, and growing organizations cited public service and good products as objectives far more often than did managers of small, unsuccessful, and nongrowth firms. Healey polled 445 firms and made similar findings. Levitt (1960) found that improper definitions of service objectives led to a decline in the market position of several American industries, including the railroad, film, and oil industries.

2. If the organization operates in ways that consistently offend society in general or some of its members in particular, undesirable consequences will follow. The survey by Bowen (1953) and the case studies by Nader (1965) support this contention. Bowen studied the concern of businessmen about their sense of social responsibility and

reasons for having such concern and found that when they were persuaded or forced to be concerned, conditions became favorable. Nader's study indicated sharply that American industry failed to recognize and observe social expectations.

3. Individuals' performances are directly improved when they know what is expected of them by a clear statement of organizational objectives.

   Work of such men as Raven and Rietsema (1957), Tomekovic (1962), Cohen (1959), and Kahn and co-workers (1964) also supports this position. They found that, in addition to improved performance, workers who understood their company's objectives experienced greater feelings of group belonging and greater commitment to group goals, and they became more highly motivated.

4. When the achievement of an organizational objective is seen as a simultaneous achievement of one's own objective, motivation to work and the satisfaction with one's job will be high.

   The survey study of Thomas and Zander (1959) showed that air force trainees who understood that their survival depended on what they learned scored significantly higher than others in motivation, performance, vigor, and morale and showed a decline in tension. They were motivated to achieve organizational objectives because they saw their contributions as a means of achieving their personal objective, survival. Georgopoulos, Mahoney, and Jones (1957) had similar findings.

These studies all indicate that systems in which individuals and groups contribute to the primary objective of the organization as a by-product while in pursuit of their own objectives were more successful than those systems in which employees subordinated their personal objectives to the primary organizational objective.

A SAMPLE OF ORGANIZATIONAL AND INDIVIDUAL OBJECTIVES
Central organizational objective

At the end of a designated period of time (year, month, day, or shift) and given (1) system of the health care organization (structure, community, and environment), (2) the institution's policies, procedures, and constraints, and (3) appropriate resources (financial and personnel), the nursing service department of a hospital or any other health care institution will be able to provide (1) direct and indirect quality of care to all patients 24 hours a day and (2) a conceptual and a physical environment that is conducive to the fulfillment of both organizational and individual objectives. We have set the criteria of acceptable performance for this central objective at 85%.

This cut-off point was selected because we believe in performance at the mastery level. The concept of mastery level learning or performance was initially conceived by Carroll (1963), Bloom (1971), and Block (1971) and was applied to a model of school learning. The concept of mastery performance or learning postulates that, given sufficient time and appropriate kinds of help, 95% of students distributed on a normal curve basis (the top 5% plus the next 90%) can learn a task or a subject matter up to a high level of mastery. We are not so optimistic as these researchers and therefore have decided on the mastery level of 85%.

Before we point out the contributory objectives, we will operationally define the specific terms used in the central objective.

Direct patient care refers to situations in which care given to each patient is on a first-hand basis—patient and nurse are in direct contact with one another, such as giving a bath to a patient, giving medication, and talking with the patient.

Indirect patient care refers to situations in which tasks are performed away from the patients on their behalf and for their welfare, such as giving a report to another nurse about the patient's physical and mental conditions, calling the x-ray department to ensure that they are ready to receive the patient for x-ray treatment, calling the laboratory to find out blood results, or cleaning the patient's environment.

Quality care refers to the standards of care patients receive every day. It is the situation in which safe care is given and the patient's physical, social, and psychological needs or problems are met. Quality care can also be measured in terms of numbers of hours of direct care patients receive every day. It is also the situation in which patients can verbally express their satisfaction or dissatisfaction with the type of nursing care they receive every day.

Contributory objectives

For the sake of specificity and clarity the contributory objectives are classified under five headings. These objectives by no means constitute an exhaustive list, but they can serve as a sample. Each organization has to adapt its own objectives and tailor them in accordance with its own needs. These objectives are set forth for the nursing service department of a health care institution, so it is the responsibility of the nursing administrator to see that they are achieved.

1. Contributory objectives for delivery of patient care
   a. Delineate and design people structure through which coordinated planning for meeting patient care needs can be achieved.
   b. Develop and implement the program for providing quality nursing care to all patients and set up the standard for the delivery of quality care, which includes the following:
      (1) Establish written policies and procedures to implement the program for nursing care.
      (2) Implement a program in which the professional nursing staff develops, implements, and evaluates a written plan of care for each patient. The plan of care is kept current with the patient's changing needs and is recorded in the patient's record.
      (3) Plan and staff each clinical unit with qualified nursing (professional and nonprofessional) personnel; each patient receives op-

timum care with regard to proportion of number of hours of professional versus nonprofessional care given to each patient per day.

(4) Plan and implement a program in which the registered professional nurse determines (a) nursing care requirements, (b) assumes the responsibilities requiring professional skill and judgment, (c) assigns and supervises the care that can be safely performed by the practical or vocational nurse and the activities that can be carried out by other personnel.

c. Plan and secure adequate resources (people, money, and technology) to enable delivery of quality care to all patients.

d. Plan and maintain the equilibrium of the system of the nursing department and its components by controlling and balancing the inputs (such as patient load, personnel, money, and changes required) and outputs (such as care or service given to patients and employees) of the nursing department.

e. Plan and implement a research program to investigate problems of patient care and nursing services.

f. Utilize the evaluation of the administrative process of nursing services in assessing the effectiveness of the department and utilize these evaluative data as a feedback mechanism to forecast, modify, and further develop additional objectives to improve delivery of health care service to patients and to meet the needs of the employees more effectively.

2. Contributory organizational objectives for the establishment of physical environment

a. Estimate the needs of the nursing service department and plan a system of operation for control and use of the plant, equipment, and supplies. To achieve this objective the nursing administrator needs to do the following:

(1) Develop plans and policies that are effective in securing, maintaining optimum use of facilities, equipment, and supplies in support of patient care.

(2) Provide sufficient monetary resources for the nursing service to ensure the operation of its system (provision for supplies, equipment, salaries, and educational facilities).

(3) Periodically evaluate the adequacy of facilities to meet patient and personnel needs and for educational programs.

(4) Provide and maintain optimum levels of physical working conditions (lighting, heat, safety, and ventilation) with special emphasis on prevention of accidents by patients and personnel maintenance of health and rehabilitation practices.

b. Establish *people structure* that is consistent with the objectives of patient care and the total organization of the health care facility, since people structure is an important aspect of the physical environment of an organization.

c. Develop a written organizational chart* that is current and defines the responsibility, authority, and relationships of all positions within the nursing department, delineates and defines intradepartmental relationships (line and staff relationship), and defines interdepartmental and interagency relationships.

d. Develop written policies and procedures to implement the organization-

*An organizational chart is a visual aid symbolic of design of *people* or *position structure* indicating responsibility, authority, and accountability.

al plan for intradepartment, inter-departmental, and interagency re-lationships.

e. Establish a system or a channel of communication (written or verbal) that is consistent with the total or-ganizational plan and disseminates accurate information vertically and horizontally to the right people and at the right time.

3. Contributory organizational objectives for the establishment of conceptual en-vironment

a. Create a climate (by providing the individual employee with the time and the place) in which the personnel can meet with the nursing service ad-ministrator and their immediate superiors to express personal opin-ions, likes, dislikes, satisfaction, con-cerns, and recommendations that will affect patient care and their own wel-fare and work conditions.

b. Create acceptance and tolerance of valid view points of others on mat-ters related to patient care or things specific to their job situations.

c. Establish an environment that is re-warding to the individual employees when they have demonstrated a de-sirable behavior; the nursing admin-istrator, supervisor, or head nurse can positively reinforce the employee by praising or acknowledging the person who has perhaps performed duties exquisitely and met the organization's objectives.

d. Delegate responsibility for decision making at the lowest level possible.

e. Consult with the employees in ex-pressing their views, perceptions, and expectation of the specific role and those of the organization and determine how compatible the two are.

f. Provide the opportunity for the in-dividual employer to utilize the em-ployee's potentialities.

4. Contributory organizational objectives

for the achievement of individual objec-tives

a. Develop nursing personnel policies that are in accordance with the over-all personnel policies of the health care facility that (1) specifically de-fine and delineate areas of responsi-bility and accountability in each position and (2) protect and safe-guard the employee from external pressure groups.

b. Explain to each employee the objec-tives and the policies of the organi-zation and the employee's role in ac-complishing these objectives.

c. Give each employee a written copy of the job description and the objec-tives that are inherent in that specific position.

d. Explain the job description and the objectives to the employee.

e. Utilize these objectives in the fair evaluation of the employee's per-formance of duties and in upgrading and promoting the employee.

f. Provide appropriate orientation, on-the-job training, and opportunity for continued education and learning so the employees can maintain their competence, keep abreast of current advances in nursing technology, and continue to improve themselves.

g. Provide the opportunity for the dif-ferent levels of nursing personnel to participate in planning, conducting, evaluating, and revising policies, pro-cedures, and programs of in-service education that influence the achieve-ment of both organizational objec-tives (quality patient care) and in-dividual objectives (self-fulfillment and self-actualization).

h. Place employees in roles that are con-gruent with their personality charac-teristics, their potentialities, and their capabilities.

i. Provide job security and financial re-wards that are comparable to those prevailing in similar positions elsewhere.

j. Provide for health, welfare, and safety programs in the interest of each employee.

5. Contributory individual objectives
   a. Each employee shall secure a written copy of personnel policies that have a direct bearing on matters such as hiring, firing, sick leave, vacation allowances, and fringe benefits.
   b. Each employee shall secure a written copy of the organizational objectives that affect patient care, the maintenance of the physical and conceptual environment, and individual employees.
   c. Each employee shall secure a written copy of personal objectives.
   d. Each employee shall secure a written job description with the following expected specifications: responsibilities, specific roles, task, duties, and salary ranges.
   e. Each employee shall demonstrate knowledge and understanding of pertinent personnel policies.
   f. Each employer shall demonstrate either orally or in written form knowledge of organizational objectives that affect patient care, physical and conceptual environment, and the individual employee.
   g. Each employee shall demonstrate knowledge and understanding of personal objectives, expectations.
   h. Each employee shall demonstrate knowledge and understanding of the job description with regard to responsibilities, specific roles, tasks, duties, and salary ranges.
   i. The employee should be able to apply acquired knowledge of both personnel and organizational policies in work situations.
   j. The employee should be able to apply aquired knowledge in fulfilling such organizational objectives as optimum delivery of care to all assigned patients and to efficient utilization of hospital facilities and equipment.
   k. The employee shall be held responsible and accountable for the fulfillment of personal objectives.
   l. The employee should be able to utilize aquired knowledge in performing the specific functions that are delineated by the job description, for example, assume responsibility and authority invested in the position and assume specific roles (team leader, team member, or head nurse) in the performance of tasks and duties.
   m. Each employee should feel free to express feelings about (1) policies, personnel and organizational, (2) organizational objectives, (3), individual objectives, (4) job specification, (5) opportunities for self-improvement, and (6) satisfactions and dissatisfactions experienced on the job.
   n. Each employee shall attend and participate in orientation programs, workshops for continuing his education, and planning and decision-making sessions when invited.

We realize that setting forth these definitions of goals and objectives and indicating how they can be utilized by organizations and individuals is one of the most complex and time consuming tasks. But all the planning, effort, and perhaps even struggle necessary to establish such procedures as we have outlined in this chapter are really worth it all. To put it simply, the setting of goals and objectives, if done well, *works*.

REFERENCES

Argyris, C.: The individual and organization: some problems of mutual adjustment, Admin. Sci. Q. 2(1):1-24, 1957a.

Argyris, C.: Personality and organization: the conflict between system and the individual, New York, 1957b, Harper & Row, Pubs.

Barnard, C.: The functions of the executive, Boston, 1938, Harvard Business School Division of Research.

Block, J. H., editor: Mastery learning: theory

and practice, New York, 1971, Holt, Rinehart & Winston, Inc.

Bloom, B.: Learning for mastery. In Bloom, B., Hastings, J. T., and Madaus, G. E., editors: Formative and summative evaluation of student learning, New York, 1971, McGraw-Hill Book Co., pp. 43-57.

Bowen, H. R.: The businessman's view of his specific responsibilities. In Richard, M. D., and Nielander, W., editors: Readings in management, ed. 2, New York, 1953, South-Western Pub. Co.

Carroll, J.: A model of school learning, Teacher's College Record **64**:723-733, 1963.

Cleland, D. I., and King, W. R.: Management: a systems approach, New York, 1972, McGraw-Hill Book Co.

Cohen, A. R.: Situational structure, self-esteem and threat-oriented reactions to power. In Cartwright, D., editor: Studies in social power, Institute for Social Research, Ann Arbor, 1959, University of Michigan Press.

Davis, R. C.: Fundamentals of top management, New York, 1951, Harper & Row, Pubs.

DeCecco, J. P.: The psychology of learning and instruction: educational psychology, Englewood Cliffs, N. J., 1968, Prentice-Hall, Inc.

Dent, J. K., Organizational correlates of the goals of business management, Personnel Psychol. **12**:365-393, 1959.

Drucker, P. F.: Practice of management, New York, 1954, Harper & Row, Pubs.

Filley, A. C., and House, R. J.: Management process and organizational behavior, Glenview, Ill., 1969, Scott, Foresman & Co.

Georgopoulos, B. S., Mahoney, G. M., and Jones, N. W., Jr.: A path goal approach to productivity, J. Appl. Psychol. **41**:345-353, 1957.

Georgopoulos, B. S., and Mann, F. C.: The community general hospital, New York, 1962, Macmillan Pub. Co., Inc.

Goddard, H. A.: Principles of administration applied to nursing service, World Health Organization, Monograph Series #41, Geneva, 1958, Palais des Nations.

Healey, J. H.: Executive coordination and control, Bureau of Business Research, Columbus, Ohio, 1956, Ohio State University Press.

Kahn, R. L., Wolfe, D. M., Quinn, R. P., Snock, J. D., and Rosenthal, R. A.: Organizational stress: studies in role conflict and ambiguity, New York, 1964, John Wiley & Sons, Inc.

Kast, F. E., and Rosenzweig, J. E.: Organization and management: a systems approach, New York, 1970, McGraw-Hill Book Co.

Levitt, T.: Marketing myopia, Harv. Bus. Rev., July-August 1960, pp. 45-56.

Lonsdale, R. C.: Maintaining the organization in dynamic equilibrium. In Griffiths, D. E., editor: Behavioral science and educational administration, the 63rd Yearbook of the National Society for the Study of Education, Chicago, 1964, The University of Chicago Press, pp. 142-177.

Mayo, E.: The social problems of an industrial civilization, Cambridge, 1945, Harvard University Press.

McGregor, D.: The human side of enterprise, New York, 1960, McGraw-Hill Book Co.

Murray, H. A.: Exploration in personality, New York, 1938, Oxford University Press, Inc.

Nader, R.: Unsafe at any speed, New York, 1965, Grossman Publishers.

Raven, B. H., and Rietsema, J.: The effects of varied clarity of group path upon the individual and his relationship to his group, Hum. Relat. **10**(1):29-45, 1957.

Taylor, F. W.: Principles of scientific management, New York, 1919, Harper & Row, Pubs.

Thomas, E. J., and Zander, A.: The relationship of goal structure to motivation under extreme conditions, J. Individ. Psychol. **15**:121-127, 1959.

Thorndike, E. L.: Animal intelligence, New York, 1911, Macmillan, Pub. Co., Inc.

Tomekovic, T.: Level of knowledge of requirements as a motivational factor in the work situation, Hum. Relat. **15**(3):197-216, 1962.

ADDITIONAL READINGS

Dimmock, M. E.: A philosophy of administration, New York, 1958, Harper & Brothers.

Duce, L. A.: A philosophic dimension of administration, Hosp. Admin. **11**(3):6-22, 1966.

Hicks, H.: The management of organizations: a systems and human resources approach, ed. 2, New York, 1972, McGraw-Hill Book Co.

Mager, R.: Preparing objectives for programmed instruction, Belmont, Calif, 1961, Fearon Publishers.

McGregor, D.: The human side of enterprise, New York, 1960, McGraw-Hill Book Co.

Moore, M. A.: Philosophy, purpose and objectives: Why do we have them, J. Nurs. Admin. **1**(3):3-14, 1971.

Palmer, J.: Management by objectives, J. Nurs. Admin. **1**(1):17-23, 1971.

Selznick, P.: Leadership in administration, New York, 1957, Harper & Row, Pubs.

Skapura, J. A.: Management by objectives: a systematic way to manage change, J. Nurs. Admin. **1**(2):52-56, 1971.

Tosi, H. L., and Carrol, J. S.: Management reaction to management by objectives, Acad. Man. J. **11**(4):415-426, 1968.

ADMINISTRATIVE COMPOSITE PROCESS: CONCEPTUAL AND PHYSICAL ACTS

This chapter deals with the two administrative acts that comprise the composite administrative process: (1) conceptual (planning and organizing) and (2) physical (directing and controlling) (Fig. 4-1). These two acts delineate the functions of the nursing service administrator. The functions essential to creating an organizational design and to formulating a plan of action are stating the purpose and the objectives of the organization in view of its resources and the requirements of the job; determining the kind of planning the administrator must do to provide for growth, an intelligent strategy, and answers to the "what," "how much," and "when" of the service to be provided; determining the kinds of organizational structure, personnel, and education required; establishing the kinds of control the administrator should exert if the institution is to stay current and capable of adjusting to unforeseen and changing circumstances; and setting mechanism for periodic reappraisal of all of these functions, particularly when control information shows unusual discrepancies. The all-pervasive element in the composite administrative process is coordination.

It is possible to attain a viable health service by focusing on the basic design of a care facility, the direction it is taking, its scheme of operation, and the interconnection of its parts. The key to success lies in the administrative process.

PLANNING

"No age ever viewed planning with the respect and familiarity of the twentieth century," wrote Finer in 1952, and now, almost 25 years later, the emphasis on planning is paramount to successful operation. One may well ask why. Health care organizations are complex, dynamic structures and are always subject to external environmental pressures imposed by funding sources, governmental and community agencies, professional groups, unions, suppliers, and scores of others. In addition, internal adjustment persuasives are created when the personnel and procedures of the organization respond to these environmental pressures.

As Lawrence and Lorsch (1969) suggest, when an organization exists in a highly differentiated and turbulent environment marked by complex interdependencies between and within many organizations, it must maintain a low degree of formal organizational structure. Less formal and less differentiated structure allows an organization to respond to constantly shifting environmental pressures. Modern health care organizations exist in such turbulent, evolving settings. They cannot function with a codified structure. They must remain flexible, and this requires planning at all levels of administration. The planning may be formal or informal, may be accomplished by a variety of mechanisms such as committees, professional planners,

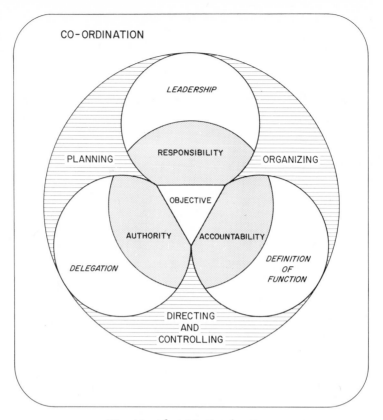

Fig. 4-1. Administrative functions.

or individual administrators and their staffs, and may differ from organization to organization. Each nursing service administrator will be situated in a unique organizational structure, challenged by continually changing demands for planning input. Therefore, our emphasis is on the process of planning based on principles underlying administration.

Nature of planning

According to Henri Fayol (1947:43): "if foresight is not the whole of management, at least it is an essential part of it. To foresee, in this context, means both to assess the future and make provisions for it; that is, forecasting is itself action already." Planning is the act or process of interpreting the facts of a situation, determining a line of action to be taken in light of all the facts and the objective

sought, detailing the steps to be taken in keeping with the action determined, making provision to carry through the plan to a successful conclusion, and establishing checks and balances to see how close performance comes to the plan.

Planning is a prerequisite for the successful operation of the nursing service department and the first conceptual skill required of the nursing service administrator. Without planning, the administrator cannot possibly meet the requirements and standards of the organization. If delays in nursing service are to be avoided, waste of professional skills and equipment eliminated, effective use of physical facilities realized, and personnel efficiently utilized in patient care, planning is essential. The ability to plan is an essential qualification of an administrator. Administrators are not entitled to the confidence of personnel unless they are willing to plan for and with them.

A variety of criteria may be employed to classify the process and output of planning. Scope, level, time, subject, degree of detail, purpose, and degree of control are useful concepts for delineating a specific planning problem (Levey and Loomba 1973). Such classifications are relative and seldom mutually exclusive. For example, nursing service administrators may differentiate four areas of planning for which they are responsible: (1) extension and expansion of nursing services, (2) improvement of patient progress, (3) increased effectiveness of staff utilization, and (4) heightened staff satisfaction. Long-range, medium-range, and short-range plans will probably imply different time scales on each of the planning areas, and the scope of these subject area definitions will obviously overlap.

Types of planning: strategic and tactical

There are many criteria for classification of types of planning, but one classification is notably useful, the differentiation of strategic and tactical planning (Levey and Loomba 1973). Strategic planning is the process by which basic organizational goals and directions are determined. Strategic planning is long-range and encompasses ends as well as means. In contrast, tactical plans look at shorter time frames, have a narrower scope, and focus in more detail. They are also more flexible, whereas strategic plans require large allocations of resources and are not easily altered once implementation has begun. Tactical plans are always created in support of some larger strategic plans. A chief administrator may withhold approval of a plan if it does not provide evidence of soundness and stability. The administrator's plan may be unacceptable as being out of touch with reality. Those called upon to implement such a plan may be equally critical and confused by the am-

biguity of an all too open-ended proposal. Examples of strategic planning in the health field are choosing the location and design of a new health care facility and deciding on the degree of interinstitutional affiliation or the scope of health services of the period. Tactical planning includes staffing for patient care on the clinical units, budgeting, determining patient admission and scheduling, purchasing, controlling inventory, and maintaining equipment.

Process of planning
FORCES

Nursing service has always been concerned with planning, but each year new forces make themselves felt, demanding more and better planning.

The forces for planning can be classified conveniently into two groups, namely, external and internal forces. External forces work from without the institution; they are beyond the control of the nursing service administrator. Internal forces operate inside the institution and are generally within control of the administrator.

External forces may be listed as (1) the patient, consumer, in a new role, (2) the community obligation, and (3) area-wide planning associations. Internal forces emanate from the nursing service administrator's responsibility for planning.

In recent years the patient has assumed a new initiative and a new influence in health care planning and in the evaluation of its quality. The means previously open to patients for judging care in the past were severely limited. Most patients now admitted to the hospital have anticipated their need for care through some form of prepayment. The potential patient is no intruder in health care. It is the prospective patient who has entered into a continuing relationship with hospitals and physicians. The hospital now finds itself in intimate, uncomfortable, but crucial contact with more demanding patients, with state insurance departments, and others. The public is asking more questions, demanding more explanations, participating more fully, and challenging the policies set down in the past.

Jenkins (1964) describes the public, with its change in attitude toward hospitals, as more sophisticated and more acutely aware of what it wants in health services. The public has come to accept the hospital as the health center of the community.

Hospital planning agencies have come into existence in some cities. It is the function of a hospital planning agency to achieve more effective use of total health personnel and facilities in the area in which it is established. Coordinated health planning is considered essential to the economic and cultural development of a community, as is an efficient transporta-tion, public safety, educational, or welfare program.

Internal forces of planning demand fixing responsibility for planning and delegating it through line administrative personnel. Another demand made is that planning be evaluated; this in turn directs further planning.

The process of planning starts with an analysis of the system and the setting of organizational objectives (goals) and culminates with implementation and control of strategic and tactical plans (Fig. 4-2). It is a continuous process characterized by seven phases, all interdependent and many of which may occur simultaneously. To undertake a planning program, the nursing service administrator considers each of them, either explicitly or implicitly.

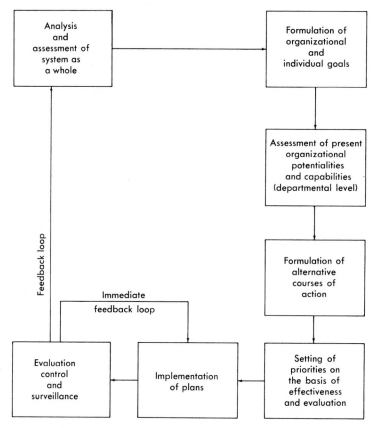

Fig. 4-2. Systems approach to the process of planning.

STAGES

Stage 1—analysis and assessment of system. The analysis of the existing system is the first step in formulating strategic plans. According to Churchman (1968) there are five basic considerations inherent in an analysis of the system as a whole. They are (1) objectives and performance measures, (2) environment, fixed constraints, (3) resources, (4) activities, goals and measures of performance of its subsystems, and (5) operation.

The administrator can rely on this general survey as a background against which to make quick decisions and plans when necessary. Systematic thinking can then begin to be habitual, and the time required for a systematic survey will not be a problem when sound and immediate decisions are required.

The general survey, if kept current, will mean that the detemination of objectives and policies and the measurement of the general existing situation will be phases of the planning process that are not turned off and on again but rather are relatively stable and reliable. This shared perspective will permit the nursing service administrator and co-workers to concentrate their attention on the design and redesign of operations as needed.

In general, the implications of this phase analysis and assessment of the system are threefold: (1) the implications make the administrators aware of the system as an open system so their sights are lifted from tactical to strategic planning, (2) they force the administrators to define the purpose of the system and the particular measures of performance that must be assigned to the system, and (3) the analysis of the resources and constraints of the system yields the information and data to develop organizational strategy.

As Levey and Loomba (1973:279) point out, this step answers the question, Where are we at the present time? This is a question that must be faced if concrete answers for two other important questions, Where do we want to go? and How do we get there? are to be satisfactorily answered.

Stage 2—formulation of organizational and individual goals. The second stage helps identify the ends toward which the administrator would like the system to move during a specific period of time. This stage requires that a schedule of achieving those goals be established. To create the schedule, one must evaluate goals along three dimensions: priority, time, and structure.

Priority of goals not only implies that at a given time the accomplishment of one goal is relatively more important than others, but also says something about the relative importance of certain goals regardless of time. Once objectives have been determined they should be clearly and precisely stated.

If the nursing service administrator states her creative ideas in terms of specific objectives, for example, (1) a greater outreach of services, more patient care, (2) improved patient progress, better patient care, (3) more effective staff utilization, to achieve 1 and 2, and (4) greater staff satisfaction, that is, reduced turnover, especially among the organization's professional nursing staff and if the nursing service administrator has a clear concept of the strategic goals of her organization, she can then begin to ask questions such as Are team nursing and the health team desirable to accomplish the goal? and she will be able to measure the possible answers against these specific objectives.

Stage 3—assessment of present organizational potentialities and capabilities. A nursing service administrator cannot establish realistic goals and objectives without knowing the current capabilities of the organization and specifically those of her own department. A complete self-assessment must occur in every subsystem and level of an organization so that an accurate picture of the entire system is available. This calls for cooperative planning with all department heads. As each functional department within the organization undertakes a self-appraisal the emerging information will indicate the current capabilities of the system. The data will describe (1) available resources, (2) strengths and weaknesses, and (3) opportunities and constraints present in the external and internal environment.

The nursing service administrator may generate information on personnel, equipment, and physical space resources and on the strengths and weaknesses in intrastaff communication patterns, home care programs, and scheduling procedures. Information concerning the relationships between her department and other departments as well as professional groups, unions, or estimates of public demands for nursing care may also be generated by the nursing service administrator.

At this stage all forecasting must begin to correspond to the realities of the organization. It is easy to produce the ideal plan, but that plan is useless if the resources necessary to implement it are not available. True planning takes into account all the limitations as well as the resources of the situation, and factors such as shortage of equipment and personnel or lack of adequate funds become at once a challenge and an imperative to the improvising powers of the planner.

Stage 4—formulating alternative courses of action. This stage considers specifying means by which organizational goals and objectives are to be achieved. The nursing service administrator may conceptualize (1) the addition of professional nurses to her staff, for example, those with public health background may work as home care coordinators, and (2) the expansion of team nursing to include the health team. Alternative courses must be considered at this stage. This may mean generating different methods for meeting patient and community demands and needs, perhaps by soliciting staff ideas. Alternatives should be evaluated for their feasibility and their

impact on health status. Various alternatives such as transfer of clerical work from nurses to secretaries, grouping of patients who need continuity of care, and instituting the use of nursing aides may all be considered during this phase of planning. In the selection of these alternative courses of action, certain factors should be weighed, such as (1) degree of relevance to the purposes and obligations of the organization, (2) anticipated cost-effectiveness ratio, (3) acceptability to the public, (4) acceptability to staff, (5) urgency, time ratio, and (6) extra dividend factor, which operates when the involvement of the Visiting Nurse Association or other groups in the work of the organization may lay the groundwork for other cooperative efforts.

Once particular proposals have been designed, plans must be formulated specifying the type and amounts of various resources that must be employed, their method of acquisition, and the necessary programs and procedures to support the implementation of these courses of action.

If the administrator is considering creating a position of professional nurse home care coordinator, it will be necessary to catalogue the professional and support personnel, equipment, supplies, and bookkeeping necessary for such a program. The administrator is then ready to evaluate the effectiveness of this plan.

Stage 5—setting of priorities on the basis of effectiveness and evaluation. In this stage the consequences of the various plans enumerated in stage 4 are projected. This phase is largely concerned with the establishment of priorities. Because the desired program will almost always outdistance the staff and facilities available, it is usually desirable to establish priorities in the various aspects of the service being planned. The degree of priority assigned will depend on the following:

1. Expected impact of the service in relation to saving lives, improving health, preventing illness or disability, improving health

practice, and by implication, raising the health level.

2. The accepted obligations of the health care organization, as defined by law or incorporation statements and as applied or stated by the philosophy of the policy-making body.
3. Community readiness.
4. Public relations impact.

Another important aspect of setting priorities is the recognition of time as a crucial element. The organization of time is often referred to as phasing, time planning, or target setting. When the consequences of a plan are projected it is helpful to take into account the four sequences of program activity, that is, (1) lead time, (2) initial trial period, (3) peak load adjustment, and (4) evaluation and replanning point. Plans that remain acceptable after this series of considerations and are not discarded as unfeasible or unviable can then be carried by the nursing administrator into stage 6.

Stage 6—implementation. This phase is concerned with resource allocation commitment. If the nursing service administrator has decided to add a professional home care coordinator to her staff, for example, the task of implementation requires that decision-making procedures affecting the home care coordinator now be spelled out for all parts of the organization.

This is the action and direction stage. Time and scope now play an important part as detailed questions of what, who, how, and when are answered.

Stage 7—evaluation control and surveillance. Evaluation or provision for measuring the outcomes of service against the objectives should be built into every plan. It should be planned for at the initiation of the service to assure such periodic progress checks as may be required as a basis for modification before the next planning period. An evaluation component also ensures that records be kept to provide the data necessary for appraisal at the same time. The administrative staff can be assured that the program is being implemented in accordance with the plan,

and they can promptly locate any breakdown. Review and assesment of patient care plans, supervisory visits, and leadership conferences may be needed to check on qualitative phases of the work. Statistical and narrative service reports will provide varying degrees of specificity.

Results from total evaluation and control measures are then fed back through the feedback loop and can be taken into consideration in future planning.

Criteria for evaluation

With the variety of plans made by the various levels of administration, the classification of plans, as good or poor, risks oversimplification and overgeneralization. There are, however, certain characteristics that can be used as yardsticks in qualifying a plan as good or poor. Table 3 summarizes the major characteristics of a good plan, which may be described as follows:

1. The plan should be based on clearly defined objectives. The intent of the plan should be described in terms that are clear not only to the planner but also to all who may be concerned with the implementation and operation of the plan.
2. The plan should be clear and simple. If the statement of a plan is ambiguous, there is danger that it may become complex and lead to misdirected effort and unnecessary expenditure. Therefore, the simpler the plan, the more chance of success it has (Urwick 1947).
3. The plan should have stability while providing for flexibility. Since planning premises, internal requirements, and external influences can change with time, the elements of flexibility must be built into the very design of a plan. In nursing, perhaps more than in any other field of work, flexibility is essential, and the plan must be capable of adaptation to meet emergencies or changing situations. On the other hand, stability of plans is also very crucial. If the plan is too fluid it will create distrust.
4. The plan should be economical and realistic in terms of the resources needed to implement it. Whenever possible, a plan should provide for the utilization of existing equipment, supplies, and personnel. It should be emphasized that economy in the use of personnel, material, and authority is as im-

Table 3. Major characteristics of good planning as seen by various authors

Characteristics of planning	Authors				
	Urwick (1947)	Levey and Loomba (1973)	Seckler-Hudson (1957)	Watson (1958)	Our selection
Based on clearly defined objectives	X	X	X	X	X
Clear and specific	X		X	X	X
Provides for stability and flexibility	X	X	X		X
Economical and realistic	X		X	X	X
Provides for analysis classification of action and outlines standards of operation	X	X	X	X	X
Anticipates and forecasts the future		X	X	X	X
Purposeful, rational, balanced, and justifiable in terms of needs	X	X			X
Allows for the sociopolitical environment of the organization		X			X
Specifies the dimensions for which it applies		X			X

portant as economy in the use of funds. Furthermore, if existing organizations and staff are qualified to do the work required, it is demoralizing to personnel if they are disregarded when a new plan is implemented.

5. The plan should provide for a thorough analysis and classification of activities and for determination of the evaluation criteria, which become the basis of the control system. A study of the various activities needed to accomplish the work will nearly always show some opportunity for simplification of work. In making a plan operational, it is important to take into consideration the following points: (a) Are the scheduling, sequencing, and coordination of activities and plans congruent and realistic? (b) Are the priorities set up appropriately? and (c) Are the target dates set up in realistic terms? If the means and evaluation standards of operation are missing, the plan is likely to be considered too theoretical or unfinished, and in reality, it is unfinished until some plan of operation is provided.

6. The plan should anticipate and forecast the future. No person or group engaged in preparing a plan can afford to deal only with the here and now. Planning deals with the future and as such requires an input of forecasts of economic variables, patient needs and demands, utilization of health services, social environment, and direction of political forces. It should be emphasized that, in the last analysis, the true worth of a plan is measured by the accuracy with which the future has been anticipated and the degree to which the specifics of the plan have been based on such forecasts (Levey and Loomba 1973; Seckler-Hudson 1957).

7. The plan should be purposeful, rational, and justifiable in terms of organizational and individual objectives.

8. The plan should allow for the unique sociopolitical environment of the organization. An important point of reference for planning is the current capability profile of the system (Levey and Loomba 1973).

9. The plan should be based on clearly defined dimensions and objectives.

ORGANIZING

The second conceptual act required of the nursing service administrator is that of organizing, the carrying out of plans to meet the objectives of the total organization and of the nursing service department. Organizing is for the purpose of creating relationships that will minimize friction, focus on the objective, clearly define the responsibilities of all parties, and facilitate the attaining of objectives. This means creating a structure, or a working arrangement of positions, jobs, and organizational roles, spelling out responsibility and lines of authority in terms of decision making, setting regulations, and procedures, all of which will guide the entire personnel within the nursing service department. Even though creating this structure is a massive piece of work, it would vastly simplify the work of the administrator if that was all there was to the organizing function. The inevitability and need for change in any complex organization do not disappear, however, simply because a department is structurally well organized. If the nursing service department is to be responsive to the needs of its patients, it must be flexible, adaptive, and innovative in addition to being well organized; it is for this purpose that creating problem-solving mechanisms is a central part of organizing. The unique limitations and talents of any group of workers has to be taken into account here. Interdepartmental and intradepartmental communication needs to be established and nurtured.

Also to be considered is the need for coordinating with other departments within the health care system and with the community. In carrying out their work, nurses cooperate with personnel from other parts of the organization and from other disciplines. A nursing service administrator who oversees the organization of her department without consulting other departments is shirking her responsibility to her nurses and breeding interdepartmental misunderstandings with which the nurses may not be able to cope.

Thus organization may be defined as the process of grouping activities, delineating authority and responsibility, and establishing working relationships that will enable both the institution and the employee to realize their mutual objectives. Or one may agree with Appley (1952:2): "Or-

ganizing is determining, assembling, and arranging the resources by function and in relation to the whole to meet the planned objective."

When successful organizations are studied, all are found to have the following common characteristics that are essential if they are to function efficienctly: (1) strong resourceful leadership, (2) clearly defined responsibilities, (3) a carefully selected, trained, and placed working force, (4) standardized methods, (5) adequate cost and other records, and (6) cooperation. The development of an effective health care organization requires proper observance and application of a series of fundamentals of organization.

Nature of organizing

A helpful guide to organization planning stems from Stieglitz (1972), who lists four elements containing 11 principles of organization:

1. Objectives. (a) The objectives of the enterprise and its component elements should be clearly defined and stated in writing. The organization should be kept simple and flexible.
2. Activities and grouping of activities. (b) The responsibilities assigned to a position should be confined as far as possible to the performance of a single leading function. (c) Functions should be assigned to organizational units on the basis of homogeneity of objective to achieve most efficient and economic operation.
3. Authority. (d) There should be clear lines of authority running from the top to the bottom of the organization and accountability from bottom to top. (e) The responsibility and authority of each position should be clearly defined in writing. (f) Accountability should always be coupled with corresponding authority. (g) Authority to take or initiate action should be delegated as close to the scene of action as possible. (h) The number of levels of authority should be kept to a minimum.
4. Relationships. (i) There is a limit to the number of positions that can be effectively supervised by a single individual. (j) Everyone in the organization should report to only one supervisor. (k) The accountability

of higher authority for the acts of its subordinates should be absolute.

SETTING OF OBJECTIVES

Conceived in the largest terms, the basic objectives of an organization are stability, growth, and interaction, or more simply the ability to maintain itself over time. These prime objectives are obtained by achieving the more concrete objectives of producing quality service and effectively utilizing resources. In health care organizations more specific objectives are determined by answering such questions as Is it a single, specialized health service, or is it a diversified service? What community is being served? Is the community stable or temporary? and What is the total patient care provided?

The objectives thus defined by a health care organization will then be colored by a host of environmental factors, such as the degree of competition in the health care industry, the relative degree of change in the technology involved, the legal environment, and the availability of personnel. These factors will all affect the type of organization at the departmental level. They will delimit or expand and influence the structure of authority, responsibility, the social system, and the relationships between various units of the organization.

The first and one of the most important functions of an administrator, such as the nursing service administrator, is to establish clear, workable departmental objectives that are congruent with the larger organizational framework. When designing these objectives, the administrator can be guided by their utility in helping her fulfill her role and responsibilities. The administrator can use the following four functional criteria for choosing and defining the objectives for her department:

1. Objectives should provide the basis for co-operation in the organization. Thus the subunit goals must be compatible with and contribute to the overall goals. This is what is meant by *unity of direction*. In addition, the relationship between each subgoal and the ultimate goals must be made apparent to all concerned, otherwise the organization runs the danger of going adrift.

2. Objectives should help determine proper courses of action. They should be practical evaluative criteria that facilitate the decision-making abilities of organizational members. Measuring particular activities and procedures against a well-defined objective should ease the elimination of those who are least important to the organization.

3. Objectives should establish standards for control. Well-defined goals that are broken down into nursing service targets, quality standards, time deadlines, and other similar quantifiable specifics result in invaluable yardsticks for measuring accomplishments and progress. At the same time they provide incentive and motivation toward work accomplishment.

4. Proper definition of objectives will make effective the *exception principle*. In this administrative approach, feedback is required only when actual performance is different from planned performance. Attention is directed to significant deviations, whether especially good or bad. Deviations are then analyzed for possible corrective action or for the redefinition of an objective. A simple example of administration by exception is the elimination of daily time sheets and the substitution of less frequent reports showing only absenteeism or overtime.

The specific objectives that the nursing service administrator identifies will determine the balance between quantity and quality of patient care and will indicate means by which the output of patient care can be measured. They will also determine the ways that people will relate to each other in the course of accomplishing their work and whether the personal objectives and development of individuals will be provided for or disregarded. Any objective that is formulated will have personal implication for each individual who works in support of it. Thus, once an objective has been identified, it must be conceptualized so that it contains qualitative as well as quantitative criteria. The quality of the work life as well as patient care in the department should always be a central concern for the administrator, especially when activities are designed and grouped to meet specific objectives.

DESIGNING AND GROUPING ACTIVITIES

Having set objectives, one must organize to put them into action. The nursing service administrator has to organize her department for patient care through the conduct of nursing practice. Nursing practice is the actual performance or application of knowledge, the exercise of an occupation. In this context, nursing service is primarily an administrative mechanism with the function of providing the conditions, including both staff and material equipment, for optimum nursing practice. The nursing service administrator is the servant or the spokesman for the practitioners of nursing. At the same time, she is held responsible to her employer, the health care administrator, for the quality of nursing practice.

The activities involved in nursing practice are determined by the unique setting in which they take place. The community served and the types of services offered to patients will set definite boundaries around the kinds of tasks the nurse will need to undertake, as will her physical surroundings and the number and type of her co-workers, from physicians to other professional disciplines and maintenance staff. Thus, the environmental setting of the nurse determines what she will and will not do professionally. Nurses gain further definition of their tasks from the specific technology that they practice. Nurses have different technical requirements to fulfill, whether in the operating room or the cardiac intensive care or the pediatric clinical unit. Each implements a different body of specialized knowledge and skills. Along with the environmental determinants, these technological components are the aspects of work that are least likely to change through administrative intervention on the part of the nursing service administrator. Nursing technology is the raw material of nursing practice.

In grouping together activities to design jobs, the administrator is creating a social support for nursing practice. The social system will be composed of the work-related interactions between people, and each activity so identified and structured will have a social and technical component. It is up to the administrator and her staff to find the most effective use of both the social and technical components of activities.

The job of planning a nursing service organization is becoming more demanding for the administrator because of the increased complexity of health care facilities and operations; more specialized services; further refinements in the *division of labor*, specialization; and the changing goals of the health care facilities in the field.

Functional approach. One way to view the nursing requirements that determine activities is to identify a functional unity that the tasks are serving. This functional approach looks at what needs to be done for nursing practice to take place and is concerned with the functions of the health care facility from the standpoint of the purpose of the institution as a whole, analyzing each department or component of the broad functions pertaining to nursing services and then deciding, on the basis of administrative principles, how the nursing service should be organized to accomplish these functions at the level of skill required. This approach analyzes what needs to be done before a plan of organization is designed, instead of starting out by deciding what professional nurses and other nursing personnel should do.

Utilizing the functional approach, the nursing service administrator sets about to (1) state the function, (2) review the principles and activities that comprise a stated function, that is, outline what needs to be done, (3) determine the kind and level of knowledge, skill, and competence required to do what needs to be done, and (4) provide for doing what needs to be done by personnel at the required level of skill consistent with good administration, communication, coordination, and control. In other words, the professional nurse's knowledge and competence is matched to the needs of the patient. Functions are assigned according to competence not according to positional or hierarchical authority.

By analyzing the function first, one can lay a basis for determining the kinds of personnel needed, where decision making should take place, what supporting services may be required, and what relationships need to be created. All of these factors can influence the organizational design.

In 1968 the American Hospital Association issued a statement on functions in health care organizations that require the competence of a registered nurse. Using that statement as a point of departure, the AHA made the following comments in a pamphlet in 1970 concerning the functional approach for providing nursing care of patients:

1. Plan nursing care pursuant to the medical care plan of the physician. Assess patient needs for nursing and establish objectives for nursing actions on a continuing basis.
2. Implement plans of nursing care in accordance with objectives of the nursing care plan. Organize, direct, and supervise nursing personnel in giving nursing care. In the assignment of nursing personnel, registered nurses give care to patients whose conditions require their professional competence and skills.
3. Evaluate the quality of nursing care in terms of the extent to which objectives of the nursing plan are met. Appraise the quality of nursing care, the performance of nursing personnel, and the proper use of equipment and supplies in rendering nursing care.
4. Coordinate patient care activities. Registered nurses, by virtue of the strategic position they occupy as the most constant figures relating and communicating both with the patients and with members of the professional staff providing patient services, are responsible for the coordination of activities to achieve to the greatest extent possible a unified approach to the care of the patient.
5. Teach nursing personnel the nursing care of patients in relation to the objectives of the nursing care plan. Determine specific nursing knowledge and skills that need to be learned by the nursing personnel.

The planning function may include communicating the physician's plan to the nursing staff, initiating that plan by the nursing staff, developing the nursing care plan pursuant to the medical care plan, consulting with other staffs, and placing authority for adopting the plan. The implementing function may involve placing authority for implementation, creating controls for standard of performance, and coordinating with other departmental staff providing services to patients. The evaluating function requires determination of standards of measurement and performance expectations and the placement of responsibility for appraisal. The coordinating function determines the relationships between patients and all segments of the professional staff as well as community-based agencies such as the Visiting Nurse Association. The teaching function may include many forms of in-service, continuing educational, and on-the-job training.

The nursing functions may not always be mutually exclusive or in any way independent of each other, but they do form one criterion for grouping tasks together to form specific job descriptions. The administration can then decide on the kinds and levels of knowledge and skills required for these jobs. These will be not only nurse practitioner skills but also administrative and interpersonal skills. Activities that are grouped together by function will require interdependency among personnel, that is, in choosing her personnel to fit a particular job, the administrator will need to match the social and nursing requirements of the work with the personal qualifications of each worker. Nursing as a profession does not believe in rigid definitions in terms of isolated tasks or activities. Nurses are concerned with the total care of patients, the individual patient's response, and interdependence of the physiological and psychological responses to potential or actual interferences. This meshing of the social and technical aspects of activities can be seen in the variety of ways in which nursing units can be structured to provide the same services and undertake the same activities. The choice of any one of these nursing methods will depend on the unique situation of the nursing department, the requirements of the patient, the philosophy of the organization, the physical environment, and the knowledge and skills of the personnel. The variety of approaches to taking care of patients are exemplified by the methods of assignment of personnel. There are several such methods in nursing, the team method being talked about as one of the best or most usable. The *team method* utilizes all nursing personnel at various levels of skill. The professional nurse has the responsibility for patient care and is assuming the role of leadership. She must know how to give skilled nursing care, but she must also be capable of directing and supervising the work of other team members. The less favored *functional method* tends to compartmentalize nursing skills, and the nurse-patient relationship is hampered, if not minimized, in many instances. The *traditional case method* of assignment is often considered impractical as it requires an all-professional staff; however, the professional nurse carries full responsibility for the care of the patients on an eight-hour basis. *Primary nursing* is a fairly new method of caring for patients whereby the professional nurse is assigned full responsibility to care for a patient from the time that patient enters the health care facility until release. It makes for excellent continuity of individualized care, since the nurse is responsible for total care, and nurses report it is a very satisfying service to the patient, to the nurse, and to the physician. Primary nursing fixes responsibility, authority, and accountability. Like the case method, though, primary nursing requires an all-graduate nursing staff. A *combination* of these methods is employed by some organizations.

It is understood, of course, that the preceding nursing functions are not isolated from one another and that nurses do not carry out their functions in isolation. A nurse takes care of more than one patient.

While planning and writing the care plan, the nurse may also organize that care. The five functions mentioned relate specifically to the nursing care of patients and do not include all the functions of the department of nursing, such as staffing, budgeting, continuing education, research, evaluation, and personnel administration. If, however, primary attention is focused on the plan of organization of the patient care unit (the basic unit of management, that is, patient, nurse, and physician), a nucleus or foundation is laid for designing a plan of nursing service organization. The overall plan is devised to support the basic units consistent with the goals and functions of the health facility.

Form follows function, or need determines form. In other words, the way a nursing service organization is built is determined by the uses to which it will be put. As we see it, the users decide what an organization will look like; that is, the system that will receive the output of the organization (families and community) and use it as its own input is the real designer of a nursing service organization. The human architect, the nursing service administrator, is seen in this view, not as the determiner of the character of the organization, not even as the planner of its configuration, but as an interpreter of the requirements of the user (patient), whose needs form the organization structure.

Decentralization. Decentralization is the term for grouping activities on the basis of service, product, or function. The term relates more to authority than to the grouping of activities, and the inference has been that authority to take or initiate action should be delegated as close to the scene of action as possible (Stieglitz 1972).

The advantages of decentralization are usually quicker and better decisions, administrative development, reduced levels of organization, and the freeing of supervisors to concentrate on broader responsibilities. How far down in the organization can authority be delegated? What limitations, if any, should be placed on decentralized authority? The following three criteria can be isolated on which the delegation of decision-making authority is dependent:

1. Competence. The person to whom authority is delegated should be competent to make decisions, and the superior should have confidence in that competence.
2. Information. The decision maker requires adequate and reliable information pertinent to the decision. Decision-making authority, thus, cannot be pushed below the point at which all information bearing on the decision is available.
3. Scope of impact of the decision. If a decision affects units outside a certain sphere of responsibility, the authority to make the decision rests with the administrator accountable for the several units. Thus, authority can be decentralized to the level at which the impact of the decision is local. Certain decisions affecting the total organization, for example, institutional objectives, policies, and budgets, are usually not decentralized at all.

To a large extent this point concerning scope of decisions also answers the question, What limitations, if any, are there on decentralization? For, in a real sense, the decisions made at the top of the organization, which take the form of objectives and policies, delimit decentralized authority. And authority grants freedom to act or make decisions only in conformity with overall organizational objectives and policies.

To return to the term itself, decentralization, something must be centralized before it can be decentralized. To prevent decentralization from becoming complete fragmentation, it is necessary that part of the control core remain as the unifying element.

Thus, decentralization, in practice, becomes a matter of degree, with the degree being determined by how far down authority has been delegated and how stringent the limits are that have been placed on the authority. It is this fact that leads organizational analysts to declare that no organization is completely decentralized, only more or less so.

STRUCTURING AUTHORITY, RESPONSIBILITY, AND ACCOUNTABILITY

Authority has its base in responsibility, which is derived from the objective. Authority makes itself felt through leadership, which is multiplied through delegation and clarified by functional definition (see Fig. 4-1). Accountability is always associated with responsibility and authority.

The position vested with authority is the universal building block of all organizations. Authority defines which position will be superior and which subordinate. These authority relations are institutionalized; that is, they are characterized by explicit rules, predictable behavior, and continuity of relationships. Incumbents may come and go, but authority of position remains.

Definition. Authority is defined by Webster as "legal or rightful power; a right to command or to act; domination; jurisdiction." Mary Parker Follett (Metcalf and Urwick 1941:104) distinguishes between authority and power: "We can confer authority; but power or capacity no man can give or take." And again: "I do not believe that power can be delegated because I believe that genuine power is capacity." Rather than seek external and arbitrary authority, Miss Follett suggests that our efforts be used in seeking the "law of the situation." Another definition of authority is given by Chester L. Barnard (1968:15-17):

Authority is the character of a communication (order) in a formal organization by virtue of which it is accepted by a contributor to or member of the organization as governing the action he contributes; that is, as governing or determining what he does or is not to do so far as the organization is concerned. According to this definition, authority involves two aspects: first, the subjective, the personal, the accepting of a communication as authoritative, and, second, the objective aspect—the character in the communication by virtue of which it is accepted.

Authority is the right to command or to act (Tannenbaum 1949). Thus, a person having authority has the right not only to act himself but also to expect action of others. But what is the source of this right?

Source. The various levels of divisional activities in health care organizations are a direct result of the size and complexity of modern institutions. At the top level is the poilcy-making body, that is, the employing authority. At the next level is the operating authority, that is, the chief executive officer or administrator of the organization. Theoretically this individual takes the place of the employer in the superior-subordinate relationship; but, as it is manifestly impossible for the chief executive officer to know and give directions personally to all the employees, this person, in turn, delegates responsibility to a group of individuals who exercise that delegated authority in supervising the work of others. This level is that of supervisor. This is authority based on legitimacy and position. Authority when viewed in this customary manner is referred to as formal authority. At the end of the chain of responsibility the point is reached at which responsibility is delegated for the performance of specific functions. Such activities are known as operations, and they cover a range that extends from the performance of duties requiring a high degree of skill to those that are simply repetitive. This is functional authority, and it is based on technical knowledge and personal skills, in other words, competence and influence. Both types of authority are necessary for achieving goals and satisfying individual needs through organizational activity, but the appropriate combinations and the effectiveness with which they are exercised remain matters requiring further empirical inquiry.

The divisions of authority give rise to various types of relationships between officials. Four main types may be distinguished as follows:

1. Line relationships between a superior and the subordinate immediately and directly responsible to that superior.
2. Lateral relations between positions in various parts of an undertaking in which no direct authority is involved.
3. Functional relations that arise when duties are divided on a functional basis, that is, when an individual exercises authority on one particular subject by reason of special skill or knowledge. They can, and should, exist side by side with line relations.
4. Staff relations that arise when individuals are acting as representatives of superiors. These individuals are not vested with authority in their own right but are acting "for and on behalf of" the persons in whom the authority is vested. Their function is one of transmission and interpretation coupled with the duty of seeing that the orders given are executed. The following are examples of relationships that may be found among individuals in a health care organization:

Relationship	Health care organization personnel
Line	Nursing service administrator to head nurse
Lateral	Head nurse with physician, social worker, and dietitian
Functional	Nursing service administrator with finance officer, head nurse with unit manager, head nurse with clinical instructor, and night supervisor with engineer
Staff	Head nurse acting on behalf of the nursing service administration because both the director and the assistant are absent

The sources of *formal authority* need to be distinguished from the sources of *functional authority*. In general, functional authority supports formal authority. In a given superior-subordinate relationship, it is the superior's lack of functional authority or the subordinate's possession of greater competence, experience, or personal skill that tends to undermine formal authority. Competition may also occur between incumbents of equal formal rank but of different task or specialist orientation, for example, between the controller and the nursing service administrator. Finally, competition between functional and formal authority may occur where hierarchical channels are ambiguous, a condition frequently characteristic of staff-line relationships.

One of the conflicts in modern nursing service organizations is derived from the divergence of the two bases of authority: authority legitimized by incumbency in office and authority based on professional competence. Not only do subunits of organizations differ as to the importance attached to these two bases of authority, but different kinds of organizations in different times and cultures also seem to emphasize one or the other. Although a number of writers have commented on an increasing tendency toward reliance on professional competence with an attending decline in the perceived legitimacy of hierarchical authority, evidence suggests that the strategic location and influence of those in hierarchical roles often enable them to get along without specialized skills.

Delegation of authority. Having the authority to act is fundamental, but the delegation and utilization of that authority are of equal importance. Modern administration is recognizing more and more that the nursing service administrator in a health care organization must free herself of the minutia of administration and devote her energies to planning, organizing, directing, and controlling. She must save her energies for only top-level or exceptional problems of the organization. She must not only operate at her own level but at the highest possible level of her capacity. In turn, this should be true of every person in the organization. The level of an assistant may not be her potential stature, and it is incumbent on the head of the organization to see assistants not only for what they are, but also for what their potential stature may be.

If the nursing administrator in a large and complex organization operates at the optimum level and speed, she will need (1) to delegate as much work and respon-

sibility as possible to her nursing staff, always of course in terms of their capacities and environment; actually the administrator may prefer to operate at her own highest level, which may vary from time to time; and (2) to delegate responsibility and authority as close as possible to the point in the organization where problems arise and action occurs. She must appraise her personnel in terms not only of performance and progress but also of potential, so that together they can rise to higher and higher levels of responsibility and leadership. Cumulatively, therefore, all leadership in an organization should be rising to its highest tide, and as this occurs delegation can be made with greater certainty and confidence.

Delegation of responsibility and authority can be appraised fairly only in terms of the environment in which the administrator operates. The time has passed for picturing the nursing service administrator presiding at the top of a pyramid over the hierarchical structure of personnel and the clinical units or departments. The inverted pyramid with the nursing administrator at the bottom reaching upward and outward for the most important relationships is replacing that image. The climate upward may not always be without its problems, and almost surely in that climate there will be many supervisors assisting the nursing service administrator. In "plural leadership at the top" there may be frictions and tensions that condition what the administrator can do within her own organization. At the base of the inverted pyramid the administrator is subject to all of the "climate above herself."

In addition to the relationships upward in the administration environment, there are delicate relationships on a horizontal level. Especially in a complex health care facility every administrator must maintain harmonious working relationships with many other similar program leaders, whose work and organization conditions hers and vice versa. This reaching across, as well as reaching upward, takes tact, time, and judgment. Some of the relationships in the administrator's internal environment that influence her actions may be (1) program, (2) organization, (3) staff, (4) resources, and (5) mores and tradition. In summary, the factors in the nursing service administrator's environment that will condition the limits and potentialities of delegation within her immediate organization include the following:

1. Institutional conditions upward.
2. Institutional conditions horizontally.
3. Institutional conditions downward, including abilities and capacities on the part of personnel.
4. Institutional culture, including prevailing mores, workways, protocol, and expectations within the organization.
5. Legal jurisdiction and limitations of the institutions.
6. Cultural environment of the organization and the resultant pressures from the outside.
7. Ability, capacity, and philosophy of the nursing service administrator.

Line and staff. One of the main factors in dealing with authority, well described by Stieglitz (1972) and Tannenbaum (1949), is the concept of line and staff, organizational terms used to define the relationship between the work and authority components of organization. Line and staff are two of the most perplexing, ambiguous, overworked, and overdefined terms in the lexicon of the organization planner.

Some institutions have attempted to dispense with them, substituting operating for line and auxiliary or service for staff. But substitution of terms is of doubtful value in clarifying the organization relationships involved.

Generally the terms are used in two quite different settings: (1) to distinguish or characterize types of work and (2) to distinguish and characterize types of authority. The confusion arises from the general conclusion that staff work implies staff authority.

In terms of work, line connotes the tasks,

functions, or organizational components that are accountable for fulfilling the service and economic objectives of the organization. This is not to imply that any unit of the organization does not contribute to the income of the organization. But line units are explicitly concerned directly with producing the values in the form of goods and services that the customer or client will pay for.

In terms of work, staff connotes the tasks, functions, or organization components that are required to supply information and services to the line components.

The nature of the staff work performed is of three types:

1. Advice and counsel. The staff gathers and disseminates information, often of a specialized nature, to other elements of the organization that require information. The staff unit advises and counsels its superiors on procedures, methods, and systems that will most effectively accomplish the objectives of the organizational unit. When the organizational unit is the institution as a whole, staff units advise and counsel the administrator in the planning of overall institutional objectives and policies.
2. Services. The staff supplies to other units services that can be provided more economically by centralizing them. A unit may be created, for example, to recruit and screen new employees rather than have the several components recruit and screen separately, or a purchasing department may be created to handle the buying for several departments. In such situations the staff may be viewed as relieving the line unit of chores.

   In other situations, however, the services required are of a more specialized nature and cannot be adequately performed by line units. For example, the special skills and knowledge required to negotiate a legal contract or to provide medical attention give rise to staff units providing these specialized services.
3. Functional control. The staff acts on behalf of its superior to see that certain controls, in the form of objectives and policies, budgets, plans, and procedures, are being adhered to by other units. On behalf of its superior, the staff inspects, measures, and evaluates performance within its sphere of functional competence, relative to the standards and controls that have been estab-

lished. In this respect, the staff is working within the area of its superior's reserved responsibility to plan and to control.

In regard to the staff, consideration is often restricted only to the staff's work as an advisory and counseling unit. This leads to the contention that when staff performs certain services or exercises functional control it is actually line. Very often, too, the traditional role of staff is said to be that of merely providing advice and counsel. This neglects the historical fact that the need for special services gives rise to some of the earliest types of staff units: finance, purchasing, legal, and medical departments. Functional control, too, is a traditional role, so traditional that when control is mentioned, one automatically thinks of a financial controller.

In many organizations there are staff units whose work is primarily to advise and counsel, for example, a long-range planning unit; there are other units that are primarily service units, for example, units in charge of purchasing or press relations; and there are units that are solely functional control units, for example, the auditors or controllers. But it has been increasingly recognized that staff units perform all three types of work. The personnel administration, for example, advises and counsels top administration and other units on effective personnel programs and procedures; provides services in the form of recruitment, selection, and testing; and exercises functional control on behalf of its superior in overseeing adherence to organization-personnel policies.

This distinction between line and staff, when used to characterize different types of work, may confuse the relationship between the two units when they are characterized in terms of authority. It is generally assumed, for example, that units doing line work automatically have line authority and that units doing staff work have no authority over the line and, thus, no line authority. Or, more to the point, line work is often believed to be synonymous with line au-

thority, and staff work synonymous with staff authority. Possibly the simplest way to clarify the authority relationship between staff and line is to express it in terms of accountability for results. In any organizational relationship the unit or person held accountable for the specified result has authority to make the necessary decision. Line, in this authority context, connotes authority to take action, authority to make decisions.

Staff, on the other hand, connotes the unit, or units, that supply facts and information that will enable the accountable administrator to make the best decision. Staff supplies services designed to help the line administrator achieve the best results. But the staff cannot impose its judgment or its services on the administrator with line authority.

These distinctions between line work and line authority and staff work and staff authority become more evident in a given situation. The head of a department doing staff work, finance, for example, is accountable for the effective preformance of that unit. To increase effectiveness, the head of the finance department may call on the organization planning department to analyze the organizational setup (a request for service) and recommend a better structure (a request for advice). In accepting or rejecting the recommendation of the organization planning department, the head of finance is exercising line authority. To further improve the finance department's effectiveness, the head of finance may seek the advice of the nursing service department on measures that will simplify accounting problems. Again, it is possible to accept or reject the suggestions that the nursing department makes. In this case the nursing department, though labeled line in terms of work, is operating in a staff capacity to a unit conventionally labeled staff, in terms of work, that is now exercising line authority.

Thus, when the question of authority is at issue, it is the accountability for results that determines where the line authority resides. The most obvious example of a situation under which a department doing staff work apparently assumes line authority occurs when the department exercises functional control relative to overall organizational objectives or policies. According to one organization (Stieglitz 1972:26-27):

When standards have been developed for (organization-wide) application and have been incorporated in an official statement of policy or where (the executive) has made it clear through other media or methods that certain standards are to be observed, the role of the staff department is no longer advisory but becomes one of inspection and reporting.

Span of control. The principle of span of control generally used today is: There is a limit to the number of positions that can be effectively supervised by a single individual. This is quite different from the somewhat arbitrary statement still used by relatively few: The number of people supervised should be no more than five. The modification is attributable to institutional experience. There is recognition that a number of very practical factors affect span of control, all interdependent.

1. The competence of both the superior and the subordinates.
2. The degree of interaction between the units or personnel being supervised.
3. The extent to which the supervisor must carry out nonadministrative responsibilities and the demands on her time from other people and units.
4. The similarity or dissimilarity of the activities being supervised.
5. The incidence of new problems in her unit.
6. The extent of standardized procedure.
7. The degree of physical dispersion.

This brief list by no means exhausts the factors that affect a supervisor's span of control. But consideration of them has led institutions away from attempts to set arbitrary limits on the number of people that can be supervised at any level. One large institution, for example, states its span of control principle in these terms:

The employees responsible to one supervisor should not exceed the number which can be effectively directed and coordinated. The number will depend largely on the scope and complexity of the responsibilities of the personnel or patient care.

Another institution puts it this way:

There are no fixed rules for determining span of control; the number of personnel reporting to one executive should be determined by the capacities of the individuals involved and the nature of their responsibilities.

CREATING WORKING RELATIONSHIPS WITHIN THE SOCIAL SYSTEMS

The extent to which people in an organization fit the requirements of the organization significantly determine how well it functions.

Determinants of working relationships

Problem of size. The nursing personnel of a small health care facility come into easy contact. Within minutes one member knows what anyone else is doing at any particular time and what one member is doing is observed by most of the others. Their jobs in caring for patients are interchangeable, since most of the workers are capable of performing a wide array of functions or jobs as the needs arise. Formal organization is absent, or at least invisible. In brief, personnel in small health care facilities know what has to be done, know each other's capabilities, and can quite easily find a place for themselves and acquire an understanding of how the handling and care of patients are managed.

In the large health care organization the personnel are not all in plain sight of one another. Persons employed in a large facility sometimes never learn to know others or discover what jobs or functions the others perform in the care of patients. One seldom knows what activities are being carried on elsewhere in the hospital. Each does a certain job knowing that somehow it is coordinated with other activities so that patients can be admitted, treated, and released.

Unless the members of a large health

care facility are performing the same kind of functions or jobs it is difficult for them to shift functions and responsibilities among themselves. Coordination of activities becomes formalized and "coordination" or "administration" specialists crop up among the job titles. Nurses usually become known and addressed by job title rather than by name. One is likely to know intimately only those "who do the same things I do" or "who do things closely associated with what I do."

The size of operation and the degree of specialization of function all but prevent the personnel in a large health care facility from comprehending the nature of the whole organizational pattern. It is difficult for them to find a satisfactory way to take part in its activities.

This comparison of small and large hospital organizational problems leads to a number of inferences (Goodson and Jensen 1956:60-62): (1) as a hospital grows in size the coordination of its activities shifts from simple, concrete, spontaneous human interaction to abstract, ordered, careful management of the ways in which personnel are related to one another; (2) personnel are less able to check the effectiveness and the rightness of their contributions, giving rise to the specialist; (3) the specialist in coordination, often an administrator, becomes the person who determines how well the personnel are doing, how the hospital is organized, and what its accomplishment or state of progress is; (4) distortions or false perceptions are apt to occur over what other members do and how important they are to the work of the institution; and (5) it becomes increasingly difficult for individual members to know whether their tasks are worthwhile and important to the process of treating and rehabilitating patients.

Sooner or later in the growth of an organization a pattern of problems begins to take shape, and nursing service administrators must then address themselves to the careful design and maintenance of a social system that will minimize the alienation of individual persons from their colleagues.

When attempts are made to examine the effects of the human organization of a health care system on the treatment of patients, another problem arises: how to achieve the balance of formal and informal relations between personnel. Although there is no set formula for determining this balance, provision must be made for both kinds of relationships in any health care system.

Formal and informal aspects of social systems. The tasks that need to be done and the need of the individual members to share their experiences with one another determine the degree of formal organization required. Given the exacting nature of those tasks, there must be sufficient formal relations to assure their accomplishment, but no more than that. Flexibility is the key.

If the organization is structured formally beyond this point, the opportunities for personnel to share their personal and professional experiences with one another are being curtailed unnecessarily. Their chances for disturbed feelings, for professional discussions, or for sharing joys have been reduced. The balance between formal and informal relationships contributes to the member's security and to a high level of work efficiency. The need for informal relationships will vary depending on the type of illnesses that the personnel encounter in that institution's jurisdiction, the length of stay of its patients, and physical surroundings. These informal relationships develop around the formal structure of the facility. The members of the organizational systems (formal) are also members of many smaller, interlocking groups (informal) held together by bands of common interest. Changes that disturb or upset social relations within these groups reverberate throughout wide areas of the organization.

Social systems give an individual support and add meaning to the world of work. Group norms are an effective measure of control over individual behavior. The social system is pivotal in any organization because the members may develop a strong identification with their work and hence with the organizational goal assigned to them.

When the nursing service administrator thinks of individuals within her organization she is usually judging their adequacy in performing specific jobs, yet she will also find it impossible to ignore a person's ability or inability to relate to herself and to others. The administration is aware than even though people are sensitive to the norms of the group, they also retain many individual feelings. Their behavior is influenced not only by the work environment but also by their life outside. Members of contemporary society may be conformists in such matters as dress, food, and entertainment but still remain highly individualistic in their beliefs about themselves, their motivations, hopes, and goals.

Organizational chart. The overall organizational plan in the form of a chart has been used traditionally to indicate the loci of authority functions. An organizational chart shows the relationship between the owners or sponsors of the institution and the board of directors or trustees. This is the governing body of the health care facility from which legal responsibility for the proper operation of the institution emanates. From the membership of the board, a number of standing committees are usually appointed. The function of these committees is indicated by their titles.

Up to this point the organizational chart will have great clarity for most members and will be accepted without many questions. When we reach the level of the heads of departments, we find that the director of nursing services is on the same level as the dietitian, housekeeper, and other administrators of service groups. At the same time the range of authority posi-

tions within each department will be larger and more complex than the differentiations on the upper levels of the chart. On a functional, day-to-day basis relationships may begin to get lost or confounded as problems arise and unique personality traits have their effects.

It is at such points that the relationship of authority to formal work functions requires clarification and the organizational chart should be consulted. It can help those within the department examine their formal relationships to one another to determine whether the nursing service roles have been defined and distributed in the most effective and efficient way. Because imperceptible changes take place and accumulate in every organizational department daily, examination of a department's operations may reveal that what was once an effective, formal work structure may no longer be so.

The activities, tasks, and personnel of the department may have changed gradually, so that what once was a smooth-functioning, efficient set of formal relationships between the various jobs in that department has now become most inadequate and cumbersome and may be building up needless emotional tension. Frequent study of the organizational chart helps nursing service personnel realize that changes are taking place within the department and helps them decide to reexamine and reconstruct its formal work structure in the light of existing conditions and the tasks to be accomplished.

Another way an organizational chart can be helpful to nursing service personnel is by its use to discover how the work of persons in other departments is related to their efforts. In large health care organizations especially, the nursing staff needs to develop a comprehensive perception of the institution's operations. Breakdowns in carrying out work are most often attributable to a failure to coordinate the functions attached to different jobs and offices in their proper sequential order. This failure arises whenever persons from different departments do not perceive the sequential pattern that integrates their efforts with the efforts of persons from other departments. Organizational charts can provide a picture that will enable nursing service personnel to understand the entire operation of the institution.

When new personnel join a department, their orientation to the organization can begin with the organizational chart and a precise description of their personal relationship to it. If the chart is used as a constant tool for all personnel, it will be reevaluated and updated constantly and will provide an invaluable map for anyone who requires an understanding of how the nursing service is operating.

To enrich this map, other charts can be created to represent different kinds of relationships in addition to the hierarchy of authority. For example, personnel can be drawn in relation to a particular function that cuts across departmental lines, such as direct patient care, community outreach, evaluation, and training functions. Or it may be helpful to create a chart with the patient in the center and place personnel the appropriate distance from the patient in concentric circles. Only those who have direct interaction with the patient would appear in the innermost ring, and others with less direct responsibility for the patient would be placed further out in relation to their span of control.

In short, the relationship between formally delegated work functions and responsibilities can be captured and chronicled graphically as nursing services evolve. The nature of this relationship requires especially careful monitoring devices, since it is here that morale and motivation are most likely to become issues of concern.

Relationship of formal work functions to authority functions. How supervisors or coordinators, head nurses, and staff nurses relate to one another in the nursing service department manifests the relationship of the formal work structure to the authority structure of the facility. The supervisor's or coordinator's role is one of heavy responsibility for making decisions that smoothly coordinate activities of those she supervises, and it is a role with many authority functions attached. The staff nurse's role has heavy responsibility for performing the actual nursing services needed by patients, and it is a role with many formal work functions.

A study suggested (Beard 1965) that incongruency in the head nurse's and supervisor's value judgment, which determine for each their expectations of the head nurse role, serves as a source of conflict for the head nurse and results in negative feelings (dissatisfaction) about the job and in ineffective performance. It was proposed further that ineffective performance is a consequence of job dissatifaction.

The kind of care patients receive is affected by the extent to which the supervisor's and head nurse's decision-making authority functions alters the ease with which staff nurses perform their formal work functions. The patient's recovery is therefore affected by the nature of the relationship between the two kinds of function. When that relationship becomes incompatible, the emotional tension of personnel rises and nursing productivity falls. How is that compatibility between functions to be measured? Experience with organizational phenomena has led to the formulation of a number of fairly reliable inferences about the relationships that need to be maintained between authority and formal work functions (Goodson and Jensen 1956):

1. Coordination between the two sets of functions should occur so that patient care will not be interrupted at those points where decisions about possible alternatives for implementing the work of the nursing department must be made.
2. Authority or decision-making functions assigned to the director of nursing services, supervisor, head nurse, and staff nurse should be only those that are related to and necessary for implementing the work of the department.

3. There should be no overlap or conflict in the authority functions assigned.
4. All members of the nursing service department should understand clearly what authority functions have been assigned to which nursing service jobs or roles.

Job satisfaction and distribution of authority and formal work functions. The way in which authority and formal work functions are distributed among the various jobs of the nursing department is important for determining the satisfaction that departmental members will get from performing their respective jobs. Some persons will get most of their job satisfactions from performing formal work functions. These are persons who probably like to be close to the patient most of the time and who gain a great deal of satisfaction from seeing patients recover. They like to feel that their activities have contributed to that recovery. They like to sense that day by day they are becoming more understanding of the problems of medicine and nursing and that they are becoming more able to cope with difficult nursing tasks. These persons will become dissatisfied quickly with any nursing role that does not have the greatest share of its functions directly associated with care of the patient.

Members of the nursing services department will differ as to their desire to enter into the decision-making action of the department. Some will have a strong need to take part in decision-making; others will not, so long as the decisions being made do not interfere with their performing their formal work functions.

The distribution of formal work and authority functions among the various roles of the nursing services department is significant in that each person who fills the role has personality needs that are satisfied through those occupied roles. This means that the distribution of authority and formal work functions among the various personnel must match the needs possessed by persons who fill the roles.

When department roles do not provide for the personality needs of members who fill them, the department will evidence a great deal of unrest and a drop in efficiency in the care its patients receive. This kind of situation requires either a redefining of roles or a reassignment of personnel to the roles.

In summary, the status of the human organization of a health care facility may be diagnosed by answering the following:

1. Does an analysis of the formal work structure reveal that all necessary tasks have been assigned?
2. Are various tasks carried out in a sequence that facilitates the patient's recovery process?
3. Are authority and work functions coordinated so that the patient's care is not interrupted by the need for making a decision?
4. Does each worker understand clearly what authority is attached to which role?
5. Are boundaries of responsibility clear so that the authority relationships of various personnel do not conflict or overlap?
6. Are the needs of personnel for informal relations satisfied?
7. Is each member of the work force assigned to the role or job that gives optimum satisfaction?

Communication. An administrator cannot go about creating a social environment that supports the individuals working within it unless there is an adequate communication system through which information can be transmitted. The formal communication system at work in any nursing services department is usually defined by the hierarchical authority structure of the department, with the administrator at the top of a pyramid and her assistants, unit heads, nurses, and nursing assistants occupying their appropriate spots below. Thus the formal communication system is for the most part vertical, linking these levels of authority in a well-established and highly visible network. The formal system utilizes a variety of channels, such as scheduled meetings and standardized forms, records, and memos.

In addition, any working unit will develop informal channels for communicating information. All of the unrecorded, spontaneous interactions between individuals create this informal system through which much vital work-related information is conveyed along with other data that may have social rather than technical significance. Informal communication facilitates the release of tensions and the building of emotional rapport and support. The specific characteristics of any informal system of communication are determined partly by the social and geographical proximities that have been designed into jobs and partly by the unique combinations of personalities within any job setting.

Since work relations between individuals and groups are constantly shifting in response to patient flow and changes in personnel and procedures, reliance solely on the formal communication is problematic. The formal communication system is slow in evolving and is seldom responsive to the unique chemistry among individuals. The administrator needs to recognize and utilize the informal system as well so that work can be accomplished efficiently and the morale of the staff can be maintained at the same time.

The nursing administrator and her supervisory personnel can look for ways to facilitate an overlap of the informal and formal communication systems. They can identify existing channels, or lines, along which information moves through the department, and they can then expand the amount and kinds of information that flow through them. If nurses in a particular clinical unit are able to coordinate their break and meal times through a well-established informal channel, then perhaps that group of nurses can begin to take over some other coordination and scheduling functions that had previously been undertaken independently by a supervisor and communicated indirectly to them in memos and notices. Expanding the informal system in this case would place the decision making related to patient care activities closer to those directly involved in patient

care. At the same time it would strengthen the teamwork the group has already begun to develop.

As long as formal communication systems require exchanges of information between persons with varied levels of authority, prestige, and status, the system will always be limited in the amount of information it will carry, especially in a health care setting, where interdependence and cooperation are unavoidable. It is a known fact that all communication is colored by the personal needs and motivations of the individuals involved, and these human factors often become crucial in authority-based relationships. The need for personal security, which leads to much self-protecting behavior, often defines the way we relate to someone who has more authority, prestige, or status than we do. Thus, we tend to communicate with those who can help us feel more secure. Research has shown that employees will communicate upward in an organization more readily than they will downward and that their upward communication is designed to lessen the threat of loss of position. This means that anyone with authority and responsibility for personnel will receive information that has been screened and coded so that the individuals communicating upward can feel that they have represented themselves as competent and worthy of their present positions and any higher positions they may aspire to. The same need for security will keep individuals from communicating downward, since their subordinates are not able to satisfy this need directly. In fact, for many persons, giving information downward provides a threat to personal security and authority. By withholding and censoring the release of information downward, individuals can use their knowledge to keep others in the dark and dependent on their authority and thus keep their positions secure from displacement from below.

These are constant threats to communication, and if these threats are not addressed, much information will flow only along informal channels such as friendship lines, where there is some basis for trust between individuals and the personal needs for security are not being risked. If open, nonthreatening communication is to occur along more formal organizational lines, some conscious effort must be expended. None of us will discuss problems, fears, and failures unless it is known that this candor will be appreciated and that the information will not be used against us. Fear of disclosing inadequacies at the risk of being punished is deeply ingrained in all of us from our earliest days. To overcome these human barriers and establish the communication of complete and accurate information, it is necessary for the department to address itself to some basic questions. Jackson (1964) has identified the following four problems for which faulty communication is but a symptom:

1. Lack of trust between individuals.
2. Differing goals and value systems, which place persons at odds instead of fostering interdependence.
3. The problem of distributing rewards fairly so that the free flow of ideas is encouraged.
4. The problem of understanding and agreeing on the social structure of the organization.

These organizational problems are universal and reflect the strains that bureaucratic structures place on human interaction. A nursing service administrator can provide settings in which these problems can be minimized. She can undertake staff development, human relations training, planning workshops, and similar positive steps to strengthen the social system within her department. In addition, this person can also model a communication style for her supervisory personnel so that information that moves downward is received and utilized effectively. This is a primary responsibility for any person holding authority. The following are characteristics of effective supervisory communication. They describe a working style that the nursing services administrator and her supervisory

staff can use when they are providing for the delivery of nursing services and for the human needs of the individuals to whom they are responsible.

1. The relationship between supervisor and subordinate is characterized by mutual trust and shared expectations. The subordinates can feel secure that their needs are not misunderstood or disregarded by the supervisor.

2. Supervisors are able to build support and interdependence among their groups of personnel. Information is heard and used best when it is given to a work group collectively rather than to individual members in isolation. It is known that horizontal channels of communication within a group are usually strong and fulfill the emotional needs of members. Supervisors can build on these channels and keep them open, but these channels must be filled with work-relevant information that can be used by the group to coordinate its activities. Otherwise less useful and ultimately counterproductive information, or "noise," will begin to flow through these channels.

3. Supervisors must code information into a form in which it is useful to their personnel. Policy changes for the whole department will most likely need to be reworded for application to a specific work setting and a particular group of workers. As information moves across subgroup boundaries the needs of each group receiving the information will alter the appropriate form of the message. Although they may have excellent personal relationships with the staff, supervisors or administrators who do not understand and transmit information in the code of their work unit may find that others are not acting on the information they have given them. This may prove to be a simple cognitive problem resulting from the message being coded so that its application in actual work situations could not be fully understood by those who received it. By asking for direct feedback from their staff, supervisors can begin to evaluate and upgrade

this component of their communication style.

4. Supervisors have several kinds of information that they can direct to their subordinates, and their effectiveness as leaders will be reflected in the richness and variety of information they make available. Katz and Kahn (1966) have identified five types of information that move downward in an organization: (a) job instructions, (b) job rationale, (c) procedures and policies, (d) feedback, and (e) indoctrination of goals. In the pressured environment of a hospital, job instructions, the directive information necessary for people to carry out the immediate tasks within their job, are a primary responsibility of the supervisor. The supervisor's concern is that people know what to do and that they are familiar with organizational procedures and policies so that they can make appropriate decisions when confronted with the typical variations within their jobs. For a supervisor, it may often appear that the pace and workload make it nearly impossible to keep up with the large numbers of job instructions that must be conveyed. Thus, the supervisor may find that communication has become a steady flow of directives, policies, and procedures, and little else. Katz and Kahn (1966) suggest that if some balance is achieved between giving job instructions and job rationale, then supervisors will find themselves giving fewer directions as personnel begin to understand how their jobs fit into a larger framework. If the nurses receive a systematic overview of the interrelations between the parts of the nursing services department and other departments and of the total concept of patient care and the role they play in it, they may begin to see the broader rationale behind their individual roles and the design of their jobs. With this understanding, the amount of direction and instruction they require to do their jobs can begin to decrease. Taking time to transmit information about job rationale from supervisor to subordinate ultimately frees this channel for other functions such as feedback and goal setting. A supervisor who is always giving orders and does not have time to give feedback to personnel or undertake the setting of objectives and long-range plans is not providing the support that the staff needs to do its best work.

DIRECTING

It is through the directing function of the physical act that the grand strategy of an organization unfolds. Once a plan is conceived and organized, the directing function takes over. The purpose of this function is to put organized plans into action through the deployment of resources and the translation of strategy into tactics.

In a narrow sense, the directing function is similar or equal to supervision. In a larger sense, however, it involves the following closely interdependent elements: (1) delegation, (2) supervision, (3) coordination, and (4) control (Dimock 1958).

The relationship of these four essential elements of directing can be described as follows: We delegate to give everyone an appointed task and to relate the total job to a particular organization, structure and individuals. We supervise to teach others to help themselves and to see that through appropriate techniques the strategy is played out in the best possible fashion. We coordinate everything that has been delegated to guard against leaving loose ends. And we exercise internal administrative control of this unfolding program to see that everything is being done according to plan, on time, and with predetermined effectiveness to achieve unity and symmetry. These interwoven elements constitute the process of directing and are tied together by the philosophy of administration by objectives.

Process of directing
DELEGATION OF AUTHORITY

Delegation means allocating and decentralizing authority, imposing responsibility and accountability, and assigning tasks down to the lowest possible level at which there is sufficient competence and information for effective decision-making or task performance (Dimock 1958). Administration by objectives means that all people in the nursing service organization are involved in the determination of objectives, in working out plans and policies, and in formulating detailed plans of operation. The fullest use of an individual's talents is called forth under conditions that the individual has helped to determine, for example, by being included in staff meetings and consultations.

Once the objectives of the program have been made clear, the next step for the nursing service group is to spell out what each clinical unit is to do and what each individual is expected to accomplish. The staff in the personnel office formulate departmental job classifications and job descriptions. This is the one way to clarify individual objectives, delegate responsibilities, and give all employees a clear mandate with respect to their individual jobs. It entails not only analyzing positions but also looking at them in relation to the skills of the particular individual who will fill the position. This allows for the unique strength and the potential of each professional nurse to be as fully developed as possible and also takes into account individual weaknesses. All nurses in the chain of command should be given as much discretionary power as they are able to absorb, consistent with their individual preferences and state of mind and with the good of the organization as a whole.

By assuring that each and every person is treated fairly and equally, the nursing service department will avoid the charge of favoritism and promote congenial work relationships. For example, when there are two nurses at the same level and the administrative supervisor wishes to give one more latitude than the other, the superior ought to adhere to principle and give the more professionally developed nurse the enhanced authority; but at the same time, the supervisor should take pains to explain to everyone concerned, and especially to the one who is denied comparable authority, why it was decided to increase the other nurse's responsibility and authority. The indispensable condition for making a success of administration by objectives is that the nursing administrator and her supervisory staff be completely objective and sympathetic at all times.

There are two major gains for a nursing service administrator who employs this style of delegation in the direction process: she lightens her own load of detailed responsibilities so that she may use her conceptual skills by having more time for future planning, for maintaining institutional vitality, and for promoting change and research; and she is helping to develop the personal potential of everyone to whom she delegates authority. The latter is the group that is mainly responsible for the directing segment of nursing service administration, namely, the action or mediating population such as supervisors, assistant directors, and head nurses. Everyone in the nursing service oranization has a potential that can be roughly determined. If there are 20 supervisors in a nursing service organization and if the quality of the average performance is raised by ten points each, there would be a total improvement of 200 points. But if there is a short-sighted, self-centered administrator with one supervisor over all and if the quality of performance of this one administrator is raised by 20 points, there would be a net loss of 180 points. The actual gain in developing the 20 supervisors will prove to be even greater over time owing to the multiplier effect at work. Even if the nursing service administrator is near the limit of effectiveness, others, who are at different stages in their careers, may have room for growth and, thus, will continue to develop if an organization is supportive of their development (Dimock 1958).

With the objectives set and authority

delegated all along the line, the next step is to give the personnel maximum latitude in professional freedom and autonomy so that all can work out the appropriate means of attaining the ends for which they are responsible. This is necessary because it communicates to personnel that the administrator and supervisors trust them and expect them to grow on the job, that they recognize that there is more than one good way to do things, and that assigned personnel may have several different ways they prefer, dependent on their knowledge, judgment, and other factors.

If, however, the individual nurse's way is not satisfactory or costs more than it serves the patient, that is, if it does not fulfill its objective, then the nurse must be informed and a better way found through good supervision and continuing education. Nursing service administrators and supervisors should know that as part of dynamic leadership they must issue orders at times. There is no conflict between firm leadership and allowing for professional autonomy. On the contrary, the two in the right proportion give the balance that is needed, provided orders are not given in a punitive manner and with the wrong spirit or given unnecessarily when a professional nurse may be expected to use personal discretion.

To know where to find this dividing line unerringly is a chief test of administrative and supervisory capacity. It stems from a sound philosophy even more than from sound experience.

Not to be overlooked is that a nursing service organization in which individual growth is explicitly valued boasts deep, sound morale and satisfaction. The program is, therefore, more appealing to its professional nursing staff and contributes to institutional survival and excellence in patient care.

Two important factors that affect the quality of direction in nursing service are the administrative personnel's resistance to delegation and co-workers' avoidance of responsibility. Supervisory nurses who are both conscientious and have high standards of performance are tempted to take it upon themselves to perform any task that they can do better than their co-workers. They are basing their choice solely on the varying quality with which they or their co-workers will perform the specific task instead of comparing the improvement in performance resulting from doing the work themselves against the benefits to the total operation if they were to devote their attention to planning and supervisory functions only they are in a position to perform. Only after nurses accept emotionally and intellectually the idea that their job requires getting the most things done through other people will full use be made of delegation.

Lack of ability to direct is another barrier to successful delegation. Nurses must be able to communicate to their co-workers, often far in advance, what is to be done. This means that they must (1) think ahead and visualize the work situation, (2) formulate objectives and general plans of action, and then (3) communicate them to their co-workers.

Lack of confidence in co-workers is another block to effective delegation. In this situation nurses hesitate to turn things over to their co-workers because "They'll take care of details alright but miss the main point." or "They have ideas but don't follow through."

When this kind of situation is open and recognized, the remedy is clear. Either training should be started immediately or, if this is impractical, a new person should be found.

Often the situation is by no means so clear-cut. The lack of confidence in others may be a highly subjective perception and almost unconscious. When this is the case, the nursing service administrator or supervisor is likely to compound the problem by giving lip service to delegation but in fact withdrawing her confidence from a person whose perceptions she is unsure of. In such an instance, the administrator must become a model for the rest of the organization. Rather than allow a lack of confidence in a worker to go unresolved it is encumbent on the administrator to open communication, seek more information, and become explicit about her delegation of responsibility to the person in question.

Another obstacle is absence of selective controls that give warning of impending difficulties. Problems beyond those covered by the delegation may arise, and the supervisor naturally wants to avoid being caught with no warning. Consequently, the responsible supervisor needs some feedback on what is going on. Such information is also useful for staff consultation and for appraising final results.

Although care must be taken that the control system does not undermine the very essence of delegation, it is also true that the supervisor cannot completely abdicate responsibilities. Unless the supervisor has confidence in the adequacy of the controls set up, the delegation of tasks will be undertaken very cautiously.

The supervisor may be handicapped by a temperamental aversion to taking a chance. Even with clear instructions, proper co-workers, and selective controls, there still remains the possibility that something will go wrong. The supervisor who delegates takes a calculated risk. Over a period of time she expects that the gains from delegation will far offset the troubles that arise. Until the supervisor sees this characteristic of her job and adjusts to it emotionally as well as intellectually, she is likely to be reluctant to delegate.

These obstacles to effective delegation are related to the attitudes of the supervisor, the administrator, the nurse, or whoever is doing the delegating. Fortunately, there are means by which specific attitudes can be recognized and unfrozen. If lines of communication are kept open through regular conferences and consultation, there exists an opportunity for personalized counseling directed to these specific attitudes.

Or there is the possibility of assisting an entire work unit to evolve in delegation skills by offering some structured team building or human relations experience. So when faced with a situation in which authority is in fact not being delegated as it should be, the nursing service administrator can first look for the reasons why the reluctance to turn over authority exists; then a method for creating change can be determined.

Delegation is a two-way relationship. Even when the supervisor is ready and able to turn over authority, there may be reasons why the co-worker shrinks from accepting it. Something within the co-worker or in the relationship between the supervisor and the co-worker may become a block.

Often workers find it easier to ask the supervisor how to deal with a problem than decide for themselves. Decision-making is hard mental work, and people seek ways of avoiding it. Furthermore, making one's own decision carries with it responsibility for the outcome. Asking the supervisor is a way of sharing, if not shifting, this burden. Such acts, when repeated over a period of time, foster dependence on the supervisor rather than on the nurse.

Fear of criticism for mistakes deters the nurse from assuming responsibility. Much depends on the nature of the criticism. Negative criticism is often resented where constructive review might be accepted. Negative or unreasonable criticism given publicly in a way that embarrasses a person before co-workers adds salt to the wound. The impact of such criticism on a person's willingness to take on a responsibility is adverse. The nurse will be very cautious and play it safe. The person's feeling is "Why should I stick my neck out for the supervisor?"

Lack of the necessary information and resources to do a good job is another reason for avoidance of responsibility. It is possible for a person reared in a restraining web of budgetary and personal limitations to accept responsibility knowing full well there will be a battle for each step taken. Generally, however, the frustrations that go along with inadequate information and resources create in the person an attitude that rejects further assignments.

Another obstacle is simply that the co-worker may already have more work than can possibly be handled. True, such an overload may be the supervisor's own fault; for example, she may make poor use of her own time or fail to hire trained, competent assistants even though she has the authority to do so. But, from the point of view of her willingness to accept responsibility, the cause of the overwork is not the critical point. If there is already a feeling of overwork, the supervisor will probably shy away from new assignments that call for thinking or exercising initiative.

Lack of self-confidence is another reason for avoiding responsibility; for example, the supervisor believes the nurse can do the job and is willing to take the risk of the outcome, but the nurse is unsure and does not like to take the plunge. Self-confidence may be developed by carefully providing experience with increasingly difficult problems to help the person sense personal potentialities.

Positive incentives may be inadequate. As already mentioned, accepting additional responsibility usually involves more mental work and emotional pressure. There is more or less risk of failure, which is unpleasant. For these reasons there should be positive rewards for accepting delegated responsibility. These incentives may take all sorts of forms, such as pay increases, better opportunity for promotion, different title, improved status, and more pleasant working conditions. The important point is that the specific co-worker affected by delegation should be provided with an appropriate positive incentive.

So that one can analyze and evaluate the location and use of authority within an organization, the following checklist of questions is offered. The list is not all-inclusive. Many of the questions cannot and often should not be answered *yes* or *no*. Organizations and administrators within them will, and should, vary.

1. Is the delegation of authority and responsibility within the organization clear? By division, by subdivision, by individuals?
2. Is the delegation of authority commensurate with the assigned responsibility of the particular position or person? Are the limits made clear?
3. Are the separate delegations of authority within the organization so correlated and understood that responsible persons can see their role in the total plan?
4. Are these conflicts in delegations of authority?
5. Can delegations be relied on? Are they relatively stable?
6. Is the delegation of authority so made as to preserve unity of command or unity of purpose?
7. Are specific delegations of authority and responsibility related to specific aptitudes and talents of the personnel?
8. Does the delegation of responsibility tend to support homogeneous activities?
9. Is the delegation such that what is assigned can probably be accomplished?
10. Are the controls established to ensure accountability for the discharge of responsibilities assigned?
11. Do the delegations of authority all support the dominant central idea of the larger policy? Do they aid in coordinating all efforts toward that end?
12. Is there over delegation of authority and responsibility?
13. Does the delegation of authority and responsibility provide a workable span of control?

SUPERVISION

The nursing supervisor excels at shaping interests and values in such a way that a close affinity is created between the aims of the institution and the individuals who work for it. According to Tead (1951), human beings have a two-way interest: in their integrity of selfhood and in their effective relation to their total surroundings. If they can find their way of life and their selfhood in their work, then they are much happier than if they must function in two separate and even hostile spheres—

the divided world of the organization person.

Tead's solution is the key to the problem of how to make employees deeply loyal to the organization of which they are a part. Moreover, it works toward that end without regimentation, manipulation, or any of the other poor, antisocial devices that caused W. H. Whyte (1952) to contend that to protect their individualities and give the organization the criticism it needs, people ought to oppose the dehumanizing influences of institutional life.

Peter Drucker (1954) calls this blending of institutional and individual values the ultimate principle. The supervisor's challenge is to blend the full scope of individual strengths and responsibility with a common direction, create a climate in which spontaneous team work is possible, and harmonize the goals of the individual with those of the group.

The views of Tead and Drucker are borne out by modern psychological research. Daniel Katz (1950:4) of the Michigan Survey Research Center states this principle as follows:

> People are more effectively motivated when they are given some degree of freedom in the way in which they do their work than when every action is prescribed in advance. They do better when some degree of decision making about their jobs is possible than when all decisions are made for them. They respond more adequately when they are treated as personalities rather than as cogs in a machine.

These views are especially strong points among professional personnel, nurses included. Although this discussion could apply to any professional in the health care field, our focus is on the professional nurse. A distinguishing characteristic of the professional nurse is a strong need for self-determination. Professional nurses are self-motivated to enter and pursue the profession, and they conduct their daily activities so that personal objectives are satisfied. Health care organizations and their administrators and supervisors assume responsibility for the performance of professional people. Administrators and supervisors carry within themselves limitless potential of professional knowledge and motivation, yet organizational performance often does not live up to that potential. Dissatisfaction, indifference, friction, apparent irresponsibility, or downright resistance can seriously undermine the performance of an organization of professionals. Often it is supervision that is needed.

The job of the supervisor is to motivate the professional nurse to peak performance by creating the right leadership climate. The achievement of this climate depends to a great extent on the degree to which the personnel will adopt the organization's goals as their own and work toward them, and this depends on the supervisory climate in which they operate. That is, the manner in which the supervisor exercises her authority and influence, uses her system of control, and enables the members of the organization to achieve personal satisfaction on the job determines the overall effectiveness of the organization.

As organizations grow they become more impersonal and more formalized. The supervisor must then concentrate more on problems of motivation, which in the small organization, might be resolved informally through personal contact. It is assumed that when the organization itself is small enough, the day-to-day interaction of all people, including nursing service administrators, supervisors, head nurses, and staff personnel makes it possible for a supervisor to spot discontent early and to create an environment in which the members are well informed and feel reasonably secure and satisfied.

When the work is so divided that small groups or teams take responsibility for patient care, supervisors can spot discontent as early in larger health care organizations as in small organizations. Thus the type of work people do in hospitals and other health agencies and the size of the organizations give them built-in advantages that come from closely knit, small groups working together on projects they can identify as their own.

In addition, the fact that most nurses in hospitals and other institutions identify with the profession gives these organizations a distinct advantage over other organizations. Professional nurses are self-motivated to do their best, even under adverse circumstances. Good supervision of professionals means creating opportunities for the people to perform what they already are committed to perform by their choice of the nursing profession as a career. On both counts—small group activity and professional interests of its employees—health care organizations enjoy some built-in advantages, which good supervision will exploit to the fullest. But care should be taken not to take for granted the motivation of the professional nurse. An overbearing supervisory climate can destroy the wholesome benefits that come from built-in good human relations.

It is wrong to assume that communication will be automatic because the group is intimate and to assume that informal or casual relationships can be an effective substitute for good supervision and organization. The self-perceptions of professional nurses can be badly shattered by experiences that they perceive as being not professional; for example, too many non-nursing duties, too much clerical work, close supervision rather than freedom of action, being expected to give blind conformity rather than reasonable compliance, and limited information about the system as a whole all are supervisory practices that directly contradict the professional self-view that is so basic to motivation.

In addition to the right leadership climate are two important factors that influence motivation to perform and depend on the quality of supervision. One factor is organizational objectives. Employees will commit themselves to objectives in the achievement of which they find rewards, and they will exercise self-direction and self-control in the service of objectives to which they are committed. The need to earn a living certainly induces people to seek a job, or to stay on one, but it rarely motivates them to do their best. Motivation stems from psychological rather than logical foundations. Whether a person will work for a particular health care facility depends on the take-home pay, but how devotedly that person will work depends on feelings about how worthwhile the work is. To the motivated, devoted person the work is worth more than money.

Health care organizations have been quite successful, especially during the last several years, in improving wage and salary systems and other fringe benefits and in tying these financial compensations to performance. But the real challenge today is to provide a conceptual and physical environment in which professional nursing can be practiced. How the supervisor deals with the less tangible, but seemingly more powerful, needs of each individual person remains to her a constant supervisory challenge.

The other motivating factor to perform effectively is concerned with satisfaction of social and personal needs. They manifest themselves in the attitudes and sentiments of people who consider their organization a good place to work because it is just and considerate (especially through efforts of the supervisor) and because it offers a good work group and a winning team. What they express basically is satisfaction of social needs (to be a part of a satisfying organization and work group) and of personal needs (self-respect, recognition, reputation, creativeness, achievement, reasonable freedom, and human dignity). Good performance must be earned; and given legitimate and worthwhile objectives, it is the quality of supervision that determines the degree to which personnel will commit themselves to the objectives of an organization.

Since the organization's objectives are given and each individual differs in personal needs, it is unreasonable to suppose that every member's total needs can be satisfied through work in the organization. Nevertheless, the more "professional" a person is, the more this work becomes a way of life. Therefore, in an organization of health care professionals there are vast opportunities to help a person get many of life's satisfactions through work. To the extent that the organization fails to channel this motivation into job performance, it fails in achieving its own objectives.

In view of individual differences, motivation is still situational and requires good judgment of the supervisor in each specific situation. Also, health care professionals as a group are not entirely different from the professionals in the general population. As a general proposition, however, the preponderant needs of the professional person at work are limited to those that compelled that person to enter the profession, and these may tend to put greater emphasis on finding gratification of needs beyond economic security, such as the egoistic needs for self-esteem and recognition, than may be true for employees who avoid the profession.

There are no set rules on how to motivate professional people, whether they work in the health care field or some other area entirely, but a few guidelines may be useful.

The effective supervisor pays more attention to developing competence in personnel by giving them continuing education and experience, rather than expending energy to give orders and keep people "under control." The supervisor should satisfy the professional's need for knowing the rational reason for doing things by communicating freely, formally as well as informally.

The supervisor should satisfy the professionals' need for creativity and achievement by giving personnel challenging assignments and permitting them to exercise judgment and individuality in deciding how to fulfill the assignment. The supervisor should set goals and objectives in consultation with her personnel; impose quality standards; set deadlines; and require routine feedback on performance. But the personnel should be given much discretion in structuring the approach and pacing the efforts toward the goals.

The supervisor should satisfy the professionals' needs for psychological and social satisfactions that make life worthwhile to them by developing congenial and compatible work groups and by recognizing both formally and informally the work accomplished and goals achieved by both groups and individuals. The supervisor should offer constructive help and support where breakdowns occur and encourage other recognition through off-the-job professional association and personal development.

Since the professional thinks of the work relationship as a colleague-relationship, not as a superior-subordinate relationship, the supervisor should recognize the interdependence of superior and subordinate and consult freely with the personnel, well in advance of the action itself, on matters that will affect them. Furthermore, the supervisor should encourage free and honest upward communication of feelings and attitudes and encourage constructive criticisms and suggestions. The colleague-relationship can come about only through long experience of consistent supervisory action that convinces the personnel that they need not fear reprisal even though they know that the supervisor is the overall person responsible.

Whatever the route by which a person moves into supervisory responsibilities, whether from the ranks of the profession itself or from outside the organization as a specialist in supervision, the supervisor assumes the obligation of getting maximum performance from the other members of the organization for whose work that supervisor is ultimately responsible. When the other members are professional people and specialists, the supervisor is faced with some challenging problems and some unusual opportunities. To neglect these challenges and to be insensitive to the human needs of the human organization means not only that the supervisor is not supervising, but also that the organization is not gaining the utmost from its human resources. To face these opportunities and to develop leadership that motivates the professional person can result in marked improvement in organizational performance, bringing satisfaction to the supervisor at the same time.

COORDINATION

If administration and supervision are to be effective, coordination of specialized effort is imperative. Having achieved cooperation, the nursing supervisor has an excellent basis for achieving coordination. If the fruits of the specialist are to be preserved, then at some points in the organization there must be a careful collecting and combining of the particles to give them meaning and pattern.

There are many coordinating factors in organizations, most of them classifiable as division of labor, specialization, or interdependence. The division of labor, accompanied as it is by specialization of functions, creates the initial basis of coordination, but it is the condition of functional interdependence that constitutes the basic need for coordination in organizations. Each specialty in a system, as Hawley (1950) points out, contains its own unique set of functions and rhythms. But only when the various sets of specialized functions are linked together according to an organizing principle or for the purpose of contributing to fulfilling the objectives of the system do they gain meaning and utility. This linking together illustrates the concept of functional interdependence.

Functional interdependence means that the various roles, skills, and activities in an organization must come into play at the appropriate time and place and in a certain order if the organization is to achieve its objectives. The various sets of func-

tions of specialized parts in the system must complement or supplement one another in a manner that maximizes the convergence of diverse efforts on a given target and minimizes interference or disruptions in the process. When one considers the steps involved in processing an emergency case in the hospital from admission to discharge or all that is involved in performing an operation on a patient, one immediately realizes both the fact of interdependence and the sequence of events such interdependence entails, a sequence that demands timing and ordering of workflow, with certain things taking priority over others and all things being articulated into a coherent pattern.

In industrial organizations much of timing, spacing, and articulation of activities is accomplished by the use of machines, that is, through mechanical coordination. Organizations with lower levels of routinization and mechanization, such as hospitals, however, require the expenditure of considerable and continuous human effort to achieve and maintain adequate coordination. In these organizations it is difficult to evaluate how well the system is functioning, even more so if coordination is not well developed. The motivation to evaluate the effectiveness of the system and its parts constitutes a rather subtle basis of coordination. In many cases the only way to evaluate the performance of various parts of the system is to relate and compare them with one another and to evaluate the relative contribution of each. This process implies coordination. Another basis for coordination arises out of the inevitability that certain parts in the system come to be more influential than others. As Hawley (1950) suggests, differential influence among organizational parts or groups is characteristic of most organizations, which stems from the fact that certain parts in the system have greater control than others over the allocation of resources and facilities. But when such a hierarchy of parts is developed on the basis of the type and amount of resources each part controls, an accompanying tendency by the less dominant parts to align themselves with the more dominant parts also develops. This tendency, coupled with the motivation of the dominant parts to structure the system so as to maximize their own objectives, results in a need for organizational coordination to avoid throwing the system out of equilibrium. This need for checks and balances entails coordinative activity.

The range of methods and mechanisms by which coordination may be attained in large organizations is almost infinite. The process of coordination may be formal or informal, and in either case, it may be intentional or unintentional. Health care organizations create administrative and liaison positions and committees whose main purpose is coordination. In fact, some hospital organizations have gone much further in this direction by establishing the position of coordinator of clinical units. Similarly, some hospitals have a so-called joint conference committee, consisting of members of the board of directors, physicians, and hospital and nursing service administrators whose main functions include coordination. In other cases various functional roles in the organization are assigned a good deal of coordinative responsibility, such as the role of the registered nurse in the hospital. Sometimes, as previously suggested, parts of the system will also align with a more dominant segment without any intentional effort at coordination.

The constitution, bylaws, and other written documents of an organization also serve as instruments of coordination. Formal and informal meetings, conferences, and exchanges among organizational members whose activities are in some way related illustrate additional means of coordination. The system of superior-subordinate relationships in organizations constitutes, among other things, a mechanism for coordinating activities. Finally, one of the less obvious but more important means

of coordination is found in the attitudes and values of organizational members. The development of common norms, shared expectations, and mutual understanding among different people in the system is probably the best guarantee that adequate coordination can be achieved and maintained. Alongside the administration plans and directives, the written rules and regulations, and all other aspects of the formal organizational structure are these extensive and often forgotten important informal aspects.

Regardless of the coordination methods employed in a given organization, coordinative behavior may vary according to its particular scope or according to the objectives to which it is directed and the motivations underlying it. For example, coordinative activity may be initiated in response to an existing problem; it may be initiated to prevent certain problems from arising at all; or it may be initiated without any reference to a particular problem, for instance, to implement a new plan. Accordingly, it is possible and convenient to group coordinative activities into various types. In their study, Georgopoulos and Mann (1961) distinguished four major types: corrective, preventive, regulatory, and promotive coordination. Regardless of which is the prevalent type in a particular organization, most organizations at one time or another engage in all four types. The four types are intended to serve as convenient devices for organizing data, not to suggest that all coordination phenomena in an organization are purely corrective, preventive, regulatory, or promotive. As analytical devices, they may be important tools, for what makes good coordination of a given type may not necessarily make good coordination of another type. Adequate promotive coordination, for example, may require certain things not needed by adequate corrective coordination and vice versa.

We have differentiated coordinate activities into four types, but other kinds of differentiation are also possible and are already receiving attention in the literature. All coordinative activities in an organization may be divided into two broad categories: those that involve programming and those that do not (see Georgopoulos and Mann 1961).

Programmed coordination concentrates primarily on the means of coordination listed under planning and does not emphasize the importance of social-psychological forces such as motivation, reciprocal understanding, and complementary expectations among organizational members. It follows preestablished schedules and relies on specifying the functions associated with the various roles in the organization. Thus, activities are programmed; that is, times are regulated and role linkages in the system are established and articulated to fit the program involved.

General coordination makes allowance for adjustments required to meet organizational needs arising in the day-to-day operations of the system, needs that cannot be satisfied through formal planning in advance. Activity in most organizations is not sufficiently predictable to permit exclusive, or even predominant, reliance on programmed coordination. Thus, organizations engage in both types of coordination.

SUPERVISORY CONTROL

Each time a nursing service administrator delegates work to a supervisor or the supervisor delegates work to a nurse, the problem of knowing whether the work is performed satisfactorily is created, and so delegating inevitably raises the question of control. In certain situations a supervisor guides and observes work while it is being done. But when the delegated work increases, control by direct observation no longer remains possible. Then, when a large part of planning as well as operating is delegated, new complications are added. For if an administrator attempts to control the decisions of her personnel, does she not repudiate her earlier delegation of planning?

This question bothers many administrators. They see the benefits that can come from a high degree of decentralization, and yet they are aware that they have a continuing obligation. Often they desire full decentralization if they can do so "without losing control." Control shifts as decentralization increases (Table 4).

An administrator need not lose control when she delegates a measure of planning, but she should be prepared to change her controls. First, the types of control standards that are appropriate change. When decisions are centralized, the administrator establishes rather detailed standards for the method and output at each stage of the work. But as she delegates increasing amounts of authority to plan and decide, the administrator should shift her attention away from operating details to the

Table 4. Effect of decentralization on control

| | Nature of control | |
Degree of decentralization	Type of standard	Frequency of measurement
Centralization of all but routine decisions	Detailed specifications on how work is to be done and on output of each person	Daily for output; hourly to continuous for methods and for quality
Action within policies, programs, and standard methods; use of exception principle	Output at each stage of operations, expense ratios, efficiency rates, and turnover	Weekly to daily for output; monthly for ratios and for other operating data
Decentralization	Overall results and a few key attention-direction signals	Monthly for main results and for attention signals; quarterly or annually for other results

results that are achieved. This is not a sudden shift. As varying degrees of planning authority are delegated for each of a wide range of subjects, standards, too, cover more or less detail. As a general proposition, however, the administrator does forego her personal control over detail and relies increasingly on the appraisal of results.

The frequency of appraisals also changes. Because the administrator is no longer trying to keep an eye on detailed activities, most daily reports can be eliminated. With increasing decentralization, the administrator's attention shifts more and more toward overall results; the span of time covered by reports can typically be lengthened. For a nursing service department that operates on an established, measurable program of quality and quantity of patient care and on a yearly budget basis, monthly or biweekly statements can be obtained. The frequency is at the administrator's discretion.

Retained safeguards. The shift from frequent, detailed control reports to periodic, general-appraisal reports does not preclude the use of a few controls of the attention-directing controls. The administrator who has delegated a measure of authority may want some of these warning devices to come to her attention regularly. As decentralization of authority increases, however, it is common practice to expect a supervisor to keep her administrator informed of impending difficulties rather than bother the administrator with control data when conditions are satisfactory. An administrator may ask to be notified when deviations from standards exceed a certain norm, thus applying the exception principle to control as well as to planning.

Moreover, it is common practice to use preaction control for certain major moves, such as the appointment of key personnel or expenditure of capital. Here again, the number of proposed actions that require confirmation will decrease as the degree of decentralization increases.

Still another kind of safeguard is to insist that head nurses use specific control devices even though a supervisor herself neither sets the standards nor receives reports on performance. An associate director in charge of patient care, for example, may be vitally concerned that a reliable quality-supervisory plan is in use but may take no personal part in its operation. She expects sufficient control data to be handy if the need for determining the cause of any particular problem arises.

Increased importance of self-control. As a nursing service administrator delegates more authority to the nurses, shifting control from the details of how work is done to an appraisal of overall results, the personnel's responsibility for control increases. Details still have to be watched, but more reliance is placed on the nurses down the line. The nurses must control their own activities.

Control is partly a matter of attitude and habit. In a situation in which centralized control has been the traditional practice, general staff nurses naturally rely on supervisors and their nursing service administrator to catch errors and initiate corrective action. If authority is then passed down to them, they need to formulate a new attitude. It may also be necessary to redirect the flow of information so that the nurses down the line have what they need to do their own controlling.

Because the nursing service administrators are no longer attemping to follow the details of daily operation and are not trying to solve a multitude of on-the-spot problems, they naturally issue fewer directions.

In place of directing, the administrators cultivate a coaching relationship between themselves and the nurses. If standards have been set in terms of results, the nurses, supervisors, and nursing administrators know what is expected. Hopefully, too, they fully agree on the desirability of achieving these results and will interpret control information from the same viewpoint, especially if the nurses have partic-ipated in setting standards and the meth-od of measuring performance. In these circumstances the administrator or super-visor can easily become a coach. Instead of orders, they give advice to the nurses on how to accomplish desired results. The control mechanism, standards, measure-ments, and reports, simply points to the need, and the supervisor, acting as a coach, tries to help the nurses fulfill it.

Ideally in this situation the initiative for correction comes from the nurses. To foster a relationship in which the personnel is not reluctant to seek advice in tough prob-lems, administrators should (1) avoid giv-ing the impression that they feel an admis-sion of difficulties is a sign of weakness, and (2) be careful not to make unilateral decisions that, in effect, take authority back from the personnel.

Setting the stage. The kinds of control and their associated relationships that we are discussing grow only in a favorable climate. To create such an environment, we must think out a clear set of objectives for a task that is being delegated and de-velop ways of measuring the achievement of these objectives. Also necessary is a clear understanding about which policies, organi-zation, management methods, and other institutional rules must be followed and which may be regarded only as recom-mended practice. Moreover, those actions that require prior approval by a supervisor need to be so labeled. In addition to the substantial amount of planning and organi-zation clarification just outlined, high decentralization requires the right people. Nurses who are able to perform the delegated duties must be selected, oriented, and motivated. Supervisors themselves must be able and willing to adjust their behavior, and the two particular personalities in-volved in each delegation must be com-patible and must trust each other. If one removes or significantly diminishes any one of these aspects of an operating situation, there will be a corresponding reduction in

the degree of decentralization that is possi-ble without loss of control.

Important issues in control. Any method of measuring results will act either as a unifier or as a divider. It will act as a unifier if it embodies common expectations, if it provides each person with the tools to improve performance, if it does not attempt to increase the nonmeasurable, and if it does not become a fetish or a tyrant. The most effective control is exer-cised at the working level, where its pur-pose is to give the people working with it a boost to their performance.

But any control system will act as a divider if it is remote and mysterious, if it grinds out a deadening uniformity, and if most people have no part in devising, operating, and improving it. Under these conditions, "Control of situations by 'measur-ability' may be as inefficient as control over people by use of position" (Barnard 1968).

Another debatable issue concerns the appropriate role of rules and regulations. An excessive number of written rules and regulations militates against delegation of authority, tends to restrict areas of admin-istrative discretion and procedural flexi-bility, creates an atmosphere of legalism and timidity, and is one of the chief causes of bureaucracy in the objectionable sense.

The ideal plan, therefore, is to be as clear and as precise as possible about ob-jectives and policies but to allow decisions to be made so far as possible on the basis of these rather than on the basis of rote. Rules and regulations should be kept to a minimum, otherwise thinking is discour-aged, flexibility is made difficult, and ad-ministration by objectives becomes next to impossible.

The arguments in favor of extending rules and regulations are almost legion. This may be why the practice is so wide-spread. Rules and regulations strengthen equality of treatment by restricting dis-cretionary decisions. They may serve to protect procedural rights and even civil liberties. They reduce areas of ambiguity and, hence, make it possible for persons with less schooling or intelligence to follow a specific guide. They make work for administrators whose knowledge of these subjects becomes a priceless stock-in-trade.

The arguments do not cause us to retreat from the position staked out above. If there is a real need to protect human rights, there is justification enough for admitting such rules to the select circle of minimal needs. If employees are not motivated, they can be educated to be otherwise.

The policy that applies to rules and regulations is analogous to the policy that ought to apply to bigness: justifiable if technologically induced, otherwise to be avoided. By this we mean to suggest that some rules and regulations are not only necessary but may even be indispensable. However, such rules are really statements of policy and objective, and in most cases they could be better expressed as such.

A sense of struggle is inherent in all distinguished supervisory performances. The best administrators and supervisors are the ones who thrive on the rough-and-tumble of pressure and group competition, the unforeseen problems that test the mettle of individuals, and the chance of using acumen, personality, and persuasiveness—one's entire being—in working for objectives that are worthwhile. The administrator and supervisor use strategy analogous to political strategy. The politician attempts to win votes. The nursing service administrators and supervisors attempt to win institutional objectives. The political leader formulates policies and explains them to constituents. The administrator and supervisor formulate policies and sell them to their co-workers and chief administrators.

Tactics is like strategy except that it is one episode in a larger problem, an action along a wider issue. The skills of the strategist and tactician have much in common, although we can all doubtless think of individuals who are more successful at one than at the other. There seems to be more intuition in tactics than there is in strategy, or putting it another way, the intellectual element in strategy exceeds that of tactics. But, both must be internally consistent and of a piece. Shortsighted tactics often succeed only in alienating those who might otherwise support one's overall plans. When we talk about strategy and tactics for nursing service administrators and supervisors we mean that there is a logical intellectual pursuit in which one must set objectives and decide how to attain them. For example, when meeting with the staff to solve problems, nursing service administrators always have before them the same questions, for the problem-solving process does not vary greatly: What is the problem? What are the alternative solutions? Which seems to be the better solution? Are there any factors that are being overlooked? and Is the plan of execution entirely feasible? If all of these questions are fully considered, with each one present permitted input, a real consensus will emerge. If the nursing service administrator had a solution in mind before the meeting started, it will, in most cases, prove to be an advantage, providing the administrator is able to admit that the tentative solution can be improved upon. Under such conditions, staff meetings will be immeasurably strengthened as will the influence, affection, and respect with which the administrator is held by others.

Heavy-handed use of positional authority solves no problems; it only creates more. Cooperation is gained when the nursing service administrator anticipates the question that is invariably in the minds of the nurses, "What does this mean to me?" Nursing service administrators know they cannot do the job by themselves, and they can expect each person in their own department to look at an issue a bit differently. Their most potent solutions to these obstacles to effective supervision are to

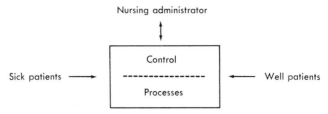

Fig. 4-3. Delivery of nursing care viewed as institutional process.

consult with their personnel and make certain that their communications are understood.

CONTROL

The fourth administrative function is control, the use of formal authority to assure, to the fullest extent possible, the attainment of the purposes of action by the methods or procedures that have been devised (Tannenbaum 1949).

The utility to nursing administrators of the systems frame of reference is in what it leads them to pay attention to in the operations they oversee. It leads them to view the delivery of nursing care as the institutional control of processes that change sick patients into well patients. Most importantly, it leads them to scrutinize the nature of the control devices they use (Fig. 4-3).

When action has been taken to achieve stated goals, it is necessary that the action be described in relation to its expected effects on those goals. Action can be described in a variety of useful ways—in accounting terms, in quantitative terms, in qualitative terms, and in behavioral terms. The nursing service administrator considers three aspects: (1) the nature of the problem, (2) the fact that qualitative as well as quantitative patient care data have to be collected and analyzed, and (3) the appropriateness of the measures to the goals selected. How is a nursing service administrator to maintain control amid a rapidly increasing flow of data? What are the vital elements in this particular service to the patient in relation

to its goals that need control by the nursing service administrator? The particular blend of service, costs, and behavioral data that are necessary can usually be supplied in whole or in part. The responsibility for choice of information rests with the nursing service administrator and is one that, if delegated improperly, can lead to less effective control.

The nursing service administrator needs to gather information about patient care and human behavior in the organization. Statistics on quantity and quality of changes in patient care, turnover of nurses, or the influx of new graduates are some of the information on service changes.

Certain nursing service administrators have great skill in assessing the patient care and behavioral patterns around them but need the assistance of experts such as the supervisors and personnel administrators, who have both the time and the skill to interpret the quality of nursing care and behavioral realities of the organization. Nursing service administrators need to stress to their coassistants the necessity for learning to measure standards of care and to hear and see the significance of the behavioral patterns in particular situations and how modifications in the pattern can be achieved by specific changes.

The control function was the emphasis of scientific management. Urwick synthesized the previous work of Fayol (1947), Mooney and Reily (1931), and Taylor (1947) to arrive at a framework for analyzing the controlling function. According to Urwick (1947), the desired effect of administrative control is a stable work force that pursues its planned activities with a spirit of initiative and a sense of unity. The means to this end include the staffing of the organization with competent administrators and selection and placement of a qualified nursing staff and other personnel, augmented by the use of rewards and sanctions. The scientific management people emphasized structural means for control, but they stressed that the competence of administration crucially determines the outcome of control efforts.

The classical concept of control was expanded by R. C. Davis (1951) and was broken down into subfunctions and each one related to the total concept. At the same time, control can be related to planning, directing, and organizing. Finally, it is possible to demonstrate the relationship of certain well-known and widely used accounting, financial, and service control methods to the scientific management form of control.

This administrative function includes all activities the nursing administrators undertake in attempting to ensure that actual operations conform to planned operations. Donnelly, Gibson, and Ivancevich (1972) and the National League For Nursing (1967) assert that successful implementation of control methods depends on the provision of three basic conditions: (1) standards must be established, (2) information that compares actual results with standards must be provided, and (3) action to bring about correction of any deviations between actual and standard must be possible. The logic is evident: without standards there can be no basis for evaluating the adequacy of actual performance; without information there can be no way of knowing the situation; without provision for action to correct deviations, the entire control process becomes a pointless exercise.

Standards are derived from goals and have many of the characteristics of goals. Like goals, standards are targets; to be effective, they must be clearly stated and logically related to the larger goals of the unit. They are the criteria against which future, current, or past actions are compared. They are measured in a variety of ways, including physical, monetary, quantitative, and qualitative terms.

Information that reports actual performance and permits appraisal of the performance against standards must be provided. Such information is most easily acquired for activities that produce specific and concrete results, such as results of patient care. In this respect the performance of the nursing department, the research and development unit, and the personnel department is quite difficult to appraise because of the nature of the activities of these departments.

Action to correct deviations results from the discovery of the need for action and from the ability to implement the desired action. The nurses responsible for taking the corrective steps must know that they are indeed responsible and that they have the assigned authority to take the action, and this should be specified in their job description.

The control function thus involves the implementation of methods that provide answers to three basic questions, What are the planned and expected results? By what means can the actual results be compared to planned results? and What corrective action is appropriate from which authorized person?

Types of control

The controlling function can be broken down into three types:

1. Preaction control focuses on the problems of preventing deviations in the quality and quantity of resources used in the institution. Human resources must meet the job requirements as defined by the organizational structure; the nursing staff must have the capability, whether physical or intellectual, to perform the assigned task. The material equipment must meet acceptable levels of quality and must be available at the proper time and place. In

addition, capital must be on hand to assure the adequate supply of plant and equipment. Finally, financial resources must be available in the right amounts and at the right times. A number of methods exist that enable administrators to implement preaction control.

2. Concurrent control monitors actual ongoing operations to assure that objectives are pursued. The principal means by which concurrent control is implemented are the directing or supervisory activities of the administrators. Through personal, on-the-spot observation the administrative nurse determines whether the work of others is proceeding in the manner defined by policies and procedures. The delegation of authority provides the administrative nurse with the power to use financial and nonfinancial incentives to affect concurrent control. The standards guiding ongoing activity are derived from job descriptions and from policies that result from the planning function.

3. Feedback control methods focus on end results. This type of control derives its name from the fact that historical results guide future action.

PREACTION CONTROL

Preaction control procedures include all the efforts of the administrator, whose purpose it is to increase the probability that future actual results will compare favorably with planned results. From this perspective, one can see that policies are by nature guidelines for future action. Yet we want to distinguish between setting policies and implementing them. The setting of policies is included in the planning function, whereas the implementation of policies is a part of the control function. Similarly, we might include job descriptions in the control function since job descriptions predetermine the activity of the jobholder. At the same time, however, we want to distinguish between defining and staffing the task structure. Defining the task structure is a part of the organiz-

ing function, and staffing the task structure is part of the control function.

The organization structure defines the job requirements and predetermines the skill requirements of the job holders. These requirements vary in the degree of specificity, depending on the nature of the task. At the staff nurse level the skill requirements can be specified in terms of knowledge, skill, and attitude as well as physical attributes and manual dexterity. On the other hand, the job requirements of administrators and consultative staff-nursing personnel are more difficult to define in terms of concrete measurements.

This preaction control is effected through procedures that include the selection and placement of administrative and nonadministrative personnel. We should distinguish between those procedures designed to obtain qualified nursing personnel and those designed to obtain qualified administrators and determine operatives (selection and placement). The basic procedures and objectives are essentially the same, yet classical theory makes the distinction because of its emphasis on administrative competence as the fundamental determiner of the organization's success.

The candidates for positions must be recruited from inside or outside the institution, and the most promising applicant must be selected from the list of candidates. The selection decision is based on the congruence of the applicant's skills and personal characteristics and the job requirements. The successful candidate must be oriented in methods and procedures appropriate for the job, an administrative responsibility that is clearly defined in classical theory by Taylor (1947). Most modern nursing organizations have elaborate procedures for providing continuing education and orientation on a continual basis.

The equipment and material used by the nursing staff must conform to standards of quality. At the same time a sufficient inventory must be maintained to ensure a continuous flow to meet the nurses' needs in patient care. The modern health care facilities have special departments for equipment and supplies with which the nursing personnel cooperate.

The acquisition of capital results from the need to replace existing equipment or to expand the institution's service capacity. Capital acquisitions are controlled by establishing criteria of potential service, which must be met before the proposal is authorized.

The principal means of controlling the availability and cost of financial resources is budgeting, particularly cash and working capital budgets. The budgets anticipate the ebb and flow of patient care activity, where equipment and supplies are purchased, nursing services are produced, and income is received. This cycle of activity results in a problem of timing, the availability of cash to meet the obligations.

CONCURRENT CONTROL

Concurrent control consists of methods that monitor the actual execution of plans. In most cases the focus of concurrent control is the work of the action or mediating population and professional nurses. The direction and supervision phases of the control function encompass all activities of the nursing personnel. The responsibility of the administrative staff when directing and supervising nursing personnel is (1) to interpret policies and to assist and instruct nursing personnel as needed in methods and procedures required and (2) to ensure that nursing personnel are following estabished policies and instructions within acceptable flexibility.

The direction function follows the formal authority line and the use of influence since the responsibility of each action supervisor is to interpret for and to her personnel the policies as set forth by the institutional authorities with personnel presentation.

The scope and content of the direction function varies, depending on the nature of the specific nursing and personnel work being supervised. We can also distinguish a number of other factors that describe differences in the form of direction. For example, if we recognize that direction is basically the process of personal communication, then we can see that the amount and clarity of information are important factors. Nursing personnel must receive sufficient information to carry out the task and must understand the information that they receive. On the other hand, too much information and too much detail can be damaging, especially to professional nurses. We should also recognize that the administrator's mode and tone of expression greatly influence the direction function.

FEEDBACK CONTROL

The distinguishing feature of feedback control methods is focusing on corrective action on historical outcomes, which then are used to correct future actions. For example, the financial statements of a health care facility are used to evaluate the acceptability of historical results and to determine the desirability of making changes in future acquisitions or nursing operation procedures. The following three feedback control methods are widely used in health care facilities: (1) quality control, (2) financial statement analysis, and (3) standard cost analysis.

Quality control. Nursing service administrators in cooperation with their staff must specify the nursing practice characteristics that are considered critical for patient care. This may be measured by the number of hours of direct care by a professional staff; by the standard that determines quality achieved; and by the degree to which physical, emotional, and individual needs have been met and specific to individual care plans.

Financial statement analysis. A principal source of information from which administrators can evaluate historical results is the accounting system of the health care facility. Periodically, the administrator receives a set of financial statements, which usually include a balance sheet, an income statement, and a sources and uses of funds statement. These statements summarize and classify the effects of transactions in terms of assets, liabilities, equity, revenues, and expenses—the principal components of the institution's financial structure.

Standard cost analysis. Standard cost accounting systems date from, and are considered a major contribution of, the scientific management area. A standard cost system provides information that enables the administrator to compare actual costs with predetermined (standard) costs. Administrators can then take appropriate corrective action or assign the authority to take action to others. The first use of standard costing was to effect control of manufacturing costs, but in recent years, standard costing has been applied to general and administrative expenses. This discussion concerns standard service costs.

The three elements of service costs are: direct labor, direct materials, and overhead. For each of these an estimate must be made of the element's cost per unit of output. For example, the direct labor cost per unit of output (per patient) consists of the standard usage of labor (nurse power) and the standard price of labor. The standard usage derives from time studies that fix the expected output per man-hour; the standard price of labor will be fixed by the salary schedule appropriate for the kind of work necessary to produce the output. A similar determination is made for direct materials.

Statement for control

The following is an outline on controlling for the nursing service administrator:

1. Determine what information various echelons of administration will require (a) to evaluate performance, (b) to relate progress to program schedules, and (c) to maintain status of funds (that is, maintain accounts), staff, plant equipment, supplies, and material.
2. Establish a system to measure work to yield required data.

3. Develop, where possible, standards of cost, quality, and production for individual work operations.
4. Set up a system of control records and reports to collect and summarize this information for administrative use.
5. Develop a system of operational audits as a continuing control device.
6. Determine what information is required about the program's effect on the community and provide for its collection.
7. Provide for the collection of intelligence and information necessary for planning.

SUMMARY

Principles and concepts are the major tools of the conceptualizer-planner contemplating the organization of a part of an institution or the whole institution. Few planners, if any, have had the opportunity to organize an institution from its beginning. Most often, an existing institution reorganizes. The move may be instigated by any of a number of external factors that contribute to changing or expanding existing facilities or by external factors having to do with personnel and their work. The move to reorganize may be an attempt to correct a poor situation or improve an already satisfactory situation. The reorganization may be large, affecting many units of the institution, or small, confined to just one department.

There are the identifiable steps, certain priorities that planners attempt to follow when approaching a reorganization. Briefly, they are as follows: (1) the setting of objectives, (2) analysis of the existing organization, (3) preparation of the long-term, ideal structure, (4) determination of the methods of change, (5) preparation of phase plans, and (6) implementation.

Implementation, of course, involves the actual personnel changes, regrouping of activities, changes in responsibility and authority called for by the phase plan. This part of the process is in the hands of the line administrators rather than the staff planning unit. In many institutions the planner-organizer at this implementation stage becomes both a teacher and maintenance person: a teacher is familiarizing personnel with the concepts involved in the organization and planning in general and with those involved in the particular plan adopted; a maintenance person in keeping the institution's organization charts, manual, and position guides current. But the administrator's role during the implementation stage is in reviewing all organization changes to see that they are in conformity with the long-term plan or will not impede the realization of the ideal.

Implementation, short-term organizing, tends to be very pragmatic. For here, the institution is confronted with adapting reality to the plans and the plans to reality. Planners for an organization, such as the nursing service administrator, find implementation to be just another step in a continuous cycle, rather than the last step in the organization process. The ideal is seldom attained. For through constant feedback, reevaluation, and adaptation, the institution may find that as it approaches the ideal this ideal too becomes another phase plan on the road to a new ideal plan.

REFERENCES

Appley, L. A.: A current appraisal of the quality of management, General management series no. 156: progressive policies for business leadership, New York, 1952, American Management Association.

Barnard, C. I.: The functions of the executive, Cambridge, Mass., 1968, Harvard University Press.

Beard, E. M.: A study of the relationships between congruence of value judgments in role expectations and job satisfaction, Master's thesis, U.C.L.A. School of Nursing, 1965.

Churchman, C. W.: The systems approach, New York, 1968, Delacorte Press.

Davis, R. C.: The fundamentals of top management, New York, 1951, Harper & Row, Pubs.

Dimock, M. E.: A philosophy of administration, New York, 1958, Harper & Brothers.

Donnelly, J. H., Gibson, J. L., and Ivancevich, J. M.: Fundamentals of management, Austin, Tex., 1972, Business Publications.

Drucker, P. F.: The practice of management, New York, 1954, Harper & Brothers.

Fayol, H.: General and industrial management, London, 1949, Sir Isaac Pitman & Sons, Ltd.

Finer, H.: Administration and the nursing services, New York, 1952, Macmillan Pub. Co., Inc.

Georgopoulos, B. S., and Mann, F. C.: The community general hospital, Survey research center and department of psychology, the University of Michigan, New York, 1961, Macmillan Pub. Co., Inc.

Goodson, M. R., and Jensen, G. E.: Organizing nursing services in the hospital, Nurs. Outlook, special yearly issue, pp. 60-62, 1956.

Hawley, A. H.: Human ecology, New York, 1950, The Ronald Press Co.

Jackson, J. M.: The organization and its communication problems. In Leavitt, H. I., and Pondy, L. R., editors: Readings in managerial psychology, Chicago, 1964, University of Chicago Press.

Jenkins, S. S.: Community obligation in planning, Hosp. Prog. **45**(3):82-6, 1964.

Katz, D., and Kahn, R. L.: The social psychology of organizations, New York, 1966, John Wiley & Sons, Inc.

Lawrence, P. R., and Lorsch, J. W.: Developing organizations: diagnosis and action, Menlo Park, Calif., 1969, Addison-Wesley Pub. Co., Inc.

Levey, S., and Loomba, N. P.: Health care administration: a managerial perspective, Philadelphia, 1973, J. B. Lippincott Co.

Metcalf, H. C., and Urwich, L. editors: Dynamic administration: the collected papers of Mary Parker Follet, New York, 1941, Harper & Brothers.

Mooney, J. D., and Reily, A. C.: Onward industry, New York, 1931, Harper & Brothers.

National League for Nursing: A self-evaluation guide for nursing services in hospitals and related institutions, New York, 1967, The League.

Seckler-Hudson, C.: Organization and management: theory and practice, Washington, D. C., 1957, The American University Press.

Stieglitz, H.: Concepts of organization planning. In Frank, H. E., editor: Organizing structuring, London, 1971, McGraw-Hill Book Co.

Tannenbaum, R.: The manager concept: a rational synthesis, pamphlet no. 8, Los Angeles, 1949, University of California at Los Angeles.

Taylor, F. W.: Scientific management, New York, 1947, Harper & Brothers.

Tead, O.: The art of administration, New York, 1951, McGraw-Hill Book Co.

Urwick, L.: The elements of administration, rev. ed., London, 1947, Sir Isaac Pitman & Sons, Ltd.

Watson, E. T.: Diagnosis of management problems, Harvard Business Review, **36**(1):69-76, 1958.

Whyte, W. H., Jr.: Is anybody listening? New York, 1952, Simon & Schuster, Inc.

ADDITIONAL READINGS

Abdellah, F. G., Beland, I. L., Martin, A., and Matheney, R. V.: New directions in patient-centered nursing: guidelines for systems of service, education, and research, New York, 1973, Macmillan Pub. Co., Inc.

Anderson, E. H., Bergersen, B. S., Duffey, M., Lohr, M., and Rose, M. H., editors: Current concepts in clinical nursing, vol. 4, St. Louis, 1973, The C. V. Mosby Co.

Banaka, W. H.: Training in depth interviewing, New York, Harper & Row, Pubs.

Bergersen, B. S., Anderson, E. H., Duffey, M., Lohr, M., and Rose, M. H., editors: Current concepts in clinical nursing, vol. 2, St. Louis, 1969, The C. V. Mosby Co.

Bernard, H. M.: Psychology of learning and teaching, ed. 2, New York, 1965, McGraw-Hill Book Co.

Bjorn, J. C., and Cross, H. D.: Problem-oriented practice, Chicago, 1970, Modern Hospital Press.

Bridgman, P. W.: The way things are, Cambridge, Mass., 1959, Harvard University Press.

Bross, I.: Design for decision, New York, 1953, Macmillan Pub. Co., Inc.

Brown, J. A. C.: Techniques of persuasion, Baltimore, Md., 1963, Penguin Books, Inc.

Bruner, J. S., Goodnow, J. J., and Aushi, G. A.: A study of thinking, New York, 1956, John Wiley & Sons, Inc.

Byrne, M., and Thompson, L. F.: Key concepts for the study and practice of nursing, St. Louis, 1972, The C. V. Mosby Co.

Costello, R., and Zalkind, S.: Psychology in administration, Englewood Cliffs, N. J., 1963, Prentice-Hall, Inc.

Deese, J. C., and Hulse, S.: The psychology of learning, ed. 3, New York, 1967, McGraw-Hill Book Co.

Duffey, M., Anderson, E. H., Bergersen, B. S., Lohr, M., and Rose, M. H., editors: Current concepts in clinical nursing, vol. 3, St. Louis, 1971, The C. V. Mosby Co.

Dunlap, K.: Habits, their making and unmaking, New York, 1932, Liveright. Reprinted 1972.

Faust, J.: Body language, New York, 1970, M. Evans & Co., Inc.

Fiedler, F. E.: A theory of leadership effectiveness, New York, 1967, McGraw-Hill Book Co.

Fulcher, G. S.: Common sense decision-making, Evanston, 1965, Northwestern University Press.

Garrett, A.: Interviewing, its principles and methods, New York, 1942, Family Service Association of America.

Guyton, A. C.: Textbook of medical physiology, ed. 4, Philadelphia, 1971, W. B. Saunders Co.

Hague, J. H., and Johnson, M., editors: Practical approaches to nursing service administration, The American Hospital Association, 9(2), Spring 1970.

Haire, M.: Psychology in management, ed. 2, New York, 1964, McGraw-Hill Book Co.

Hall, E. T.: The silent language, New York, 1959, Doubleday & Co., Inc.

Hamilton, W. P., and Lavin, M. A.: Decision-making in the coronary care unit, St. Louis, 1972, The C. V. Mosby Co.

Harvey, O., and Ware, R.: Conceptual systems and personality organization, New York, 1961, John Wiley & Sons, Inc.

Highet, G.: The art of teaching, New York, 1950, Alfred A. Knopf, Inc.

Hill, W. F.: Learning, a survey of psychological interpretations, rev. ed., Scranton, Pa., 1971, Intext, Educ. Pubs.

Hodnett, E.: Art of problem solving, New York, 1955, Harper & Row, Pubs.

Hurst, W.: Problem oriented system, New York, 1972, Medcom Books, Inc.

Johnson, M. M., Davis, M. L. C., and Bilitch, M. J.: Problem solving in nursing practice, Dubuque, Iowa, 1970, Wm. C. Brown Co., Pubs.

Kahn, R., Wolfe, D. M., Quinn, R. P., and Snoet, J. I.: Organizational stress, New York, 1964, John Wiley & Sons, Inc.

Karlins, M.: Conceptual complexity and remote-associative proficiency as creativity variables in a complex problem-solving task, Id of Personality and Social Psychol., 1967.

Karlins, M., and Abelson, H. J.: Persuasion, ed. 2, New York, 1970, Springer Publishing Co., Inc.

Katz, D.: Industrial conflict, New York, 1950, McGraw-Hill Book Co.

Katz, R. L.: Skills of an effective administrator, Harvard Business Review 33(1):33-42, 1955.

Kiesler, C., Collins, B. E., and Miller, N.: Attitude change: a critical analysis of theoretical approaches, New York, 1969, John Wiley & Sons, Inc.

Kintzel, K. C., editor: Advanced concepts in clinical nursing, Philadelphia, 1971, J. B. Lippincott Co.

Koontz, H., and O'Donnell, C.: Principles of management, New York, 1964, McGraw-Hill Book Co.

Kron, T.: The management of patient care, putting leadership skills to work, Philadelphia, 1971, W. B. Saunders Co.

Kron, T.: Communication in nursing, ed. 2, Philadelphia, 1972, W. B. Saunders Co.

Leavitt, H. J.: Managerial psychology, Chicago, 1958, University of Chicago Press.

Leininger, M.: Nursing and anthropology: two worlds to blend, New York, 1970, John Wiley & Sons, Inc.

Little, D. E., and Carnevali, D. L.: Nursing care planning, Philadelphia, 1969, J. B. Lippincott Co.

Lockerby, F. K.: Communications for nurses, ed. 3, St. Louis, 1968, The. C. V. Mosby Co.

Luck, G. M.: Patients, hospitals and operational research, New York, 1971, Barnes & Noble Books.

Macgregor, F. C.: Social science in nursing, New York, 1960, Russell Sage Foundation.

Maslow, A. H.: Motivation and personality, ed. 2, New York, 1970, Harper & Row, Pubs.

Mednick, S. A.: Learning, Englewood Cliffs, N. J., 1973, Prentice-Hall, Inc.

Mitchell, P. H., editor: Concepts basic to nursing, New York, 1973, McGraw Hill Book Co.

Nursing Development Conference Group: Concept formalization in nursing, process and product, Boston, 1973, Little, Brown & Co.

Orens, D. E.: Nursing: concepts of practice, New York, 1971, McGraw-Hill Book Co.

Peabody, R. L.: Perceptions of organizational authority: a comparative analysis, Admin. Science Quarterly 6(4):12-14, 1962.

Pohl, M. L.: Teaching function of the nursing practitioner, Dubuque, Iowa, 1968, Wm. C. Brown Co., Pubs.

Pollack, J.: The patients' new role in planning and evaluating, Hosp. Prog. 45(3):78-81, 1964.

Rorem, C. R.: Operation of a hospital planning agency, Hosp. Prog. 45:(3):87-91, 1964.

Ruisch, J., and Kees, W.: Nonverbal communication, Berkeley, Calif., 1956, University of California Press.

Schein, E. H.: Organization psychology, ed. 2, Englewood Cliffs, N. J., 1970, Prentice-Hall, Inc.

Schroder, H., Driver, M. J., and Streufert, S.: Human information processing, New York, 1967, Holt, Rinehard & Winston, Inc.

Sengelaub, M. M.: Fixing responsibility for planning, Hosp. Prog. 45(3):92-96, 1964.

Summer, C. E., Jr.: The managerial mind, mimeographed, Cambridge, Mass., Harvard University Graduate School of Business, n. d.

Traxler, R. N.: The administrator's dilemma—the need for conceptual skills, Hosp. Admin. 9(1):6-15, 1964.

Weed, L. L.: Medical records, medical education and patient care, Cleveland, 1971, Press of Case Western Reserve Univ.

Woodruff, A. D.: Basic concepts of teaching, San Francisco, 1961, Chandler Pub. Co.

Zimbardo, P., and Ebbesen, E.: Influencing attitudes and changing behavior, Reading, Mass., 1969, Addison-Wesley Pub. Co., Inc.

Chapter 5

ENVIRONMENT

Chapter 4 illustrated how the composite process of conceptual acts *(Ac)* and physical acts *(Ap)* works together and contributes to the next phase of our model, the environment.

The concept of environment seems at first to be an obvious and simple one to identify, but as with the other components of our model, there is literally more to environment than meets the eye. Part and parcel of the total environment is the much subtler conceptual environment.

After a discussion of environment in general and a brief review of the role of environment as viewed from a different perspective and from a different conceptual framework, we will define conceptual and physical environment and then demonstrate how they work together to make their effects known both within and without the system.

The dictionary defines environment as surroundings; the aggregate of all external conditions and influences affecting the life and development of an organization.

The greater the compatability between the system and its environment, the more effective the system will be, thus, the significance of our study of environment.

Gilmer (1966:383) defines an environment as "a context of conditions that has some more or less general effect on systems operations."

Location is an obvious example. Notice how different hospitals are, depending on whether they are located in an urban area, a small town, next to a major highway, or connected to a university. Each manifestation of the environment affects the number and kind of clients, the staff and its turnover, and the duration and distribution of rush times and waiting periods. How can a hospital make allowances for accidents from rain or snow? Contingency planning must consider fluctuation in input and output, depending on the location of the hospital.

External and internal aspects of environment

Environment is complex, usually changing rapidly with various interconnections and intraconnections. In discussing environmental adaptations and differentiations and ways organizations can cope with uncertainties, Thompson (1967) proposed that an organization pay strict attention to its geographical location and its social composition.

March and Simon (1958) classify environments as either benign or hostile. Dill (1958) created a distinction between environments that are homogeneous or heterogeneous and those that are stable or shift rapidly.

Emery and Trist (1965) developed a scale of environment from placid to turbulent and illustrated that turbulent environments had more influence on interorganizational integration and intraorganizational processes.

Environment includes the image or character of the organization under study. Wolf (1966), in diagnosing organization character, asserted that organizations reflect the broader environment; hence, their characters are influenced by environmental features such as climate, culture, politics, and the economic organization of society. The organization exists by cooperating with this broader environment, which provides the resources: tools, capital, land, labor, and fuel. Other aspects of the environment include established rules and trade customs, as well as legal, religious, and moral customs, which influence specialization, delegation, authority, communication, and incentives in the organization. In short, to understand any specific organization, one must relate its activities to the environment.

Formerly, it was commonplace to view the internal functions of organizations as separate and enclosed from the broader environment. Schein (1970) probed many aspects of the environment and maintained that all organizations exist within and as part of an external environment. To survive as organizations, they must fulfill some useful function, participate in certain cultural and social arrangements, and relate to various other organizations.

Schein further explained that the external environment is represented within the organization by each employee, client, and visitor. Each individual is a member of possibly several groups that, in turn, place different demands, expectations, criteria, and influences on that individual. The individual demonstrates this by discussing the way in which the psychological problems of individuals affect the internal environment and the adaptation an organization makes when faced with technical, social, and political changes occurring in the external environment.

It is difficult to identify the boundaries between the external and internal environment. This, according to Schein, poses a problem to multipurpose and polyfunctional organizations because an agency that houses separate clinics in one building probably draws specific clinic clients from different environments, for example, drug addicts and autistic children converge on the building from different areas of the community at large.

Argyris (1964) listed adapting to the external environment as the third essential core activity for any organization, the other two being achieving objectives and maintaining the internal system.

ROLE OF ENVIRONMENT AS VIEWED FROM DIFFERENT PERSPECTIVES

At one time, many writers compared organizations to machines or organisms. But unlike a biological organism, an organization lacks a built-in homeostatic mechanism. To maintain stability or equilibrium, methods have been developed for controlling and directing activities and, to some extent, for planning and organizing activities. For the best results the response of organizations to environmental forces must be dynamic, as they require constant adjustment and anticipation. The organizations must have a means for acquiring energy for inputs and a means to extract outputs. Such means may become subsystems. Thus, it can be seen that the *physical and organismic theories* are limited and are being replaced by systems theories, particularly those systems characterized as open systems.

The Tavistock Institute in London produced two important concepts: the idea of the sociotechnical system and the open systems concept. Trist's work described the mutual interaction that occurs when elements labeled as technical (goals, means, and physical environment) are combined with elements of the social system (groupings and interrelations among people) (Trist and co-workers 1963).

Rice (1963) has contributed to our considerations of input, conversion, and export to and from the environment. His open system model has been a most useful concept.

By combining these two ideas, it is possible to demonstrate the importance of multiple paths and multiple interactions between the organization and environment. The administrator must cope with demands and constraints. The preconceived notions held by employees must be allowed for, either modified by administrative acts or rendered harmless by the nature of the organizational structure.

Homans (1961) went beyond the Tavistock findings and built a somewhat more differentiated and sophisticated model based on a three-part environment: physical, cultural, and technological. Required activities and interactions are imposed on the organization by the environment. In response to them, the organization issues activities, interactions, and sentiments, which affect the people in the organization as well as the environment itself. This model makes use of two systems: the external and the internal. The mutually interdependent activities, interactions, and sentiments between an organization and its environment constitute the external system. The changes that take place within the organization, which are not specified by the environment, produce a new pattern within the organization, which Homans called the internal system.

The model described by Homans explicitly recognizes a series of mutual interdependencies, allows predictions to be made concerning the effect of changes in a given variable, and explains many of the phenomena associated with nursing teams. Teams and groups are described in more detail in the discussion of the conceptual environment later in this chapter.

If two people have positive sentiments for each other, they will have a high rate of interaction, and if they have negative sentiments, a low rate. If people are forced to interact continually over a long period of time, they will develop positive sentiments. An important implication of this is the seeming paradox that if two people hate each other and are forced into continued interaction, the hate will decrease. There is a wide spectrum of interactions between love and hate—liking, friendship, acceptance, rapport, and their opposites all exist in gradation.

Homans described how groups can build interest, share feelings, sentiments, and attitudes and how members can participate in reaching a common goal. Intrinsic factors such as irritants, curiosity, failure, laziness, and self-esteem are considered. Such sociopsychological traits in people cannot be ignored.

The overlapping-group model of Likert (1961) touches on two additional important points: that the organization is a system of interlocking groups with "linking pins" connecting the interlocking groups and that the linking pins are individuals who have dual memberships. Relationships between organization and environment are studied by means of this linking-pin concept. Supersystems, systems, and subsystems are explained in relation to one another and to their relevant environments.

Kahn and his associates extended Likert's model by using the concept of role sets. In this way, they clarify internal boundaries and the nature of the linkages. Overlapping and interlocking role sets may transcend the boundaries of the organization (Kahn and co-workers 1964). Individual behaviors are interpreted in terms of role conflict and role ambiguity.

The newer theorists, the neostructuralists, stress the importance of organizational design, member attitudes and responses, and environmental interdependencies (Lawrence and Lorsch 1967; Burns and Stalker 1961; Dalton and co-workers 1959).

A new text by Huse and Bowditch (1973) traces the history of theories of organization from the early "one best way" concept to the adaptive-coping concepts, based on technology and environment. Neostructural ideas more oriented to human relations are shown to be suited to a highly unknown and unstable environment.

Contingency organizational structure is

based on differentiation and integration, which, according to Lawrence and Lorsch, occurs in four dimensions (Lawrence and Lorsch 1967; Galbraith 1969):

1. Orientation toward objectives
2. Orientation toward time
3. Interpersonal orientation
4. Formality of structure

These concepts closely agree with our conceptual acts. Coordination and integration become more difficult as units of the structure become more differentiated.

The interdependency of the organization with its environment dictates that it must cope adaptively. Schein (1970:120) listed six stages in the adaptive-coping cycle. The organization

1. Senses a change in some part of the internal or external environment.
2. Imports the relevant information about the change into those parts of the organization that can act on it.
3. Changes conversion processes inside the organization according to the information obtained.
4. Stabilizes internal changes while reducing and/or managing undesired by-products.
5. Exports new products and services that are more in line with the originally perceived changes in the environment.
6. Obtains feedback on the success of the state of the external environment and the degree of integration of the internal environment.

Schein stressed that to increase organizational effectiveness while coping and adapting, the organization must possess good communication, flexibility, creativity, and genuine psychological commitment. These concepts are somewhat similar to our conceptual acts, conceptual environment and, in turn, the physical environment. Environmental influences are intrinsic parts of an organization and should not be ignored or omitted from consideration in planning either system or subsystem activities. Conversely, the administrator must be aware of the effects of system or subsystem activities on the environment in their internal and external aspects.

Traditional organizational theories tend to view the human organization as a closed system. This tendency has led to a disregard of differing organizational environments and the nature of the organizational dependency on environment. It has led also to an overconcentration on principles of internal organizational functioning, with consequent failure to develop and understand the process of feedback, which is essential to survival.

Formerly, nursing stability was seen as fostered by rules, integration, and coordination, which were inflexibly applied. We see this as characteristic of a closed system. To impose coordination as an end in itself is self-defeating, especially if the possibility of different paths to the same goal is not recognized. Individual or technical procedures may have a "one best way" of accomplishment, but given a specific organization with its particular needs and goals, there are many paths to a goal. We consider this view to be characteristic of an open system.

CONCEPTUAL ENVIRONMENT
Operational definitions

Conceptual environment is operationally defined as the abstract, cognitive component of a milieu that deals with the human element. It is intangible yet real. It fosters thinking and affective relationships among people. It is this aspect of the abstract environment that deals with people's feelings, attitudes, spirits, emotions, and psychosocial needs. Conceptual environment is concerned with one of the most important variables in the operation of any sociotechnical organization: people.

In the conceptual environment the individual seeks satisfaction and responsibility, the attainment of which fosters growth, stability, and interaction. The means by which the individual achieves these aims are cooperation, integration, communication, commitment, and reward.

An important, though amorphous, adjunct of understanding the human element in the conceptual environment is climate. Climate is part of any environment, but it is a more limited and more specific concept than environment. For our purposes, it refers to the ephemeral form *morale* or mood or, to use the current vernacular, the extremely applicable term *vibes*. Are the vibrations one feels in a nursing service organization good? Or are they bad? This is another way of asking whether the climate is fair or foul.

Climate reflects the norms, values, and history of the organization. Past struggles are sometimes reflected in the present environmental pressures, general task demands that are met by procedural and technical structures, the actions of which are mediated and moderated by climate.

Gilmer (1966) suggested that many factors influence climate: the type of service offered or the special care given influences the workers in their interactions with clients, waiting times for clients, cost of care, clients' ideas of quality care, and the *criterion tolerance* or the acceptable range of fluctuation and waste or nonproductive output (time, material, errors, and carelessness).

Industrial psychologists define climate as "characteristics that distinguish the organization from other organizations and that influence the behavior of people in that organization" (Von Gilmer 1966:94). It is an important morale factor relating to promotion rates, absenteeism, tardiness, profit sharing, direct accidents, and leadership. These findings are borne out by Slivnick, Kerr, and Kosinar (1957).

In short, if the climate is suitable, the organization and its members have a stronger tendency to achieve goals than if the climate is unsuitable. So, administrative perception and receptivity are very much a part of the work climate. All organizations should assess their goals in terms of the people within them. If creative growth is to take place, the organization must foster a structure and a climate that will produce enough security to overcome the anxiety that accompanies work

and change. At the same time, there must be enough motivation to recognize the need for work, change, growth, and reform.

Complacent individuals seldom make significant contributions in any endeavor. A curious nurse or administrator, unhappy with today's effort, is a nursing service's best hope for a better organized, more productive enterprise tomorrow. Satisfaction for such individuals is in a sense a product of their dissatisfaction. It is their unwillingness to accept the status quo that causes them to project organizational goals that transcend immediate personal desires. These are goals that catch their imagination and fulfill a need for a sense of achievement. Satisfaction comes through a recognition and acceptance of organizational goals and a feeling that they are worthwhile and attainable. Most individuals like to be associated with a successful enterprise.

Good nursing services doubtless have within their staffs rather high degrees of discomfort. Pride in the accomplishment of nursing service acts as a stimulus for increased personal effort and results in greater personal satisfaction. In such a context, satisfaction has dynamic quality and is far more than simply the absence of disturbing requests and demands. What we define as conceptual environment, Schein (1970) called the work organization: time scheduling, interaction, and informal groups. It is logical that informal groups emerge, for they meet psychological needs and depend on climate.

Characteristics of conceptual environment for nursing service

The optimum conceptual environment for nursing services wherein both organizational and individual objectives (Og and Oi) are fulfilled does the following:

1. Fosters thinking and the freedom to be wrong without being censured.
2. Insists on a high rate of nursing innovations and organizational effectiveness and encourages member initiative, resulting in a

higher degree of involvement and commitment to the achievement of O_g and O_i.

3. Encourages a problem-solving attitude among the staff and widespread participation of employees in the decision-making process.
4. Places a value on adaptiveness and flexibility so that necessary changes can occur with minimal resistance.
5. Fosters effective work relationships among personnel, especially among the top administrative team.
6. Places persons who are considerate and not distant or impersonal in line for the administrative position of nursing service administrator.
7. Favors experimentation over tradition, and rational analysis over traditional practices.
8. Practices the concept of relativism rather than absolutism. In other words, accepts that there is more than one way to a goal.
9. Permits personnel to reach their potential and to practice what they have been taught and are capable of doing.
10. Respects employees and promotes in them a sense of identity, feeling of belonging, and a sense of security.

Therefore, the main objective of a conceptual environment for nursing services that is conducive to the accomplishment of both O_g and O_i is the adoption and implementation of the preceding characteristics.

In building a conceptual environment, it is necessary to consider three central foci: (1) building more effective ways for colleagues to develop working relationships with one another, (2) developing skill in creating organizational climates conducive to high rates of nursing practice, innovation, and organizational effectiveness, and (3) creating an adaptive organizational structure. These administrative goals are positive in nature, and one may well ask why the changes in emphasis from the negative. Unless nursing service administrators are aware of and continually reacting positively to society's demands, they will be replaced by nonnurse professional administrators. Organized nursing services will then be without nurse leadership, and the emphasis will divert from organized nursing to organized technical services,

with nursing being, at best, an advisory role.

Several nursing research studies aimed at assessing the beneficial use of nursing knowledge in patient care and in administration of patient care services reported that the utilization of knowledge and skills depend on the organizational environment. Where there is a progressive nursing service organization characterized by (1) problem-solving behavior, (2) widespread participation and collaboration in decision-making processes, and (3) considerate as opposed to distant and impersonal administration the education of nurses seems to have beneficial results. Otherwise, no benefit is measurable. Furthermore, nursing education(al) effects were shown to be best in organizations engaged in self-conscious programs of organizational development concurrent with their administrators' participation in formal programs of administrative education (Langford 1960; Kramer and Baker 1971; Harrington and Theis 1968).

This new focus on organizational environment led to an awareness that the problems of how administrators get along with one another—how the administrative team functions—were much more relevant to organizational effectiveness than the more restricted problems of staff nurse-supervisory relations. With this new insight, human relations in administration have tended to focus much more on how administrators can build effective work relationships with their colleagues. Dynamic, complex organizations require extensive interpersonal skills within the administrative group itself. It seems to be somewhat assumed that if effective work relationships are established within the administrative team, some of the other human problems will solve themselves. This trend has resulted in a changed goal of nursing service administration from how to "handle" personnel to how to "handle" oneself—constituting a much closer look at the personal behavior patterns of the administrator (Baumgartel 1972).

Another factor accounting for the emphasis in structure and the relationship changes stems from the fact that economists and developmental analysts have demonstrated that in any nation there can be no significant improvement in per capita income without an accelerating rate of technological innovation (Baumgartel 1972). These scientists were pointing to human-organizational factors conducive to high rates of innovation.

Similarly, nursing service administrators and nursing educators have long emphasized the need for a high rate of nursing-practice and nursing-service innovations before a breakthrough in the delivery of the health care system can take place. For that to occur, the administrator must also look to the human-organizational factors in creating organizational climates and organizational effectiveness conducive to high rates of nursing innovation and change.

Nursing supervisors realize that getting a little more work out of staff nurses is a minor problem compared with creating a climate in which major nursing breakthroughs can deliver more medical and nursing care to patients overnight without expending more energy.

Effective relationships within an adaptive and innovative environment

This discussion concerns some guidelines for bringing about a conceptual environment that is innovative and adaptive and contains effective working relationships among the personnel, as well as involvement and commitment on the part of nursing personnel to achieve O_g and O_i.

Given the new directions in nursing-service structure and human relations for administrators, we can begin to specify more concretely some of the specific goals of this new thinking. A fundamental problem has been the discovery, through research, of the organizational forms and personal skills most conducive to high rates

of nursing innovation, which Elton Mayo (1945) conceptualized many years ago as the change from "traditional" organizational forms to what he called the "adaptive" form.

We postulate that entirely new styles of administration and new personal attributes are required for effective functioning in the new adaptive organizations. The task of education in nursing service administration within the framework of human relations is to develop and prepare the supply of new people needed for the optimal functioning of new organizational forms. Preparing oneself for an administrative role in an expanding, innovative enterprise involves not only acquiring skill in the new nursing practices and techniques but also making fundamental changes in personal outlook, patterns of interpersonal relationship, and organizational role taking. What are some of these changes?

We agree with Baumgartel (1972) that changes need to occur at four interdependent levels of human functioning: cognitive, motivational-emotional, interpersonal, and organizational.

1. The *cognitive level* refers to the manner in which individuals think about, believe in, and perceive the world about them. For example, social anthropologists have observed that some people do not have cause-effect relationship concepts in their thought processes. Or some people "see" human life as being determined entirely by fate or impersonal, unknowable forces. These basic thought processes structure and influence the behavior of people in organizational life as well as in ordinary social affairs (Baumgartel 1972).

At the congitive level the fundamental requirement is that the administrator adopt a problem-solving attitude toward all aspects of the working environment. First, it will be necessary to give up custom and start to experiment with new ideas. Second, traditional practices must be subjected to careful rational analysis as to their efficacy. Third, instead of relying on beliefs (things held to be true by nature), one should habitually be testing those beliefs against the hard data and facts of industrial life. And fourth, one must question the notion that happy workers mean good workers, as those in personnel management have believed for years. Recent empirical research has demonstrated this to be a myth (Brayfield and Crokett 1955). The new nursing administrator will need to understand that there are different ways of viewing things and that there is more than one correct way of viewing some things. To illustrate, empirical approaches to the classic problems of span of control have indicated that there is no one right way to formulate organizations (Porter and Applewhite 1964).

2. The *motivational-emotional level* refers to the dynamics of feelings and sentiments within the individual's personality structure. Some individuals or groups can be characterized as having basic feelings of security or insecurity or to being full of hatred or resentment. These psychodynamics or basic personality factors may be appropriate for some social structures and inappropriate for others.

The attributes of emotional makeup required for functioning effectively in the new organization are difficult to conceptualize and achieve through education. One fundamental requirement demanded by the high degree of differentiation and interdependence in a complex, expanding organization is that the individual be controlled rather than impulsive in character structure. The administrator of a family-owned firm can, on a whim, up and leave for a vacation; the administrator of a complex, highly integrated nursing organization cannot. A corollary of this principle is that the new administrator must be characterized by more highly developed internal controls on her own behavior and be less dependent on external controls. The new administrator must be able to have more tolerance for frustration, complexity brings frustration, and be able to postpone grati-

fication, years are required for the fulfillment of complex schemes. It may be necessary to forgo seeing perfect clarity and lack of ambiguity in organizational affairs and learn to live with the opposite. Finally, the new administrator's motivation will need to be oriented toward the positive goals of achievement and self-actualization and away from the negative or defensive goals of status preservation and security.

3. The *interpersonal level* refers to the prevalent and persistent styles and forms of face-to-face interaction. To what extent people communicate with each other and how much people trust each other are examples of interpersonal phenomena. A leader's interpersonal style may have a great influence on the organizational unit. Interpersonal patterns can be discussed independently of personality concepts.

New patterns of interpersonal relationships are required. More openness is required allowing information on ideas and feelings to flow freely. Distrust must give way to trust, for dynamic organizations are too complex and skills too specialized for a climate of distrust to prevail. People with skill in interdependence-collaborative patterns among peers will be more efficient than those who base interpersonal relationships on who is "above" or "below" in the pecking order. The traditional, hierarchical patterns may function effectively in organizations with routine tasks, but they can hamper the effectiveness of growing innovative organizations. Finally, the effective member of an adaptive organization will be closer and more considerate in interpersonal relations rather than aloof and unconcerned about others.

4. The *organizational level* refers to the structural and dynamic properties of the relationship among individuals and groups in larger social units. Just as there are many structural differences among different chemical compounds, so are there differences among social organizations, and these differences can be analyzed abstractly.

We believe that nurses can learn new

attitudes and patterns of behavior if the organizational environment is supportive of these new patterns and that benefits will be derived from this change. To the extent that the administrative team creates this climate, it is possible to identify the dimensions of change to be sought at the organizational level. Size alone makes it imperative and inevitable that organizational patterns change from paternal or authoritarian to participative or consensual. A large complex, specialized, new organization is beyond the capability of one person or a small special group to manage and oversee. Administrative and staff specialists can only perform their functions optimally when they can effectively influence decisions and where they themselves are consensually, not acquiescently, in agreement with the decision. Attitudes of self-reliance and achievement whether in a paternalistic or autocratic structure. The complex adaptive organization must, of necessity, rely more on internal controls, self-created through identification and other socialization processes, than on a system of external controls. Rigid external controls may be required in military and paramilitary organizations, but they are dysfunctional in innovative work organizations such as nursing. The driving dynamic force in the creative organization is long-term organizational growth and development rather than short-term personal goals of key people. The paramount functions are goals of problem solving and achievement, with power struggles and status preoccupation pushed into the background.

To have an effective working relationship among personnel that will foster an adaptive and innovative response to the organizational environment, it is necessary to open certain options. Those who work together should be able to form a commitment to organizational objectives, to communicate with one another, and to experience rewards in an atmosphere of cooperation, motivation, and movement toward involvement with one another and with the organizational objectives.

When a new program directs nursing personnel away from a situation that is known and comfortable and toward one that is ambiguous and threatening, the antidotes to the unrest that may ensue are individual commitment and a spirit of cooperation through staff involvement. Creating these forces poses a major challenge for the administrator.

COMMITMENT

As forces begin to be exerted to energize the directing process, the demand for commitment, the pledging of self or resources to the success of an undertaking, becomes more widespread. Without the pledge of commitment by a majority of the staff, basic changes cannot be accomplished, and resistance may impede progress (Cofer and Rosenthal 1948). Firm commitment makes it possible to operate under the principle, What will further the cause will be done.

How can a nursing service administrator win staff commitment? Only when an individual is intellectually and emotionally spurred to action by a motivating force will commitment occur. Motivation is the administrator's first, continuing, and most important concern. People perform best when motivation is high. It may be any inner striving, such as a wish, a desire, a need, or a drive, which activates the individual to move toward certain goals (Berelson and Steiner 1964). Knowing this, the administrator keeps in mind the human elements involved in the work and change process; specifically, she will make it her business to do the following:

1. Inventory the individual needs of the staff.
2. Acquire and protect material objects.
3. Express ambition or willpower and to achieve prestige or recognition.
4. Exert, resist, or yield to the expression of power.
5. Be aggressive or self-abasing.
6. Give and receive affection as expressed by the desire for affiliation with or protection of another human.
7. Engage in social activities, such as play and nursing service interaction.

These are universal needs, and satisfying

them is a prime mover in getting people to become involved in an endeavor. An administrator embarking on change should assess her staff in terms of their exhibited needs and take accordingly such actions as making individual staff apppointments to committees and delegating authority.

Research suggests that the energy expended on specific tasks is closely related to the strength of an individual's motivation and that highly motivated inidviduals will strive with vigor to circumvent, remove, or otherwise overcome any barrier between themselves and the objective. The recognition and assessment of human needs go a long way toward preventing problems in work and in change.

COMMUNICATION

Communication is the means by which the administrator builds motivation. Its prime purpose is to inform the staff of what the program goals imply and particularly of what these goals will demand of each person.

To move toward an objective, an individual has to perceive a relative value in doing so, a value congruent with that of the organization. This mutual acceptance of an objective will not be achieved unless free flow of information occurs between the administrator and her nursing staff. The traditional structure of our health system militates against a free exchange. Too often the communication flows in one direction only, and proper channels for feedback are not created; an administrator attempting a new program may find it helpful to design a communication system incorporating a two-way system (Novotney 1966). It should be frequent, concise, and professional in tone.

If nurses are apt to be affected adversely by a new program, every attempt should be made to deal with it openly to avoid discontent later. It may be anticipated, for example, that some nurses will find a team nursing situation threatening because duties and decision-making responsiblities that have traditionally been centralized in

a self-contained situation will now have to be shared. This fact should be recognized, communicated, and aired. The nurses to whom a program is being suggested should be helped to see and understand that they have it within their power to implement it and that they have the ability to successfully manipulate the factors involved in the proposed program. A nurse's negative attitude of indifference and even obstructionism over a proposed change can often be traced to the fact that the nurse was never informed of what the proposed change would demand in terms of skills, attitudes, or knowledge. An example of this is observed in nurses who rebel against care plans because they have no understanding of what the individualization of patient care plans means and because they see it as completely opposed to traditional nursing. Had they been helped to see that the new approach still demanded utilization of many traditional nursing skills, their unwillingness to attempt the change might have been radically altered.

One cautionary note: nurses do not leave their prejudices, thoughts, feelings, or hates behind when called upon to launch out into the unknown. For this reason, a nursing service administrator has to be sure of herself and her objectives so that she can be informative and supportive as the program is initiated and progresses. A wavering administrator broadcasts uncertainty; an unfeeling one spurs hostility. Firmness of purpose and understanding should characterize every communication.

REWARD

In our society, rewards tend to be measured in terms of money, but research suggests that psychological rewards are frequently more powerful. In the nursing situation, the reward must come not so much from the nursing administrator or from the community as from the patients. The satisfaction that committed nurses feel when they see their patients doing better in a changing nursing situation is likely to be sufficient reward, and this is not translatable into dollars and cents. There is a definite reward implicit in the very process of accomplishing a new program. If other rewards are utilized in the change process, such as an increase in prestige or an increase in pay, they should be communicated to those involved and be made realistic and permanent so that expectations for them are not crushed once change has been achieved.

ATMOSPHERE OF COOPERATION

In a health care facility when the staff is united for the achievement of mutually derived goals and there is an atmosphere of cooperation, work and planned change can occur. Careful program planning is essential to control effects that a new, or any, program inevitably exerts on the institution and on the community. A new program demands input from numerous sources, including members of the staff. Cooperation is essential.

Cooperation encompasses human interaction and group cohesion. Human interaction implies a give and take on an interpersonal basis, whereas cohesion refers to the welding of isolates into a group. The quality of human interaction that takes place within a group reflects the freedom and sense of acceptance felt by the group as it moves ahead in its task; group cohesion is indicated by how well the group is organized, whether members are mutually supportive, and whether or not the group experiences any degree of success in its efforts (Hare 1962). Interaction and cohesion are measurable and interdependent. They are at a maximum when group members in a given situation are led to perceive the achievement of their own goals as interrelated with the achievement of the goals of others. Regardless of how difficult work or a change may appear or how onerous the tasks necessary to achieve it, if the individuals in work or the change team take their strength from one another and feel free to exchange or deal with common problems in an atmosphere of acceptance,

the possibility of successful work and change will be increased. Clearly then, to create a cooperative spirit, the nursing service administrator must express the goals and values that can be held in common by those being asked to work in a new program, all the while keeping in mind the emotional as well as the intellectual reactions of the staff. People are not rational calculating machines moved by ideas and concerned only with their correctness. Work and change decisions sometimes fail because they have been devised on the assumption that feelings can be laid aside or ignored; yet nurses may reject change goals because of anger, resentment, or fear.

It follows that in any attempt to influence the staff, administrators must be aware of their own feelings, biases, and prejudices. An administrator must know where she stands in relation to a new program before she can successfully involve nurses. For example, an administrator will find it difficult to move nurses in the direction of team nursing unless she recognizes her own strong intellectual and emotional commitment to the idea and, at the same time, understands at the outset that others may not be so committed. She must also be aware of how much she is willing to give of herself to accomplish the goal. The best of a well-planned program is not whether it was made with cold rationality but whether the emotions of all involved have been recognized and provided for.

MOTIVATED TEAM

To achieve objectives, the administrator will find it useful to adopt a motivated cooperative system, or team, that meets to strengthen and reinforce motivational forces by supplementing and utilizing favorable attitudes (Likert 1961).

The task of the administrator is to build a new work group for the accomplishment of a program. Research in various occupational situations suggests that the mark of a successful administrator is a highly coordinated and highly motivated cooperative social system (Likert 1961). Individual staff talents are utilized to form a strong force aimed at accomplishing mutually established objectives. This suggests the use of the team approach to test accomplishment based on the assumption that the complexity of most program situations demands the application of a variety of talents.

An administrator cannot make equal demands on all nor can she expect that all will be similarly satisfied. For an effective team endeavor, tasks are assigned not on a random basis but according to who can do what best, the staff having participated in the work distribution decisions. Openness and acceptance are the prime characteristics of an ideal team situation. People have the opportunity to direct their own destinies and to work together to make wise decisions. Consensus rather than decree determines the direction of the group's movement. People feel free to air their ideas without fear of retaliation or criticism. Group members support one another and their leader because all are mutually responsible for the objectives and subsequent action. In these situations, teams tend to become closely knit groups. One nursing administrator remarked that "the extent to which change has occurred is the extent to which nurses feel free to control their own decisions."

If, in a new program, nurses are allowed to participate in the decision-making process, Goodwin Watson (1967) concluded that resistance will be less if (1) participants in the work, or change, process have worked together to diagnose a situation, to agree on a basic problem, and to feel it is important, (2) the goals are adopted by consensual group decision, (3) proponents are able to empathize with opponents, to recognize valid objections, and to take steps to relieve unnecessary fears, and (4) individuals experience acceptance, support, trust, and confidence in their relations with one another.

Nurses, like everyone else, have the need to sustain a sense of personal worth. An important source of satisfaction for this need is the response they receive from colleagues whose approval and support they are eager to have (Likert 1961). This fact is relevant to the administrator's attempt to introduce a new program. She should take note of what her staff is doing and recognize with appreciation those deeds that contribute to achievement of the objectives of the sought for work and change.

TOWARD STAFF INVOLVEMENT

To involve the staff in a program is basically a leadership or administrative problem. The findings of administrative research, therefore, offer a rich source of guidance in the area of staff involvement.

Administrative leadership may be exhibited in an authoritarian, a democratic, or a laissez faire manner, or in a combination of the three. Each leadership pattern requires cooperation and some degree of commitment, but the effects of each vary; the authoritarian approach often results in low staff morale. The laissez faire approach makes the achievement of objectives a matter of chance rather than of choice, frequently resulting in independent activity. The democratic pattern, although not significantly higher in production outcomes, creates a healthier work climate, which is particularly important for a nursing situation.

In jobs such as nursing, which cannot be highly functionalized and for which time standards cannot be set, there is a direct relationship between the productivity of workers and their attitudes toward all aspects of the work climate including supervision. Likert (1961) points out that administrators who are highly productive tend to exhibit the following common characteristics:

1. They are guided by the fact that any new practice must give promise for improving both attitude and productivity.
2. They rapidly sense any unfavorable shift in attitude among their subordinates and promptly change or stop the activity responsible for the undesirable shift.

3. They avoid putting greater hierarchical pressures on workers to increase production.
4. They tend to use principles and practices of administration that yield better communication and better decisions.

This list appears to state the obvious, yet it makes eminent good sense for an administrator. In essence it states that effective leaders are acutely concerned about staff. The study by Bellows, Gilson, and Odiorne (1962) has shown that when accountants, engineers, or teachers enter their respective fields of work, 80% of their job revolves around their technical background and 20% around their ability to get along with people in the organization. As they move into the ranks of the supervisory hierarchy the technical component decreases and the human relations component increases. In the case of the nursing service supervisor the requirement for human relations increases even more. For the nursing service administrator, the conceptual skills are of the greatest importance, followed closely by human relations skills.

It seems that work or new programs will meet with little resistance in health care organizations in which the individual is motivated (1) to accept the goals and decisions of the group, (2) to seek to influence these groups and decisions so they are consistent with his or her own goals and experience, (3) to communicate fully to the members of the group, and (4) to behave in a way calculated to receive support and recognition from members of the group and particularly from persons whom that individual sees as having more power and status. In such health care organizations the administrator serves as an important resource person for a team effort. By her contribution and conceptual inputs she exercises her leadership role. Good work, change, and acceptance occur because she has opened new perspectives to her staff by involving them. She finds her gratification not in the fact that she is directing and solely responsible for the work and change, but in the fact of its accomplishment.

Means of accomplishing staff involvement
The art of decision making. Nursing is the main activity in health care facilities, and since nurses are the ones who know the most about themselves and the patients to make the most intelligent judgments, all nursing decisions should be made by them. A nursing service administrator stated it succinctly as follows:

> Let's face it. I am a better than average nursing administrator, and I know quite a lot about nursing practice and so forth, but there is at least one nurse on the staff who knows more than I about any single area. It is not always the same nurse, of course, but the fact is that I am not the best data source for any nursing area. I am always saying, "I believe in so-so, but be certain to check with Nurse—, she's the expert in pediatric nursing"; or "See Nurse—, she really knows orthopedic nursing!"

Nursing decisions include not only those that nurses make on the clinical units while practicing nursing or directing nursing activities, but also those concerning how to group patients for a particular activity more effectively and how to organize the staff more effectively. Nurses should be permitted to decide how they are to work together, such as in teams, or by case method, because the method of organization affects decisions about nursing activities, often to a marked extent.

What guarantees do administrators, physicians, and families have that nurses will make rational nursing decisions? How can the board of directors of the health care facility be assured that rational decisions are being made? Assurance can come from the nursing administrator who oversees all decisions and blocks those that appear inconsistent with their goals and values, or the nursing administrator can take responsibility for communicating the goals and values of the board of directors of the institution to the nurses and then monitor their decisions to ensure that they have followed appropriate procedures. The latter approach seems the more appropriate.

The idea that the nursing service administrator should not make direct nursing care decisions has often been erroneously interpreted to mean that the nursing administrator has no voice in the decisions of patient care. What is the administrator's role, then, if nurses make the patient care decisions? Her role is procedural; that is, she is a procedural task master who monitors procedures in two areas: decision making and group processing.

Decision-making monitor. Griffiths (1959) contended that:

> It is the function of the executive to see to it that the decision process proceeds in an effective manner. . . . In fact, the executive is called upon to make a decision only when the organization fails to make its own decision. To put this into other words, if the executive is personally making decisions, this means that there exists malfunctioning in the decision process.
>
> The effectiveness of a chief executive is inversely proportional to the number of decisions which he must personally make concerning the affairs of the organization. It is not the function of the chief executive to make decisions; it is his function to monitor the decision-making process to make certain that it performs at the optimum level.

For example, it is customary for most nursing service administrators to decide how they are going to deploy nurses and how the patients will be grouped. Sometimes nurses are consulted and sometimes they are not, but the ultimate decision is the administrator's.

The position that Griffiths espoused is that the administrator should not decide how to organize the nurse's patient care work on the clinical or specialty units. Assuming the role of a decision-making monitor, the administrator insists that nurses follow appropriate (established) procedures that will assist them in their efforts to make rational decisions. Once nurses have followed these procedures, the administrator is obliged to accept the nurse's decision whether the administrator agrees with it or not.

Procedures are practices that should be followed before making a decision. The source for procedural steps in decision making can be found in the scientific method, whereby a person making a decision typically does the following:

1. Recognizes, defines, and limits the problem
2. Analyzes and evaluates the problem
3. Identifies a number of action alternatives relevant to the problem
4. Predicts the consequences related to each alternate being considered
5. Exercises a choice from among the alternatives

These five steps constitute the prevailing conception of the decision-making process. Although they describe what does occur as a decision is made, they do so in terms that are too general to derive specific guidelines for staff involvement.

At present, nurses seldom have procedures to serve as guidelines for decision making. What are the appropriate procedures for an administrator to promulgate if, for example, the nurses are to make decisions about organizing into a nursing team? The nursing service administrator would do well to advise the nurses to (1) read what scholars and informed practitioners have written on the subject, (2) experiment with several systems or methods, (3) seek advice, (4) become familiar with the experiences of other health care institutions, (5) compare their nursing biases against the nursing philosophy expressed by the board of nursing education, (6) place the system within a long-term plan and consider the implication that it will have on the total community, (7) visit hospitals that are experimenting with different types of staff utilization, and (8) pilot test aspects of the plan.

Procedures appropriate in one decision area may not always be appropriate for another, but they could be similar. They would not necessarily be identical because they have a different character. For example, when a staff coffee break should occur requires a different decision approach than establishing a procedure for the care of a particular patient.

To function as a decision-making monitor, a nursing service administrator must be a capable resource person. A nurse has a right to expect the administrator or members of the support staff to serve as sources of information. The administrator need not be knowledgeable about all areas of nursing but should know what information is available and where to find it. For example, an administrator may not know the results of the latest research on the nursing practice program but should know who does or which journals cover it. She should know if an adjacent community with a new health care facility that experimented with a program is welcoming observers this year, that research proposals to study improved health delivery systems are being sponsored by the Department of Health, Education, and Welfare, or that the administrative interdisciplinary library has journals devoted entirely to the systems approach in organizations. If a nurse's interest continues, the administrator, as a good resource person, might offer to write to the institution producing sample material, request that a consultant visit the institution, or propose discussing the topic at the next staff meeting if the nurse thought it would be useful.

As a resource person, the administrator finds herself in a position similar in responsibility to that of the librarian. No one expects librarians to understand everything about photosynthesis and protozoa, but everyone expects them to know where the information can be found. A resource person not only acts as a source of data for nurses, but also serves as a source of promising and innovative ideas. The administrator is often the only person in the health care organization who has the flexibility of time to gather resource ideas. She visits other organizations in which various federally and privately financed projects are in progress or completed, meets with other administrators and their staffs, and attends regional and national conferences. As a result, she can keep abreast of developments in the field and know about a

variety of nursing service and practice resources available in the health care facility district and the community.

Group process monitor. As nurses become more involved in making nursing decisions, there are systematic procedures to be followed that will tend to maximize more rational decisions. How likely are nurses to follow them?

There is ample documentation to support the view that if personnel are motivated or given the opportunity to participate in decision making, desirable consequences are the result. Studies in industry dating from the famous Western Electric Studies (Roethlisberger 1939) to more recent studies by Coch and French (1948) and by Guest (1960) attest to the results. In the field of nursing, the work of Kramer (1970) and Kramer and Baker (1971) indicated that nurses who report opportunity to participate regularly and actively in making policies and nursing people are enthusiastic about their work in comparison with those who report limited opportunity to participate or practice within the professional role. Social science research since 1935 indicates that the problem in health organization exists not so much in the area of scientific management as in the area of human relations. Mayo, Roethlisberger, Dickson, Levin, and many others had a similar message—that human motivation, participation, decision making, and acknowledging feelings of liking and empathy are central factors to the productivity of a group or organization.

It appears then that participation by nurses in decision making has desirable consequences as far as morale and services are concerned. What characterizes staff involvement? should be asked rather than, Does staff involvement have desirable consequences?

Staff team work. What role does goal definition have in decision making? Are decisions made by a chairman, by majority vote, or by consensus? Who participates in decisions? Do all decisions that are reached result in an action program? How are decisions evaluated? Is leadership diffused or centered in one person? What channels of communication exist between members of the group? How do members feel about the progress of the group? It is important to know what factors contribute to a productive group and which are the most significant.

When a group of nursing supervisors and administrators began to list characteristics of good staff involvement (Western Interstate Commission For Higher Education in Nursing Conference 1972-1973), they thought in terms of teams. In a good team, nurses (1) attend courses at colleges and universities, (2) read literature in nursing, (3) discuss issues in depth, (4) make periodic visits to other health care facilities and other clinical units, (5) experiment with a variety of new methods and procedures, (6) attend local and state conferences, and (7) are constructive members of a group.

The list reveals that the nursing service administrators see a clear relationship between staff involvement and nurses' attitudes toward their work and that good nurses are of inquiring minds. Bennis (1966:47) suggested that a spirit of inquiry serves as a model for organizations. It involves a "hypothetical spirit," and an "experimental spirit." The first includes "a feeling of tentativeness and caution, the respect for . . . probable error." The second includes "the willingness to expose ideas to empirical testing, to procedures, and action." The administrators seemed to identify a good team, that is, a model of organization, with the spirit of inquiry that Bennis described.

The administrator's responsibility to monitor the group process is a difficult task, but it is of critical importance because even the most dedicated group of nurses will possess weaknesses in some category. Some staffs may be so disorganized that the administrator will find it necessary to seek an authority in group

process outside the organization, but she cannot abdicate responsibility in this area.

Another major responsibility the nursing administrator faces, as Bridges (1967:49-61) pointed out, is deciding the "constitutional arrangements" of a group. The three major types of arrangements are "the participant-determining, the parliamentarian, and the democratic-centralist." In the participant-determining and the parliamentarian arrangement, each group member can theoretically exert the same amount of influence on a decision. The difference between the two is that the participant-determining group demands consensus, whereas the parliamentarian demands a plurality vote. The democratic-centralist group places authority in one persons and that person's decision is binding.

In decisions regarding nursing, whether to use a participant-determining or parliamentarian arrangement would vary to fit different types of problems; however, this decision should be left to the nurses.

What constitutes a productive staff involvement? Meyers (1968:55-57) listed the following ten categories that are representative of the thinking of many scholars in the behavioral sciences:

1. Goals. Explicit goals guide the nurses' participation. The staff must begin its group work with some notion of objectives or goals. Both administrative and nursing theory have stressed the need for explicit goals. Systems analysis has recently convinced many persons of the desirability of explicit goals.

2. Shared leadership. A characteristic of productive groups is functional leadership; that is, leadership diffused among the group members so that different persons can assume a leadership role, depending on the function that needs to be performed. It is rare for one person to possess all of the capabilities necessary to lead a group at all times. The problem of leadership is one of the largest stumbling blocks to effective staff involvement because many administrators believe that they must retain the leadership of a group regardless of the function to be performed, and unfortunately, many nurses agree and thus are

unwilling to accept leadership roles that they believe the administrator should perform.

3. Communication. Nurses feel free to engage in an open and frank discussion of all issues. With the gradual demise of the practice of one nurse working with one patient, the interaction between nurses increases. The resulting cooperative arrangements require that nurses relinquish part of their autonomy. This necessitates an open and frank discussion of objectives, methods, and patients.

4. Cooperation and competition. Nurses cooperate with one another and deal openly and realistically with conflict. The combination of cooperation and competition may seem paradoxic, but competition is essential for good group interaction and can provide a vehicle for making progress. Some even claim that it is an inevitable vehicle for progress. Although competition tends to breed conflicts within the group, the nature of group life makes these unavoidable anyway. What is important is that conflicts be dealt with openly and not ignored simply because they are unpleasant.

5. Productivity. Committee meetings as a whole are productive; one meeting may be productive because it generates many new ideas and another because it completes a task. Brainstorming groups are different from task force groups. It is a mistake to evaluate them by the same standard. The accomplishment of a meeting can be evaluated only in terms of whether it reached its stated goals.

6. Evaluation and feedback. Methods for evaluating member behavior and for communicating this information have been developed. Regardless of the processess employed by a group, there is still a need for feedback from member to member. Effective group communication depends on understanding member behavior. Research indicates that individuals will not usually change their behavior unless feedback tells them how their behavior is seen by others.

7. Structure. Nurses form into several types of subgroups to accomplish goals. A group is productive if it is able to change its structure to accomplish its goals. If it is not successful with one structure, it will divide and create two subgroups or it will dissolve for a time and reconstitute itself along completely different lines.

8. Cohesiveness. All members have a sense of belonging to the group and feel free to participate in each meeting. Perhaps members will not contribute verbally because they do not enjoy or feel competent in verbal exchanges, but those members can contribute in many other ways, such as writing reports of the meeting, compiling research findings outside the meeting, or meeting with persons who need to be kept up to date on the progress of the group. The important factor is the cohesiveness of the group, which is generally reflected in the attendance at the meetings.

9. Satisfaction. Members gain satisfaction from their own performance. Individuals like to feel that they have contributed to the success of the group. This sense of worth and satisfaction comes from their own contributions, which is different than the type of satisfaction that comes from seeing a group succeed.

10. Atmosphere. The atmosphere appears constructive and friendly. The atmosphere of a meeting is difficult to measure; consequently, it is difficult to determine its effect on a productive meeting, although it appears to be positively correlated to productivity. When meetings are dull and heavy or when persons appear to withhold their true feelings, the atmosphere is charged and productivity is reduced.

The nursing service administrator and her staff should consider these ten areas of staff involvement as they work in groups. The role of the nursing administrator in the group process is procedural. She does not set goals but insists that the nurses do so. She does not assume leadership or protect it for someone else but encourages those with particular talents to assume leadership when it seems appropriate. She does not take responsibility for all communication but allows an open forum for all to contribute. She does not discourage competition but maintains that conflicts arising from it be dealt with openly. She does not establish all tasks but requires that the nurses clarify the nature of the task. She does not evaluate all activities but encourages frequent feedback from nurses. She does not establish the structure for each group but requires that nurses consider alternate structures. Finally, she personally enters into discussion to encourage cohesiveness, satisfaction, and a constructive and friendly atmosphere.

PHYSICAL ENVIRONMENT
Planning process for physical environment

The conceptual environment developed the realization that the human organization within a health care facility affects personnel functioning and patient recovery. This discussion is devoted to some aspects of the physical environment and its effect on personnel and patients. The health care facility that the architecture will shelter or enclose is composed of groups of people and facilities that can best be described in terms of an operational organization; that is, as subsystems of an overall medical care system.

Because the nursing department reaches into and depends on all other health care facility areas, any trend or criterion that affects the total health care facility affects nursing. Even though the need for a health care facility, the rate and type of construction, and the way in which the hospital is utilized vary widely from community to community, several trends in planning a health care facility are clearly discernible.

The nature of planning is broadening; rather than focusing on merely the building itself, it is looking at factual data or at patient and community needs for specific and general health care. Today, instead of involving only the architect and administrator, planning brings in many competencies, such as community representatives, sociologists, social anthropologists, physicians, nurses, members of the hospital board, and public health experts. Careful coordination of the recommendations of these diverse interests and capacities is essential to produce a health care facility that meets the needs of all for good patient care.

Difficulties arise in a planning problem when new conditions or requirements have no parallel in past experience or when a new factor makes the traditional solution inappropriate. This is indeed often the case in contemporary hospital architecture because changing and broadened concepts of patient care and highly specialized medical practices create demands for facilities that were unknown in the hospitals of the past. Further, the progress in building construction, especially in mechanical equipment systems for building (for example, conveyor systems and air conditioning), allows a wider variety in forms of buildings to accommodate specific needs. All these complications suggest that some statement of guiding principles should be useful in planning, even though a full theory is not possibe at present (or perhaps ever).

We mentioned that the hospital planning process utilizes the skills and expertise of not only design professionals, hospital administrators and medical consultants, but also hospital department heads and a variety of staff members including nurses. The success of the end product, the health care institution, depends on combining the diverse requirements of each department into a coherent arrangement that will satisfy the range of institutional and individual needs.

Souder and co-workers (1970) developed a model in which the planning process is divided into three separate phases. These are the phases of investigation, synthesis, and evaluation. This coincides with our planning model in Fig. 4-1. In the investigation phase, information is collected concerning the functional requirements of the health care facility. Departmental needs are assessed along with cost information and the availability of materials and equipment. Constraints such as budget and site limitations are considered along with all known previously successful planning and design solutions. The synthesis phase is the design or creative process phase. The objective in this phase is to arrive at a number of alternative physical arrangements that will satisfy operational and organizational requirements. The number of alternatives is dependent on the amount of information that has been gathered in the investigation phase. In the third phase, that of evaluation, decisions are reached based on the capacity of a plan to fulfill as many of the requirements as is possible.

In the planning and design of any hospital or other health care facility there is no adequate substitute for mock-ups of the subsystems of the proposed total health care system to test and predict operational quality. Both mock-ups and field studies may conveniently be carried out in existing hospital clinical units or wards without disturbing people unduly. These simulation exercises are low in cost and may include tests of surfacing and other building materials, equipment, and furniture, as well as new patterns of work and organization for staff.

This approach, although idealistic, permits an understanding of the planning process as one that is dynamic rather than static. Within the health care facility, planning for one section may be at the investigation phase while another section is being considered at the evaluation phase. This is especially true when remodeling occurs within an existing facility. At the same time, it is possible to reach one stage only after having completed the preceding stage. For example, it is necessary to collect sufficient and pertinent information to arrive at a plan that offers the most successful arrangement of facilities.

The purpose of the hospital as an institution has traditionally been to return those who are ill to the place they occupied in the society before hospitalization. All the hospital resources, both material and human, are organized to perform this service to society. Talcott Parsons (1958, 1959*a* and *b*) maintained that there are many types of social units and that each possesses a discernible social structure. He divided these units into three levels of social organization: the institutional, the managerial, and the technical.

At the institutional level are the members of the boards of directors and trustees. Their responsibility is to act as the intermediary between the community at large and the managerial and technical levels of operation. This responsibility is fulfilled when they explain organizational operations, solicit financial support, and provide emotional support in guiding the two levels toward congruence and achievement of broad community health care objectives.

It is significant that members of boards of directors are usually selected from the community. Providing for this group within the internal environment of the hospital expresses the symbolic act of bringing the community into the building. It requires the least amount of floor area in proportion to the spatial needs of both the managerial and technical levels. A board room satisfies the requirements associated with the function on this level of the organization.

The managerial level is occupied by administrative and executive officers who coordinate and control the hospital service functions. Decisions on spatial allocation are made at this level and responsibilities of persons who occupy this position include assessing physical environmental needs for staff satisfaction, monitoring daily operational procedures, regulating staffing patterns, and achieving a balance among the various hospital functions.

The primary hospital functions are carried out at the technical level, in which the nursing, medical, and paramedical groups are found. Functions on this level of operations require the largest proportion of floor area within any health care institution. To construct a physical environment that will facilitate and support all functions connected with patient care, it is necessary to have the specific knowledge derived from detailed information about everyday activities, information that is more valid if it emanates from persons who either observe or carry out these functions every day. The type of information that is necessary pertains to action and social structures that surround activities. Specifically, it is important to know which activities are connected to one another, which vary from one another ranging from simple to complex, and which require either combination or separation. For example, patient meals have traditionally been prepared in the hospital kitchen and transported to the nursing units, where they are served by dietary aides. In planning for a changeover to the installation of microwave ovens, the administration (managerial level) needs to consider how this change will affect the existing activity structure from the technical aspects of operating the oven to deciding which person in the hospital social structure will heat the patient's food. Including persons from the day-to-day working level in the decision-making process will aid administrators in the successful implementation of planning decisions. Waiting room activity, although it does not require a large amount of space, is an important part of the hospital experience for the patient's family, and as such, it is now receiving direct planning attention.

The hospital, when viewed from a number of different perspectives (the systems approach and the social organization approach), presents a variety of information, all of which is valuable in relation to the

Table 5. Phenomena associated with physical environment*

Functional concept	Requirements	Criteria of physical environment—unity, flexibility, and economy
Functions of utility, relative to technical objectives	Sufficient space for equipment and personnel Internal arrangement of spaces Communication between related spaces Control of movement Control of environment	1. Minimum distance from nursing station and work area to patient beds 2. Visual access from nursing station to all corridors for efficient monitoring of patients, floor activity, and visitor control 3. Centralized access to the clinical unit and centralization of highly utilized services 4. Separation of specialized traffic to avoid cross-contamination and congestion at highly utilized areas
Functions of amenity, relative to individual satisfaction	Safety and health protection Personal comfort Ease of access and movement Provision for privacy and relaxation	5. Separation of high noise level areas from patient corridors 6. Adequate circulation space in administrative and care centers
Functions of expression, relative to symbolic values of hospital complex	Aesthetic value Conformity Advertising value	7. Spatial layout responsive to changing techniques of professional practice 8. Departmental layout that permits ease in alteration 9. Provision for departmental additions and subtractions 10. Utilization of color 11. Adequate windows 12. Adequate acoustical and temperature control 13. Functional but not expensive 14. Permits adequate provision for the delivery of good medical care 15. Legibility in circulation system for efficiency and convenience 16. Operational efficiency 17. Convenient location and site plan

*Adapted from Souder and co-workers (1970).

main concern of medical practice—the recovery of persons who are sick or injured. The building plays a supporting role because it establishes the container or physical frame for patient care activities. To facilitate the patient's recovery it is necessary to scrutinize the physical arrangements of activities along with staffing and operations patterns to determine the effectiveness of the patient care environment.

The concept of systems and subsystems is a convenient frame of reference for our consideration of hospital problems. The various services in a hospital can be defined as subsystems. Further, a separate subsystem can be defined that is concerned solely with the communication between elements of the hospital.

Objectives for the physical environment of the health care facility

The physical environment of a health care facility needs to meet the criteria of functions, that is, the function that the architecture of health care facility is expected to provide and ways of assessing the performance of these functions or of the operations they shelter (Table 5).

FUNCTIONS

The three functions of the hospital facility—functions here being the broad purposes served rather than the individual patient care operations—may be labeled as utility, amenity, and expressions (Souder and co-workers 1970). These are common words with many shades of definitions, but for present purposes, we assume a restricted definition for each function as follows:

utility the working of the hospital to provide health care services to its community. Special rooms, equipment, and a clean environment for surgery are examples of the utility function of the facility.
amenity the satisfaction of individual or personnel requirements of all those people working and staying in the hospital, as distinct from the health care objectives of the hospital. An attractive and comfortable working environment

for the skilled personnel, who are a vital part of the hospital, is an example of the amenity function.
expression the impact on the community at large of the hospital facility as a public institution and a haven for the ill of the community. In this sense the aesthetic spirit of elegance and quiet contemplation of an art museum, the air of sophistication or power (the corporate image) reflected in a Park Avenue headquarters building, and the suggestion of low overhead cost in the plain brick of a discount store are manifestations of design for expression (Souder and co-workers 1970).

These are still abstract notions. Obviously, planning and design features that contribute to a pleasurable and comfortable working environment can influence work performance; thus, an overlap between utility and amenity functions occurs to some extent. Accommodations for the public, the sense of repose in the environment, and the aesthetic character of the hospital building and site enabling people to recognize it as a community institution are examples of expression.

In a slightly different sense it might be said that utility relates to the hospital's main technical nursing objective, that is, patient care, that amenity relates to individual satisfactions, and that expression relates to the symbolic values of the hospital complex.

PROPERTIES AND MEASURES

There are some specific requirements for a hospital facility, and these may be classified as properties of the three general functions as follows:
1. Utility
   a. Space sufficient for equipment and personnel
   b. Internal arrangement of space
   c. Communication between related spaces
   d. Control of movement
   e. Control of environment
2. Amenity
   a. Safety and health protection
   b. Personal comfort

c. Ease of access and movement

d. Provision for privacy and relaxation

3. Expression

   a. Aesthetic value

   b. Conformity

   c. Advertising value

If a set of properties characterizes architecture, then is assessing those properties a way of finding out how to measure utility, amenity, or expression? The concept of measurement is fundamental in theories of science, and ideas that have been evolved for these purposes can be used (Parsons 1958*b*). Measuring the properties of things —the thickness of a beam, the floor area of a room, or the comfort of an office—rather than the things themselves, is one concept. A subtle distinction is necessary here. The thickness of a beam or the length and width of a floor area can be measured with a yardstick. In these cases one is actually measuring the property of interest, the measure of thickness or area. But how can the property of comfort be measured? Comfort can be measured by identifying one or more indirect measures—air temperature and humidity, noise level, and brightness contrast. Stevens (1951) and Torgerson (1958) differentiate these indirect measures by calling them indicants.

Properties of architecture, then, are either measured directly or indirectly. In a hospital the staff man-hours per day of interdepartmental travel is a direct measure of that property called *relation between spaces*. There are indexes that measure distance, time, and traffic as functions of nursing unit design (Freeman and Smallet 1968; McLaughlin 1964; Pelletier and Thompson 1960).

Intangible properties such as aesthetic values and comfort require indirect measures. For example, it is possible to calculate the amount of time required to transport a patient from one place to another in a hospital, but there is no direct way to measure the patient's comfort in relation to the transport time.

How can the properties of utility, amenity, and expression be measured? Nurses are quick to agree with the common argument that administration and staff are more important than architecture. It is true that one can practice brilliant surgery in any army tent. The vital question is, How much better and more economical a job could be done for patients with the same staff in a well-planned, functional, and stimulating environment? (See Table 5.)

First, a look at the functional concept of utility.

The criterion of unity in the facility is paramount to design and function.

1. Minimum distance from the nursing station and work areas to patient beds.

2. Visual access from nurses station to all corridors for efficient monitoring of patients and floor activity and control of visitors.

3. Centralized access to the clinical unit and centralization of those service areas most highly utilized.

4. Separation of specialized traffic to avoid crosscontamination and congestion at highly utilized areas.

5. Separation of high noise level areas from patient corridors and employment of new soundproofing techniques.

6. Adequate circulation space in and around administrative and care centers.

The functional concept of flexibility or "looseness of fit" is of importance to design. Looseness of fit between the problem and its solution is appropriate to the facility's design to allow for (1) changing techniques of professional practice, (2) the layout of departments to be easily altered to meet such changes, and (3) the addition of some new departments if necessary in the future.

The functional concept of economy deserves much emphasis.

1. A structure need not be expensive to assure a functional facility or hospital.

2. Economy of construction must not lead to the exclusion of essentials for safe and good medical care. The average health

care facility spends as much for operation in three years as was spent on initial construction.

3. Consider possible hidden costs such as personnel turnover due to inconveniences sustained from factors associated with the physical facility, such as physical exertion from walking long corridors.

4. Plan for economy of operation to save a few steps a day and promote other conveniences and safety to achieve continuing economy.

The requirements for creating design alternatives reinforces the notion that no one design will fulfill needs for all situations and acknowledges that there is a need to be apprised of available options from which a selection may be made.

1. Health care facilities come in all forms and shapes, any of which can be functional.

2. Structural details are the architects' responsibility, based on the needs pointed out to them by the nursing staff.

The requirement of quality of safety flows throughout all the other criteria and at the same time is a clearly identifiable entity—protection from such items as (1) cross-infection, (2) patient and employee accident, (3) explosions, and (4) fire.

This discussion concerns the concept of amenity. The process of collaboration is of design concern because it creates a requirement for adequate conference rooms in which nurses may (1) plan for patient care and discuss professional problems, (2) share their knowledge, skills, and attitudes with nursing team colleagues and other professionals of the interdisciplinary health team, and (3) feel motivated to interpersonal exchange within their relationships with one another. Changes in work patterns have influenced the nurse's ideas of comfort. Nurses report that they (1) think more, (2) have become more educated, (3) have taken on more responsibilities, and (4) make a greater contribution because the job and the situation provided an opportunity to do so and not because a superior gave the orders.

The standard of living has improved at home and nurses expect more of the environment in which they are asked to work. The nursing functions of supervision and control call for design solutions that not only facilitate (1) supervision, (2) assignment of personnel, (3) teaching of patients, (4) staffing patterns, and (5) visibility, but also consider the comfort of the nursing staff. Nursing stations manifest constant activity, and the addition of cheerful and bright colors to the picture enhances attractiveness of the nursing station to both patients and nurses.

Aesthetic surroundings bring comfort to nurses, and a pleasingly decorated station will promote a pleasant place to work, thus assisting nurses in their never-ending task of being cheerful and helpful to patients. The physiological needs of individuals places emphasis on comfort for nurses in terms of adequacy of windows, humidity and noise control, some sunshine for all rooms, and a smoothly functioning intercommunication system.

Using carefully selected environments, which were termed beautiful, ugly, and average rooms, Maslow and Mintz (1956) experimented to show the effects of aesthetic surroundings on the individual. Ten negative print photographs of faces were rated by 32 undergraduate men and women. The dimensions rated were energy and well-being; the ranges were from fatigue to energy and from displeasure to well-being. Results showed that the group of subjects commenting in the environment of the beautiful room gave significantly higher ratings, that is, more energy and well-being, than the groups in the average and ugly rooms.

Their rider experiment is of equal relevance to hospital planning and design. The examiners of the subjects themselves were observed over a period of three weeks. The examiner in the ugly room finished testing more quickly than the examiner in the beautiful room and had reactions of monotony, fatigue, headache, discontent, irritability, and avoidance of the room. The beautiful-room examiner, in contrast, had feelings of comfort, pleasure, enjoyment, importance, energy, and a desire to continue the activity.

The conclusion drawn from the two experiments was that visually aesthetic surroundings can have significant effects on persons exposed to them and that these effects are not limited to laboratory situations but may be found under natural circumstances. Knighton (1955), a researcher concerned with hospital planning and design, termed the contribution a hospital building may make through the use of color in its decor as "architectural nursing."

Basic to every design decision is the need for clearly defined goals and objectives (expression). Design of the physical space and design of the methods of operation are two sides of the same coin, but both are meaningless unless associated with a specific goal.

To date, the purpose of a hospital has been to isolate the sick from the community. This was true of the mental institutions built in the country and the now obsolete tuberculosis hospitals as well as the city hospitals.

The image of the hospital before 1880 was an alms house, a place for the needy and the poor. A place not to live in but to die in. With the influence of Florence Nightingale the image of the hospital as a place in which to die was slowly transformed into the image of a place with nursing care. The nursing hospital that should do no harm developed slowly into a hospital whose goal was to do some good. A complex array of technical services and equipment was added to the nursing center. The demands on the diagnostic and therapeutic departments of the hospital to be both expandable and have proximity to one another, to serve both the bed patient and the ambulant patient, coupled with the technological developments of the elevator and air-conditioning, made possible the hospital form so common today, that is, the large diagnostic base topped by the nursing tower. The private room with private bath has become the prototype of the hospital patient room.

Today there is a new hospital goal. Those in the health care field view the hospital as a dynamic force for health education and for preventive medicine as well as a place for curing the sick and injured. The problem is to weave the hospital or health care facility into the surrounding urban fabric. The advent of new technology generates new forms of spatial organization.

What criteria can be used to measure the aesthetic qualities of the health care institution and the architectural planning of the life space? Together these factors constitute a significant principle of patient care approach, since these aspects deal essentially with human qualities. To an affluent society with rising standards of living, health becomes one of the most important factors to be dealt with, and the people of the community measure the aesthetic value of a physical building by the following criteria: (1) *Medical security* or relief of stress. The community expects the health care facility to be conveniently located to every member of the public whose medical condition requires the use of resources provided in the community's hospital, even though this means fragmenting its hospital system into uneconomic-sized units; the community expects to utilize its hospitals at its convenience rather than in the most efficient manner. (2) *Site selection.* Is the site large enough and properly located? The important point made is that the facility be located near important and other impressive governmental buildings and that it be made an integral part of the environment. (3) *Knowledge and technology.* The health care facility is judged by its spatial organization, generally made possible by the advent of new technology. It expresses the function of the hospital and directly affects the patient's recovery. (4) *Education and research.* Is the facility an educational institution? Does it contribute to the education of medicine, nursing, and paramedical personnel and, by its research, contribute to better health? This determines the character of the organization, which distinguishes it from other institutions. The community points to new facilities and community services of high quality so that the educational effort will not prove abortive. (5) *Investment and cost.* A price tag is placed on the facility, and the information is public knowledge. The aesthetic value is often measured by its social significance, known to the community as functional significance, a quality about which there is likely much agreement. Aesthetic significance is one environmental quality about which there would likely be less agreement.

CONCLUDING COMMENTS AND GUIDING PRINCIPLES

The framework for health care facility planning set forth is a set of hypotheses founded on two tenets proposed by Souder and co-workers (1970): (1) the health care facility planning process is basically an orderly, rational endeavor, and (2) the planning process can be viewed as a three-phase process of investigation, synthesis, and evaluation.

The hypotheses that follow are labeled as propositions, statements to be examined and tested but in the meantime serve as an adequate basis for some conditional statements.

Proposition 1. The requirements of all the levels of social organization are satisfied by architectural and operational pattern of health care organization. An item of architecture or of operational pattern may satisfy the requirements of one or more levels of social organization.

Proposition 2. The activities of various levels of health care organizations differ. The technical level is engaged in detailed, specific activities and responsibilities, the organizational level being less detailed and the institutional level being least specific. The architectural utility requirements need to be developed at the technical level, amenity requirements at the organizational level, and expression requirements at the institutional level.

Proposition 3. The majority of the objectives or performances of health care facilities are measurable in terms of either objective measures or on subjective scales.

Proposition 4. The performances of the health care facility are affected by the arrangement of physical resources and functioning patterns. Therefore, performance is influenced by planning strategy. Furthermore, the anticipated effects of alternative planning choices on health care facility performance can be evaluated.

Proposition 5. It is possible to measure the various requirements of any one function (such as that of utility or amenity or expression) in terms of a single additive composite score or criterion. However, the requirements and measures of the three functions are not mutually interrelatable in common terms; therefore they cannot be presented in one sum or in one score.

Proposition 6. Since objectivity of measurement decreases as one progresses from utility to amenity to expression, it may be wise in the planning strategy to consider the requirements of expression first, amenity next, and utility last. In this way the more abstract requirements of expression will act as constraints rather than as specific variables to be considered in the planning process. One shortcoming of such an approach is that an ill-chosen requirement for expression or amenity may inhibit the development of an appropriate design for utility.

Proposition 7. Accurate assessment of the health care facility's past performances and operational patterns should result in an improved planning process.

Proposition 8. The effectiveness of the planning process and the quality of the end product are improved by the development and examination of a large number of architectural arrangements and operational patterns of the health care facility.

Proposition 9. The nature of the health care facility and the large number of variables that need to be taken into consideration in the planning process limit the use of simple guidelines. Therefore, it is desirable to have a technique that enables the plan to handle a large number of variants in the planning and evaluation possibilities.

Proposition 10. The variables of the construction budget, quality of patient care, and location of the health care facility often act as constraints in finding an acceptable solution to the planning problem.

Proposition 11. There is more freedom in finding solutions to the planning problem if the planning of organizational and operational patterns proceed concurrently with, rather than ahead of, the initial planning of architectural arrangements.

These propositions do not include any that will help to set the proper balance among performances of the utility, amenity, and expression functions. The client's wishes go into any decision governing a project, of course, but in general the balance for any given type of architecture (such as hospitals or schools) seems to be determined by consensus of society as a whole, using suggestions from architects tempered by critical comment reflecting public reaction as a base. No one proper balance can be meaningful in the absolute sense, although as one learns more of other cultures one discovers the balance these propositions strike and correlates them with other features of one's own culture.

In concluding these abstractions—social organization, amenity, properties, and measures—the question is posed, Is the problem of planning really complex, or is the issue being confused by imposing a theory? Take, for example, the hospital project. The client and principal information source for it are a community and its medical care facility, a social organization. The hospital that the architecture will shelter or enclose is composed of groups of people and facilities, an operational organization or subsystems of an overall medical care system. Finally, the buildings themselves must embody their own architectonic organization (for example, logic of structure adaptation to site). Thus, the hospital planners are expected to juggle three complicated "organizations" of things and ideas—the client organization, the process organization, and the building organization—and come up with a functioning, yet economical, structure.

The problem is complex, and the conceptual framework suggested here should be a useful tool for coping with that complexity.

The planning process and the hypotheses concerning aspects of hospital planning can serve as a basis for computer-aided planning methodology. The hypotheses should be susceptible to proof at some future time.

REFERENCES

Argyris, C.: Integrating the individual and the organization, New York, 1964, John Wiley & Sons, Inc.

Baumgartel, H.: Changing goals of human relations training. In Bacon, R., editor: Personal and organizational effectiveness, New York, 1972, McGraw-Hill Book Co., Ltd., (U. K.)

Bennis, W. G.: Changing organizations, New York, 1966, McGraw-Hill Book Co.

Berelson, B., and Steiner, G. A.: Human behavior, New York, 1964, Harcourt, Brace & World, Inc.

Brayfield, A. H., and Crokett, W. H.: Employee attitudes and employee performance, Psychol. Bull. 4:377-395, 1955.

Bridges, E. M.: A model for shared decision-making in the school principalship, Educ. Admin. Q. 3:49-61, Winter 1967.

Burns, J., and Stalker, G. M.: The management of innovation, London, 1961, Tavistock Pubs., Ltd.

Coch, L., and French, J. R. P., Jr.: Overcoming resistance to change, Hum. Relations 1(4):512-532, 1948.

Cofer, C. N., and Rosenthal, D.: The effect on group performance of an individual and neglected attitudes shown by one group member, J. Exp. Psychol. 38:568-577, 1948.

Dalton, G. W., Barnes, L. B., and Zalesnik, A.: Organizational structure and design, Homewood, Ill., 1959, Dorsey Press.

Dill, W. R.: Environment as an influence on managerial autonomy, Admin. Science Q. 2:442-443, March 1958.

Emery, F., and Trist, E. L.: The causal texture

and organizational environments, Hum. Relations **18**:211-232, 1965.

Freeman, J. R., and Smallet, H. E.: An objective basis for inpatient nursing unit design, Atlanta, Ga., 1968, School of Industrial Engineering, Georgia Institute of Technology.

Galbraith, J. K.: Organizational design, Cambridge, Mass., 1969, Institute of Technology, Sloan School of Management.

Griffiths, D. E.: Administration theory, New York, 1959, Appleton-Century-Crofts.

Guest, R. H.: Organizational change: the effect of successful leadership, Homewood, Ill., 1960, Dorsey Press.

Hare, P. A.: Handbook of small group research, New York, 1962, The Free Press of Glencoe.

Harrington, H. A., and Theis, E. C.: Institutional factors perceived by baccalaureate graduates as influencing their performance as staff nurses, Nurs. Res. **17**:228-235, 1968.

Homans, G. C.: The human group, New York, 1961, Harcourt, Brace & World, Inc.

Huse, E. F., and Bowditch, J. L.: Behavior in organizations: a systems approach to managing, Reading, Mass., 1973, Addison-Wesley Pub. Co., Inc.

Kahn, R., Wolfe, D., Quinn, R., Snoek, O. O., and Rosenthal, R.: Organizational stress, New York, 1964, John Wiley & Sons, Inc.

Knighton, P. H.: The use of colour in hospitals, Ward, Newcastle upon Tyne, 1, April 1955.

Kramer, M.: Role conception of baccalaureate and success in hospital nursing, Nurs. Res. **19**(5): 428-439, 1970.

Kramer, M., and Baker, C.: The exodus: can nursing afford it? J. Nurs. Admin. **1**(3):15-30, 1971.

Langford, E. M.: Hospital climate which provides for research while maintaining safety and attention to human needs, Pamphlet, New York, May 5, 1960, American Nurses' Association.

Lawrence, P., and Lorsch, J.: Organization and environment: management differentiation and integration, Boston, 1967, Harvard Business School, Division of Research.

Likert, R.: New patterns of management, New York, 1961, McGraw-Hill Book Co.

March, J. G., and Simon, H. A.: Organizations, New York, 1958, John Wiley & Sons, Inc.

Maslow, A. H., and Mintz, N. L.: Effects of aesthetic surroundings, J. Psychol. **41**:247-254, 1956.

Mayo, E.: The social problems of an industrial civilization, Boston, 1945, Harvard Business School, Division of Research.

McLaughlin, H.: What shape is best for nursing units? Mod. Hosp. **103**(6):12-20, December 1964.

Meyers, D. A.: The art of decision-making, Dayton, Ohio, 1968, Institute for Development of Educational Activities, Inc.

Novotney, J. M.: What will they listen to? Cath. School J. **66**(7):84-85, September 1966.

Parsons, T.: Some ingredients of a general theory of formal organization. In Halpin, A. W., editor: Administrative theory in education, Chicago, 1958, University of Chicago Press.

Parsons, T.: A general theory of social organization. In Merton, R. K., Broom, L., and Cottrell, L. A., Jr., editors: Sociology today, New York, 1959*a*, Basic Books Inc., Pubs.

Parsons, T.: Structure and process in modern societies, New Work, 1959*b*, The Free Press.

Pelletier, R. J., and Thompson, J. D.: Yale index measures design efficiency, Mod Hosp. **95**(5): 73-77, November 1960.

Porter, D. E., and Applewhite, P. P.: Studies in organizational behavior and management, Scranton, Pa., 1964, International Textbook Company, 1964.

Rice, A. K.: The enterprise and its environment, London, 1963, Tavistock Pubs., Ltd.

Roethlisberger, F. J., and Dickson, W. J.: Management and the worker, Cambridge, Mass., 1939, Harvard University Press.

Schein, E. H.: Organizational psychology, ed. 2, Englewood Cliffs, N. J., 1970, Prentice-Hall, Inc.

Slivnick, P., Kerr, W., and Kosinar, W.: A study of accidents, Personnel Psychol. **1**:43-52, 1957.

Souder, J. J., Clark, W. E., Elkind, J. I., and Brown, M. B.: A conceptual framework for hospital planning. In Proshausky, H. M., Ittelson, W. H., and Rivlin, L. G., editors: Environmental psychology, man and his physical setting, New York, 1970, Holt, Rinehart & Winston, Inc.

Stevens, S. S.: Mathematics, measurement and psychophysics. In Handbook of experimental psychology, New York, 1951, John Wiley & Sons, Inc.

Thompson, J. D.: Organizations in action, New York, 1967, McGraw-Hill Book Co.

Torgerson, W. S.: Theory and methods of scaling, New York, 1958, John Wiley & Sons, Inc.

Trist, E., Higgin, G., Murray, H., and Pollack, A.: Organizational choice, London, 1963, Tavistock Pubs., Ltd.

Von Gilmer, B.: Industrial psychology, ed. 2, New York, 1966, McGraw-Hill Book Co.

Watson, G., editor: Concepts for social change, Washington, D. C., 1967, National Training Laboratories.

Western Interstate Commission for Higher Education in Nursing: Boulder, Colo., 1972-1973.

Wolf, W. B.: Management: readings toward a general theory, Wolf, W. B., editor: Belmont, Calif., 1966, Wadsworth Pub. Co.

ADDITIONAL READINGS

Argyris, C.: Interpersonal competence and organizational effectiveness, Homewood, Ill., 1962, Dorsey Press.

Arndt, C., and Laeger, E.: Role strain in a diversified role set: the director of nursing service. I. Role strain in a diversified role set, Nurs. Res. 19(3):253-259, 1970.

Arndt, C., and Laeger, E.: Role strain in a diversified role set: the director of nursing service. II. Sources of stress, Nurs. Res. 19(3): 495-501, 1970.

Baumgartel, H., and Mann, F.: Absences and employee attitudes, Ann Arbor, Mich., 1952, Institute for Social Research.

Bellows, R., Gilson, Th. Q., and Odiorne, G. S.: Executive skills for dynamics and development, Englewood Cliffs, N. J., 1962, Prentice-Hall, Inc.

Fleishman, E. A.: Leadership climate: human relations training and supervisory behavior, Personnel Psychol. 3:205-222, 1953.

Kahn, R. L., and Katz, D.: The social psychology of organizations, New York, 1966, John Wiley & Sons, Inc.

Likert, R.: Measuring organizational performance, Harvard Business Review 36(2):41-50(b), 1958.

Lindheim, R.: Factors which determine hospital design, Am. J. Public Health 56(10):1668-1675, 1966.

Schein, E. H., and Bennis, W. G.: Personal and organizational change through group methods: the laboratory approach, New York, 1965, John Wiley & Sons, Inc.

Souder, J. J., Clark, W. E., Elkind, J. I., and Brown, M. B.: Planning for hospitals: a systems approach using computer-aided techniques, Chicago, 1964, American Hospital Association, pp. 31-37.

Steiner, G.: The creative organization, Chicago, 1965, The University of Chicago Press.

U. S. Department of Health, Education, and Welfare: Public Health Service Publication No. 721, Washington, D. C., 1960, The Division of Hospital and Medical Facilities Public Health Service.

Chapter 6

EVALUATION AND MEASUREMENT

The process of evaluation is essentially the process of determining to what extent the organizational and individual objectives are actually being realized. Scriven (1966:40) views evaluation to "consist ... of the gathering and combining of performance data with a weighted set of goal scales to yield either comparative or numerical ratings, and in the justification of (a) data-gathering instruments (b) the weightings and (c) the selection of goals." Tyler (1951:48) defines it as "the process of appraisal which involves the acceptance of specific values and the use of a variety of instruments of evaluation, including measurements, as basis for value judgments."

Our purpose in this chapter is to provide the nursing service administrator and others in charge of evaluation with a theoretical framework for effective evaluation of a program, a project, an individual's performance, or a curriculum. Since a theory is a guide to action, evaluators can use this framework to evaluate the degree to which their set objectives are being reached and make decisions in accordance with these findings about revisions.

The first part of this chapter is concerned with the rationale—the purpose of the process of evaluation. Following this is an explanation of the different kinds of evaluation—their purposes, functions, and characteristics. Next we will deal with the area of measurement—the different kinds, uses, and characteristics, and finally we will present a model of evaluation for a set of objectives.

The basic purpose of evaluation for the administrator of a health care institution (or its nursing department or a given program of study) is to make decisions and judgments. Evaluation, then, is an attempt to determine whether or not an individual is "pulling his weight." The same evaluation can be made about an institution that has been set up to meet the needs of a community, such as a hospital—Is the community "getting its money's worth"?

There are two major functions of evaluation: to ascertain the nature and size of the effects of the treatment and to decide whether or not the observed effects attain acceptable standards of excellence. These two components have been termed *description* and *judgment* by Stake (1967). We cannot overemphasize the use of value judgments in evaluation. Value judgments are made at many phases in the development and assessment of the administrative and instructional systems. Too frequently value judgments, at least explicitly, are faced only at the decision-making stages (Messick 1970). Judgments determine what the anticipated behavior, product, or service outcomes are, how they are to be reached, the components and constructs to be measured, and the selection of instruments or techniques to assess the components and constructs, and at a later stage, they are used to reach decisions from the outcome data matrix.

Since evaluation is concerned with securing evidence on the attainment of specific organizational and individual objectives, methods must be found to judge the extent to which the objectives have been reached. The standards against which the evidence is appraised may be the usual type of normative data on a particular sample; it may also include absolute criterion-referenced standards. It may even include the performance of the individual learner as a standard. For example, a change in the performance of the learner over one period of time can be contrasted with the change in that employee over another period of time.

In addition to the judgmental aspect, evaluation is also concerned with interpretation of data. For example, evaluation need not be confined to a summative combination of items or scores. Various patterns of outcomes may be interpreted to determine the kinds of changes taking place in the individual performer or in the programs, the kinds of errors that are made, and the reasons underlying the attainment or lack of attainment of the specified objectives.

To effectively evaluate individual objectives, it is necessary to be explicit about the ways individuals relate to one another in terms of the following:

The individual personally
The environment
The individual's performance

This explicitness can then be extended to include more details about performance, antecedent individual behavior, and environmental characteristics. With appropriate multivariate statistical tools for this approach, cause and effect relations can then be estimated and conclusions reached about administration not possible with any other approach.

Within a teaching-learning or performance situation, evaluation involves the systematic collection of evidence to determine whether or not certain desirable changes in behavior or performance are taking place, as well as to determine the degree of change in individuals (Bloom, Hastings, and Madaus 1971).

This conception of evaluation has two important aspects:

1. Evaluation must appraise the behavior of the individual since it is change in this behavior that is sought in education or administration. If a project for improvement of patient care is being evaluated, then the behavior to be evaluated is change in improvement of patient care.
2. Evaluation must involve more than a single appraisal at any one time to determine whether or not change has taken place. Appraisals at an early point at later points identify changes that may be occurring.

Evaluation procedure

It is necessary to have evaluation procedures that will give evidence about each of the kinds of behaviors implied by each of the major organizational and individual objectives. For example, if one of the objectives is to apply the individual's knowledge of both personnel and organizational policies in a work situation, then it is necessary that evaluation give some evidence of the application of that knowledge. This means that the two-dimensional analysis of objectives also serves as the basis for planning the evaluation procedure as well as serving as a set of specifications for evaluation. Thus, in the case of objectives regarding application of knowledge about policies, the two-dimensional analysis indicates that evaluation of application of knowledge must be made for (1) behavior and (2) content heading. Content heading indicates what areas of knowledge should be sampled to have a satisfactory appraisal of the knowledge being applied by the individual in this field. In this situation the content area is organizational and personnel policies (see Table 6).

In this way a two-dimensional analysis of objectives becomes a guide to the evaluation of organizational and individual objectives of the administration in any health care institution. This also means that the process of evaluation may force persons who have not previously clarified their objectives to do so. Definition of objectives, then, is an important step in evaluation.

The next step in the evaluation procedure is to identify the situations that will give the employees the chance to express the behavior that is implied by their individual objectives. The only way one can tell whether or not employees have acquired a certain kind of behavior is to give them an opportunity to show this behavior. This means that the administrator must find situations that not only permit the expression of the behavior but actually encourage it. Nursing service administrators are then in a position to observe the degree to which the objectives are actually being achieved. For example, if they want evidence of employees' ability to express themselves orally or in written form, they must look into situations in which oral or written expressions are exhibited.

The principle is a simple one. An evaluative situation is one that permits individuals to exhibit the kind of behavior their supervisor is trying to appraise.

Before selecting a procedure to appraise a given administrative or educational program, it is necessary to first identify both the objectives of the program and the kinds of situations that would evoke the proper behavior.

Once this has been accomplished, it is then necessary to divise a means of getting a record of the individual's behavior in the test situation. In a written test, employees make their own records in writing. However, situations that require interviewing or appraisal of reaction formations to specific situations or appraisal of demonstrations of motor performances (demonstrating a catheterization procedure, for example), it is difficult to have written records. Here, a tape recording of the interview or a detailed description of the reaction recorded by an observer would be useful. The observer could use a checklist and check off particular kinds of behavior that commonly appear. The essential characteristics of evaluation tools are specification of the terms or units that will be used to summarize or to appraise the record of

behavior obtained, objectivity and the reliability of the instrument, sampling, and validity. These characteristics are discussed in detail later in this chapter.

The next step in the process of evaluation is the gathering of data. Once data are collected and statistically analyzed, they are then interpreted for the following purposes:

1. The extent to which the specific organizational or individual objective has been accomplished. For example, if the individual objective dealt with learning and application of knowledge of hospital policies, then the results of evaluation will determine the amount of learning and application that has taken place in the individual.
2. The strengths and the weaknesses that help indicate where the individual may need help or improvement.
3. Identification of strengths and weaknesses and examination of these data to suggest possible hypotheses about the reasons for this particular pattern of strengths or weaknesses.

The same type of interpretation of data and evaluative procedure is applied in evaluating any organizational objective, whether it deals with delivery of patient care or development of physical or conceptual environment.

What is implied in all of this is that administrative planning is a continuous process and that as technology and education advance, as materials and procedures are developed, they are tried out, results appraised, inadequacies identified, and suggested improvements indicated. There is replanning, redevelopment, and then reappraisal. In this kind of continuing cycle, it is possible for the administrative or instructional programs to be continuously improved over the years. In this way we may hope to have an increasingly more effective patient care and administrative program.

Evaluation procedures have other values as well. For example, the very fact that it is not possible to make an evaluation until objectives are clearly defined so that one can recognize the behavior to be sought means that evaluation is a powerful device for clarifying organizational and individual objectives, if they have not already been clarified in the planning process. (Tyler 1970).

Evaluation procedures are also very useful in the individual guidance of employees. It is not only valuable to know about their background, but also to know about their achievement of various kinds of objectives to have a better notion both of their needs and their capabilities.

Finally, evaluation becomes one of the important ways of providing information about the success of the health care institution to the institution's clientele. Evaluation results need to be translated ultimately in terms that will be understandable to consumers of the health care delivery system (patients, employees, and other clientele) and the general public. Only as the results from the health care system are described more accurately (accurate description of intended outputs in terms of achievement of organizational and individual objectives) is the health care program in a position to get support from the consumers and the community.

Thus, the nursing service administrator and others in charge of evaluation must expect to use evaluative procedures to determine what desirable changes are actually taking place in the organization's programs and in individual employees, where they are achieving their organizational and individual objectives, and where they must make still further modifications to get an effective health care delivery system.

In conclusion, therefore, evaluation is a method of acquiring and processing the evidence needed to improve the institution's outputs and the individual's performance and accomplishments. Evaluation is used as an aid in clarifying the significant goals and objectives of organization and individuals and as a process for determining the extent to which individual employees and their institutions are developing in desired ways. It is a system of quality control in which at each step in the administrative composite process it can be determined whether the process is effective or not and, if not, what changes must be made to ensure its effectiveness. Also, evaluation is a tool in administrative practice for ascertaining whether or not alternative procedures are equally effective in achieving a set of organizational and individual objectives.

TYPES OF EVALUATION: FORMATIVE AND SUMMATIVE

In this discussion two types of evaluation are presented, and their characteristics and specific uses as applied to evaluation of organizational and individual objectives are discussed.

Formative evaluation

Formative evaluation involves the collection of appropriate evidence during the construction and implementation of a new project, plan, curriculum, or a new learning in an individual in such a way so that revisions can be made, based on this evidence. Formative evaluation is applied while the project or course of study is still fluid and in the process of development. Its role is in improving the course of study or project or whatever is being evaluated and in finding the worth of a completed product. In contrast, summative evaluation is used for assessment at the end of a course, plan, project, or unit when no changes in treatment for the project will be made.

Some authorities regard formative evaluation as being not only useful as a tool in the planning and construction stage of a project, but also useful as an instructive learning device for the individual. Teaching and learning can be utilized at every phase of project planning.

When using formative evaluation methods, one must be sure to seek the most dependable evidence, to report it accurately and fairly, and to try to avoid negative or judgmental conclusions. In formative evaluation, the hope is always to use the information obtained in ways best calculated to contribute to the individual's learning process and also to the achievement of the needs of the individual and the organization.

One of the chief aims of formative evaluation is to determine the degree of mastery of a given patient care task (organizational objective) or a learning task (individual objective) and to pinpoint the part of the task not mastered. Both the learner and the teacher are thus helped.

The very essence of formative evaluation lies in the successful communication of information to the learners about their progress (with some immediacy). Summative tests can be used in this communications area as well. Such tests can be given at various times during the formation of a given project, or a large test can be given at the conclusion of the project. Generally speaking, however, summative evaluation takes place after completion of the project, course, or whatever is being evaluated, and its main purpose is to report the final output in terms of Oi and Og, resulting in judgments and decisions on the part of the evaluator.

CHARACTERISTIC OF FORMATIVE EVALUATION: SPECIFICATION OF UNIT OF LEARNING OR PERFORMANCE

Fundamental to the use of formative evaluation is the selection of a unit of learning or performance of a task. The nature of the unit may vary for different purposes, and its delineation may be arbitrary. Ideally, it should be determined by natural breaks in the subject matter or by the content that makes a meaningful whole. A unit of learning or performance can also be specified in relation to a given period of time. The task of determining specifications for formative evaluation is much the same as that of creating specifications for summative evaluation.

The first step in formative evaluation is to analyze a learning unit or performance. The *content* and *behavior* aspect of objec-

tives constitute the component of learning unit. Bloom, Hastings, and Madaus (1971) suggest that one way to do this is to determine what new content or subject matter has been introduced in the new unit. For example, in a teaching-learning situation, determination of new content may be to determine the new terms, facts, relations, procedures, or applications that have been explained, defined, illustrated, or otherwise presented in the learning material. An example of this is the formative evaluation of nursing service personnel at the completion of a six-week orientation program that would determine what new terms the nurse has learned, for example, nursing process and flow chart. What other facts, relations, procedures, or applications of policies and procedures has the nurse learned?

A second step concerns the determination of the behavior that is related to each new element of content. In other words, what is the individual's behavior expected to be and how is it expected to change in terms of each new idea or term? What is the individual expected to do with the new material presented in the learning unit?

Bloom, Hastings, and Madaus (1971) classified new material in accordance with some of the categories in the Taxonomy of Educational Objectives (Bloom 1956), which delineate a hierarchy of behavioral levels in terms of complexity levels of the learning process. This includes a knowledge of terms, concepts, facts, rules, and principles, skill in using procedures, and the ability to make translations and applications.

A unit of performance for a specific project for formative evaluation in the department of nursing can be set up in stages. For example, if the project consists of implementation of team nursing throughout the hospital in three stages, then the content aspect of the unit of performance would be, for example, knowledge of terms such as team nursing, team leader, and team conference; facts about group functioning and team composition; knowledge about principles of group dynamics and goals; and skill in using and implementing the process of team nursing. The behavior aspect would be the determination of what the nursing personnel would expect to do with team nursing. How frequently should the team leader (registered nurse) hold team conferences? In other words, what should be the behavioral outcomes? Once the unit of performance or learning is identified, then these items can be used as test items in performing the formative type evaluation for the first stage of the project. In this way formative evaluations can be done at the completion of each stage, so one can assess its progression, give feedback, and make appropriate changes before proceeding to the next stage.

Another example of the development of a unit of performance for formative evaluation could be the organizational objective that is set up to ensure optimum delivery of care to all patients. This can be done by assessing each patient's physical and psychosocial needs and determining the degree to which they have been met at the end of a given period of time, perhaps three months, six months, or a year. Outcomes in the form of feedback from these formative evaluations are incorporated in future planning of care to improve the delivery of care. This cycle continues until the accomplishment of that specific patient care objective has reached the standard of care maintained in the specific health care institutions. Our goal is 80% to 85%.

PURPOSES AND FUNCTIONS OF FORMATIVE EVALUATION

One of the major functions of formative tests is learner *diagnosis* or, in the case of a patient care project, diagnosis of the degree of achievement of patient care objectives. Formative tests should reveal particular points of difficulty. For example, if an employee lacks mastery of a particular unit, formative tests should point out in which area the employee went wrong. Diagnosis shows the elements in the learning or performance situation that the individual has not mastered. It has been observed by Bloom, Hastings, and Madaus (1971) that individuals undergoing difficulties respond best to the diagnostic results when they are referred to particular instructional materials or remedial learning situations. The supervisor should next provide the employee with a very specific prescription. Formative evaluation tests should be regarded as part of the learning process and should in no way be confused with the judgment of the capabilities of the employee or student or used as a part of final evaluation for grading purposes.

The second major function of formative evaluation is for *feedback* purposes. In a teaching-learning or performance situation, formative evaluation provides feedback to the learner (staff nurse) and to the teacher (supervisor) as well. A score on a formative evaluation test has little value in the learning process other than to reassure some individuals and to make others aware that they have more to learn. What the individuals need is feedback regarding the mastery of the various objectives in a given unit of learning, or performance, and what they still need to learn. The location of their difficulties provides a useful kind of feedback for the individuals, especially if they are motivated to do the additional learning necessary to master the cognitive or motor skills that they did not master originally.

Obviously, feedback is valuable to the teacher or supervisor in that particular points in the instruction or orientation programs can be pinpointed as being in need of modification.

What is also implicitly indicated is quality control. Comparing the performance of one group of students or employees with the results achieved by an earlier group provides a means to judge that performance, assessing whatever changes that may have been incorporated in the instruction process with the overall objective of improvement.

The third major function of formative evaluation is *pacing*. Frequent formative tests pace the learning of the individuals and help motivate them to put forth the necessary effort at the proper time. Appropriate use of these tests enables and assures the individuals that they will have mastered each set of learning tasks before embarking on new tasks. Similarly, formative tests pace the progress and the timing of projects.

The fourth function of formative evaluation is its *reinforcing effect*. For individuals who have thoroughly mastered the subject or unit of learning, the formative evaluation should reinforce this learning and assure them that their present strategy for learning and performance is on target. Knowledge of results in this form of feedback and the resultant feeling of achievement become very satisfying, motivating, and reinforcing for the individuals.

A fifth function of formative evaluation takes place at the outset and concerns *initial assessment,* which has to do with the behavior of the individuals as they enter the learning unit. Here the teacher or supervisor will give a formative evaluation test as a pretest to determine what the learners are relevantly bringing to their learning task and what are their strengths and weaknesses to make appropriate judgments and decisions.

For example, an experienced professional nurse will manage a nursing team much more efficiently than will a recently graduated nurse who has had no experience with team managing other than observation.

In this situation, a formative evaluation test is given as a pretest to find out where the individuals are at and give feedback information to the teacher or supervisor with regard to employees' capabilities, their state of readiness, and the areas that need strengthening. With this information in mind, the supervisor can make necessary

decisions about individual learners and their learning needs. Part of this initial evaluation can be obtained by previous records of the individual and from special diagnostic placement or aptitude test or both.

Such initial assessments can also be applied in evaluation of any organization objectives. For example, if the nursing service administrator wants to improve or change the number of hours and quality of care patients are receiving every day, she must first examine the situation at the given moment, pretest it to establish a baseline so that she will have a point of comparison in terms of the goals and the achievement of them.

Forecasting comprises the sixth function of formative evaluation. This is the situation in which both formative and, a few months later, summative tests are administered to the individual. Since there is some overlap between the tests with regard to area of content, behavior, and even evaluative procedures, it is likely that the two types of test results will be related. Bloom, Hastings, and Madaus (1971) have found that, with such a combination, certain predictions can be made, that is, one can anticipate results of summative tests. Thus, if leaders and learners wish, they can change the direction of a given forecast.

Summative evaluation

As indicated earlier, summative evaluation takes place at the end of a term, a course, or a project for purposes of *judgment of progress.* Certification or accreditation may be involved here. This kind of evaluation is more comprehensive than formative evaluation.

In addition to some of the differences between these two kinds of evaluations already mentioned, there are obviously differences in timing. Formative evaluation tests are given at much more frequent intervals and are utilized whenever the preliminary instruction on a new skill or concept is completed or at the completion of a first stage of a project. In other words, formative evaluation is the gathering of information in the early phases of the development of a system of instruction or administration, and summative evaluation provides information to the potential consumer of administrative products.

MEASUREMENT AS A METHOD OF EVALUATION

Measurement is the process of assigning quantitative values to observed phenomena. Scientific measurement is "a matter of counting units that are agreed upon as being generated by the same operation" (Gagne 1970:106). Unlike the situation in the evaluative process, in measurement no judgment is passed; essentially the essence of measurement is, Here is the data; do with it what you want.

Two very simple questions are the concern of this subject, What is to be measured? and How much?

In the case of the first question, obviously everyone concerned with a given project would have to agree on a definition of the unit and a common label. This is easy enough when measuring something universal such as liquid. But in more indirect measurements, such as performance, learning, and patient care, common agreement can be much more difficult.

Likewise, How much? can be tricky because of the difficulties of the varying sizes of the unit as well as standardization. What if the unit were "apple"? How would one determine "standard apple"? Therefore, indirect measurement requires that there is an operationally defined set of operations as a basis for agreement on the inference as to what is measured.

Two primary criteria of measurement are *distinctiveness* and *freedom from distortion*. Distinctiveness is a function of how the outcome of one level of learning or performance is distinguished from another, and freedom from distortion deals with a set of operations that distinguish learning

or performance from the action of other variables of various sort.

An overall goal of measurement is to completely account for variables in the total unit by the use of a small number of units of measurement. Measurement tests are used to classify and predict, and they are also used for experimentation.

As discussed earlier, evaluation recognizes and utilizes the effects of testing on the individual. Measurement, on the other hand, strives to limit the control of the effect of testing on the individual's performance. Evaluation is concerned with desirable change; measurement with equalizing the opportunities in that area in which the individual will be tested.

A major quest in evaluation is for the identification of condition of learning and performance and the conceptual environments that produce significant changes in individuals and for the creation of instruments and methods of testing that will best reveal these changes. Some of the problems that exist in evaluation are lack of better appraisal methods for measuring cognitive, affective, psychomotor, and other types of changes. Other problems exist in the search for accurate ways of determining the types of changes, change indices that are of greatest significance in contemporary societies, and in finding ways of utilizing feedback in the promotion of the desired changes, that is, the use of formative evaluation in contrast to summative evaluation (Bloom 1970).

The great power of evaluation is in its concern for human betterment through a systematic process of relating testing to the development of desirable characteristics in individuals and improvement of the programs. Used properly, evaluation does much to lead educators and administrators to a quest for desirable changes and the means for attaining them. The means-ends approach of evaluation has considerable implications for the growth of institutions as well as the growth of individuals (Bloom 1970).

Types of measurement (evaluation methods): norm reference and criterion reference

We have indicated areas in which evaluation and measurement differ. There are two basic kinds of evaluation methods designed to accomplish different purposes that are derived from two different philosophical points of view: criterion reference, or performance, tests and norm reference, or performance, tests. Normative or criteria reference testing is determined by what is done with the data derived from the measurement, for example, whether or not the data are used to determine the individual's standing in the group or in comparison to other groups (Bevis 1973).

Norm reference tests compare an individual's performance with that of established or standardized norm groups. For example, the National League for Nursing Achievement Test is a norm test that allows the student to be compared with a national population. Evaluation on the basis of a normal bell-shaped curve is an example of norm performance testing. Also, all statistical manipulations of data that use means, standard deviation offers intragroup and intergroup comprise methods, are norm performance tests, comparing individuals with one another and with groups (Anastas 1968). Norm reference measurements give little or no information regarding an individual's degree of competence or capabilities; norm reference measurements present a comparison as to where the individual stands in relation to others. Similarly, when the outputs of an institution or department are compared with the outputs of other institutions or departments, this is also a form of norm reference testing.

Evaluation in terms of criterion reference measures, on the other hand, requires that at least minimum levels of individual performance be specified before the individual goes on to the next step in an instructional or performance sequence. Therefore, criterion reference methods of evaluations are those activities enacted by the supervisor, teacher, learner, or group that enable the individual's behaviors to be compared with the target behavioral objective. The same holds true for measuring organizational objectives. Organization outputs are thus measured against themselves or against previous outputs and degrees of change needed are indicated.

Glaser (1963) advocated norms that indicate the attainment of a particular level of skill or competence. These are not norms in the sense of distributions. Instead, they make use of definitions of a task attainment or expert judgment to determine particular standards of performance. Although Glaser recommended this type of evaluative norm, it is likely that procedures for determining such norms would be most valuable for the assessment approach.

Indications for appropriate use of criterion or norm reference method

There are specific situations in which one frame of reference is more appropriate than another. The choice of which frame of reference to use is entirely dependent on the outcome desired. If a supervisor or a teacher wants to determine how an employee or a student is performing in relation to others in the same group or other groups, then the norm reference method of evaluation is appropriate. If, however, the supervisor or teacher is trying to determine whether or not the employee or the student achieved the objective and the degree of achievement of the set objectives, the choice would be the criterion reference method.

Similarly, the criterion reference method of evaluation is appropriate if the director is interested in determining the extent to which each of the organizational objectives is accomplished. Norm reference testing is appropriate if the director is interested in determining how the organization's output (such as service and products) compares with the output of other hospitals in the same area or perhaps how it is ranked nationally.

The criterion reference means of evaluation is particularly valuable in a learning situation in which active learning on the part of the learner is stressed. This particular form of evaluation indicates how well the student has mastered a given task.

These kinds of techniques can evaluate the precise assessment in terms of target behaviors, giving the person involved a sense of personal merit, tending to decrease competitiveness with peers as well as creating the kind of climate in which cooperative learning can take place.

Process of formulating an evaluation tool

Realization of a complete evaluation system takes time. For example, evaluation techniques for all areas of the nursing service administration cannot be attacked simultaneously. Furthermore, the development of the placement, formative, diagnostic, and summative components of an evaluation system need not be initiated at the same time. There will be, of course, overlapping among these components. The same instruments and items can often be used for different evaluative purposes. For example, a summative achievement test might also serve as a preentry placement test, the difference between formative and summative items revolving more around the intent and time of its use than it does around form or substance. Although taking advantage of any overlapping, cooperating evaluators (supervisors and nurses) must nevertheless establish priorities among the various components of the system as well as among various content areas. Perhaps the first task of any group of nurse evaluators should be to establish priorities. Once these are determined, in-service training can begin as deemed necessary.

Acquiring the skills needed to specify objectives will be among the first goals of the in-service training. At the completion of the in-service program, the task of co-

operatively developing evaluation instruments can begin. The remainder of this discussion is devoted to cooperative formation of item pools, which are useful in constructing various sorts of instruments. The four characteristics of evaluation tools are discussed.

DEVELOPMENT OF ITEM POOL AND THE TOOL

Bloom, Hastings, and Madaus (1971) described an item pool as consisting of a large number of items, each coded by behavioral aims, content, and approximate level (for example, registered nurse, licensed vocational nurse, and nursing assistant levels), that can be assembled to evaluate outcomes. Such a pool can be thought of as a planned library consisting of such items as test questions, checklist items, and interview questions that can be drawn on to build an evaluation instrument. Therefore, the first step in the creation of an item pool is the development of a blueprint by nursing evaluators that outlines the specifications of the pool. These form the clear delineation of the objectives of the task or program for which the evaluation system is being developed and can take the form of a two-dimensional table as shown in Table 6, one axis containing content matter and the other behaviors. For a desired balance of items in the pool, each cell in the table of specifications should be given a value weighting. Once the table of specifications has been decided on, each nurse evaluator in the group should contribute a number of items to the pool designed to evaluate a particular aspect of the table. Each table containing a series of selected items constitutes an instrument to measure a specific objective or several objectives. Once an instrument is put together, it must be checked to see if it possesses certain characteristics.

Are the specifications of terms or units that will be used to summarize or appraise the record of behavior obtained *clear?* This method of appraising the behavior should parallel the implications of the objectives.

All evaluation involves the problem of deciding on the characteristics to be appraised in the behavior and the unit to be used in the measurement or the summarization of these characteristics. For example, in the case of the objective stating—applications of knowledge of organizational policies—the characteristics involved would be range, appropriateness, and frequency. So the methods of summarization would provide a rating for range, appropriateness, and frequency. Every kind of human behavior appraised as part of an educational objective must be summarized or measured in some terms, and the decision about these terms is an important problem in the development and use of evaluation instruments.

The second characteristics of evaluation tools are *objectivity* and *reliability;* that is, to what degree would two different persons, presumably competent, be able to reach similar scores or summaries when they had an opportunity to score the same records of behavior? If the scores vary markedly, depending on who does the scoring or summarizing, it is clearly a subjective kind of appraisal, and improvement of such a scoring method is called for. Also, reliability refers to the situation in which the same test is given to the same group of individuals under the same conditions at two different times without intervening learning and identical results occur. Obtaining an observer reliability scoring is also another method of measuring the reliability of a tool. Sometimes improvements can be made through clarifying the specifications for scoring or through getting a more refined record of the behavior itself.

The third characteristic of an evaluation instrument is *sampling.* In general the size of the sample of behavior to be obtained depends on the variability of the behavior. If the behavior varies a great deal, a larger sample should be taken. When dealing with such subjective and perhaps even emotional concepts as attitudes, which will obviously vary among individuals in different situations, obviously larger and more representative samples must be taken. The important word here is *reliability.* If a test is not comprehensive enough or a set of observations is inadequate, the sample taking must be broadened before sensible and reliable conclusions can be reached.

The fourth characteristic of an evaluation tool is *validity.* Validity concerns the degree to which a test measures what it is intended to measure. For example, does the tool measure the specific objective that it was intended to measure? Thus, validity applies to the method and indicates the degree to which an evaluation device actually provides evidence of the behavior desired. Validity can be ensured in several ways. One is *face validity,* which could be done either through literature review and endorsements or through a panel of judges. Another means of ensuring validation is by correlating a particular evaluation device with the results obtained by a directly valid measurement. If the scores are positively and significantly correlated to one another, then the new tool is considered to be valid. There are other means of obtaining validity testing that space does not permit us to mention. The reader is advised to consult either a research book or a beginning statistics book that deals extensively with these topics.

A MODEL FOR FORMATIVE OR SUMMATIVE EVALUATION

This discussion presents a model for formative or summative evaluation to operationalize the measurement aspect of the evaluation process for objectives that are expressed on two-dimensional tables.

Table 6 presents a generalized model of formative or summative evaluation. The content aspects of the behavioral objectives are represented on the vertical axis; the specific behaviors to be exhibited by the employee in the area of each of the content or items are presented on the horizontal axis. For example, item A is the first item in the content category for behavior

Table 6. Model for formative or summative evaluation

Content (items) / Employees 1 2 3 ... n	Securement of a written copy of information	Acquisition of knowledge and understanding	Performance and application of knowledge	Expression of feelings (orally or written) about:	Attendance and participation	Others (as determined by each health care facility)
A. Policies	X_{1A}	X_{1A}	X_{1A}	X_{1A}		
1. Personnel						
2. Organizational						
B. Organization's objectives	X_{1B}	X_{1B}	X_{1B}	X_{1B}		
1. Patient care						
2. Environment						
C. Individual employee's objectives	X_{1C}	X_{1C}	X_{1C}	X_{1C}		
D. Job specifications						
1. Responsibilities	X_{1D1}	X_{1D1}	X_{1D1}	X_{1D1}		
2. Specific roles	X_{1D2}	X_{1D2}	X_{1D2}	X_{1D2}		
3. Tasks	X_{1D3}	X_{1D3}	X_{1D3}	X_{1D3}		
4. Duties	X_{1D4}	X_{1D4}	X_{1D4}	X_{1D4}		
5. Salary	X_{1D5}	X_{1D5}				
E. Self-improvement (cognitive)						
1. Orientation programs				X_{1E1}	X_{1E1}	
2. Workshops for continuing education				X_{1E2}	X_{1E2}	
F. Psychosocial				X_{1F}		
1. Attitudes				X_{1F1}		
2. Satisfaction				X_{1F2}		
G. Others (as determined by each health care facility)						
Subtotal	$\sum_{A}^{D} X_i$	$\sum_{A}^{D} X_i$	$\sum_{A}^{D} X_i$	$\sum_{A}^{F} X_i$	$\sum_{E1}^{E2} X_i$	$\sum_{A}^{G} X_i$

designates *securement of a written copy of information*, and item *G* is the last item in that category. Notice that items *E* and *F* in the content category were omitted. Item *E* designates the first item designed to measure the behavioral objective *attendance and participation*, and item E_2 is the last content item in that category. It should be noted that an entry does not occur in each cell of the matrix; item *G* represents the last content item in this evaluation form, but, as this is only a model, other items could be added to the content category by each individual health care facility.

Table 6 also represents an individual employee's performance on various items in the formative tests. Employees are represented on the Z axis and the number in a particular group is designated as *n*. It should be pointed out that the number of objectives, as well as the domains from which they come, might vary both from one group of employees to another; for example, objectives for a professional registered nurse and for a vocational nurse or nurse's aide would be different. For one group (professional registered nurses), objectives may deal with high-level cognitive behaviors, whereas for another group (licensed vocational nurses), objectives may deal with lower-level cognitive behaviors and also psychomotor behaviors. Since behaviors expressed in the statement of objectives can range from highly cognitive to psychomotor to motor behaviors, the degree of concentration of each category of behavior is directly correlated with the position, responsibilities, and job descriptions of each employee. Generally, objectives written for positions with professional standing and high responsibility are more concentrated on the cognitive objectives and less concentrated on psychomotor objectives.

This conceptual model presents, then, a method of looking at the performance of a category of employees on a particular formative test through objectives included in the test specifications. Looking at the notation in Table 6, one can see that a number of different kinds of information are yielded by such a test. For example, the notation of X_{iJ1} in each cell represents the score for any employee on any item. It can be seen that the first subscript (lower case i) designates the student, the second subscript (capital J) designates the items, and the third subscript (1) indicates the subheadings under each item. For example, in the use of specific representation for the notation X_{iJ1}, X_{1A} represents the score for employee 1 on item A; X_{2A} represents the score for employee 2 on item A; and X_{1B} represents the score for employee 1 on item B. It now becomes possible to write a number of characteristics of this particular test that are important for individual employee evaluation

and for supervisor (teacher) evaluation (Baldwin 1971).

Employee or learner diagnosis

One of the major functions performed by formative tests is employee or learner diagnosis. Feedback to an employee regarding mastery of the various objectives in a given unit of learning or performance of a task provides that employee with the information necessary to either progress to the next unit or take remedial measures to obtain mastery. Using the model for formative evaluation, the supervisor can provide diagnostic information for each employee.

The most general information that could be provided for the employee would be an overall performance score on the formative test. This would be that employee's total score for this particular test and would be represented by the following equation:

$$\sum_{A}^{G} X_i =$$ The sum of all items (A to G) for employee i (If items are scored: wrong = 0 and right = 1, this quantity becomes the number of items answered correctly and can be converted to a proportion by dividing by G.)

If the employee's performance on the total test reaches the established criterion of mastery, that employee would be ready to proceed to the next unit. However, if performance does not reach this level, the supervisor should provide more detailed information concerning the area in which the employee's performance is inadequate. More specific information could be provided by reporting the employee's performance on each category of behavioral objectives contained in that particular unit.

Table 6 shows that the G items have been broken up into subgroups corresponding to the objective that they are designed to measure. For example, items A to D_5 in the content category are those items that measure behaviors classified as *securement of a written copy of information,* and items A to D_5 in the content category correspond to behaviors classified as *acquisition of knowledge and understanding.* To represent this algebraically, therefore, the supervisor would write

$$\sum_{A}^{D_s} X_i/D_s$$

as the expression for the proportion of *securement of a written copy of information* items answered or performed correctly by employee *i*.

The following five quantities represent the level of mastery for employee *i* on each category of behavioral objectives.

$$\sum_{A}^{D_s} X_i/D_s$$ = Level of mastery for employee *i* on *securement of a written copy of information* objectives.

$$\sum_{A}^{D_s} X_i/D_s$$ = Level of mastery for employee *i* on *aquisition of knowledge and understanding* objectives.

$$\sum_{A}^{D_4} X_i D_4$$ = Level of mastery for employee *i* on *performance and application of knowledge* objectives.

$$\sum_{A}^{F_2} X_i/F_2$$ = Level of mastery for employee *i* on *expression of feelings (orally or written)* objectives.

$$\sum_{E_1}^{E_2} X_i/E_2 - D$$ = Level of mastery for employee *i* on *attendance and participation* objectives.

This information provides the individual employee with a *profile of mastery* at each category of objectives. If objectives or categories of objectives are arranged in hierarchical order, in which successful performance at lower levels is necessary but not sufficient condition for successful performance at higher levels, it can be expected that lack of mastery at lower-level behaviors will prevent successful performance of higher-level behaviors.

If an employee fails to reach a criterion level in one of the categories of objectives, the next level of feedback that the supervisor should provide would include information in individual objectives that the employee has failed to master. This, of course, is represented by individual items in the formative test. Feedback at this level should be accompanied by sources for remedial work to ensure mastery of that objective. In the model, information at this level is represented as follows:

$$X_{i,J} = \text{performance of employee } i \text{ on item } J.$$

Supervisor or instructor diagnosis

A second major function served by formative tests is supervisor diagnosis. The most general information that the supervisor needs is a measure of overall success in achieving mastery of all objectives with all employees assigned to that supervisor's clinical unit. This is represented as follows:

$$\sum_{A}^{G} \sum_{1}^{n} X/Gn$$ = The average level of mastery for all employees' overall objectives.

If this value falls short of acceptable criterion performance, the supervisor should evaluate the performance of the unit in more detail. The next step would be to examine the success of the total employee census in achieving mastery for each of the categories of objective. This can be written as follows:

$$\sum_{A}^{D_s} \sum_{1}^{n} X/D_s n$$ = The average level of mastery for all employees on all *securement of a written copy of information* objectives.

$$\sum_{A}^{D_s} \sum_{1}^{n} X/D_s n$$ = The average level of mastery for all employees on all *acquisition of knowledge and understanding* objectives.

$$\sum_{A}^{D_4} \sum_{1}^{n} X/D_4 n$$ = The average level of mastery for all employees on all *performance and application of knowledge* objectives.

$$\sum_{A}^{F_z} \sum_{1}^{n} X/F_z n$$ = The average level of mastery for all employees on all *expression of feelings (oral or written)* objectives.

$$\sum_{E_1}^{E_z} \sum_{1}^{n} X/(E_z - D)(n)$$ = The average level of mastery for all employees on all *attendance and participation* objectives.

The preceding information provides the supervisor with a *profile of success* in accomplishing, teaching, or implementing the several categories of behavioral objectives. If the results of this profile suggest that the supervisor is failing to achieve criterion performance for a particular category, her next step should be to examine her success on individual objectives in that category. This can be expressed as follows:

$$\sum_{1}^{n} X_J/n$$ = Proportion of students successfully completing item *J*.

Failure to achieve a given objective by the majority of employees in a group suggests that the supervisor or the teacher should reassess the teaching strategy in terms of that objective.

The final evaluation, of course, deals with the determination of the proportion achieved of organizational and individual goals (pOi and pOg). This can be determined by calculating (1) the mean of all scores on all employees for individual objectives and changing this mean score to a percent score and (2) the mean of all scores on all four categories of organizational objectives explained in Chapter 3 and transforming this mean score into percent score.

Once the percent scores on individual and organizational objectives are calculated, then the proportion of each achieved can be calculated and compared, depending on the results of the evaluation,

judgments and decisions and recommendations for improvement and change are made. Then this information is fed back as input into the system, and in this way the cycle continues as is graphically shown in our model in Fig. 4-1.

REFERENCES

Anastas, A.: Psychological testing, ed. 3, New York, 1968, Macmillan Pub. Co., Inc.

Baldwin, T. S.: Evaluation of learning in industrial education. In Bloom, B. S., Hastings, J. T., and Madaus, G. F., editors: Handbook of formative and summative evaluation of student learning, New York, 1971, McGraw-Hill Book Co., pp. 855-905.

Bevis, E. O.: Curriculum building in nursing: a process, St. Louis, 1973, The C. V. Mosby Co.

Bloom, B. S.: Taxonomy of educational objectives: the classification of educational goals, New York, 1956, David McKay Co., Inc.

Bloom, B. S.: Toward a theory of testing which includes measurement-evaluation-assessment. In Wittrock, M. C., and Wiley, D. E., editors: The evaluation of instruction: issues and problems, New York, 1970, Holt, Rinehart & Winston, Inc., pp. 25-61.

Bloom, B. S., Hastings, J. T., and Madaus, G. F.: Handbook on formative and summative evaluation of student learning, New York, 1971, McGraw-Hill Book Co.

Gagne, R. M.: Instructional variables and learning outcomes. In Wittrock, M. C., and Wiley, D. E., editors: The evaluation of instruction: issues and problems, New York, 1970, Holt, Rinehart & Winston, Inc., pp. 105-126.

Glaser, R.: Instructional technology and the measurement of learning outcomes: some questions, Am. Psychol. 17:519-521, 1963.

Messick, S.: The criterion problem in the evaluation of instruction: assessing possible, not just intended outcomes. In Wittrock, M. C., and Wiley, D. E., editors: The evaluation of instruction: issues and problems, New York, 1970, Holt, Rinehart & Winston, Inc., pp. 183-202.

Scriven, M.: The methodology of evaluation. In Stake, R. E., editor: AERA monogram series on curriculum evaluation, Skokie, Ill., 1966, Rand McNally & Co.

Stake, R. E.: The countenance of educational evaluation, Teachers College Record, 68:523-540, 1967.

Tyler, R. W.: Basic principles of curriculum and instruction, ed. 30, Chicago, 1970, University of Chicago Press.

Tyler, R. W.: The functions of measurement in improving instruction. In Lindquist, E. F., editor: Educational measurement, Washington, D. C., 1951, American Council on Education.

ADDITIONAL READING

Layton, J.: Students select their own grades, Nurs. Outlook **20**(5):327-329, 1972.

Chapter 7

CHANGE

THE NATURE OF CHANGE

In the early 1900s, with the advent of social science and social scientists, society was confronted with two opposing ideologies regarding the process of social change: Should individuals, through collaborative and deliberate forethought, seek to mold and shape their collective future? Or, should confidence be placed in the principle of automatic adjustment operating within the processes of history to reequilibrate without human forethought, yet in the interest of progress and human welfare, the inescapable human upsets and dislocations of changing society? These two questions were an important issue then and are still creating controversy among policy makers and social practitioners (Bennis, Benne, and Chin 1961).

Lester Ward, one of the earliest social scientists in the United States, stated: "Man's destiny is in his own hands. Any law that he can comprehend, he can control. He cannot increase or diminish the powers of nature, but he can control them" (see Commager 1960:208).

In opposition, William G. Sumner responded: "If we can acquire a science of society based on an observation of phenomena and study of forces, we may hope to gain some ground slowly towards elimination of old errors and reestablishment of a sound and natural order. Whatever we gain that way will be by growth, never in the world by reconstruction of society on the plan of some enthusiastic social architect" (see Commager 1960:201-202).

Today, in the 1970s, Sumner's ideological advice has been widely rejected in practice, and social planning for change is widely utilized. Laissez faire, as he advocated, has been abandoned as a principle of social management. At the same time, advocates and students of planned change have moved from Ward's sweeping modal question "Should we seek to plan change?" to "How to plan particular changes in particular people in particular settings and situations?" (Bennis, Benne, and Chin 1961:10).

Bennis, Benne, and Chin (1961:11) identified planned change as "a deliberate and collaborative process involving change-agent and client-systems. These systems are brought together to solve a problem or, more generally, to plan and attain an improved state of functioning in the client-system by utilizing and applying valid knowledge."

Kenneth Benne (1961:154-155) perceived effective planned change as one in which there is no unnecessary incompatibility between a democratic system of values and the processes of social engineering. Democratic norms are put into operation by Benne and interpreted as requirements for a methodology for resolving social and interpersonal conflicts in such a way that an adequate, mutually satisfactory, and socially wise situation is effected. According to Benne (1961:141-148): "Educators or any other change agents must be trained in the ways of stimulating and guiding change which incorporates the democratic norms as basic elements in their basic methodology."

Benne identifies the following five democratic norms:

1. The engineering of change and the meeting of pressures on a group or organization toward change must be collaborative. Such collaboration must be between persons and groups with different interests and between *theorists* and *practitioners* (for example, the creation of sociopsychological conditions that will support a problem-solving approach).

2. The engineering of change must be educational for participants. Planning is most intelligent when it accomplishes a maximum induction from the unique contributions of all individual participants. If social engineers are working democratically, they must leave the group better equipped to solve subsequent problems of change, including the management of personal adjustments, which change in social arrangements always requires.

3. The engineering of change must be experimental. Planned changes must be seen as changes that need to be tested in use and modified in terms of their human effects when tried. Therefore, to be collaborative, all who collaborate must be trained toward an attitude of research in social problems.

4. The engineering of change must be task oriented, that is, controlled by the requirements of the problem and its effective solution, rather than oriented to the maintenance or extension of the prestige or power of those who originate contributions. In terms of social control, democratic change must be antiauthoritarian. Contributions should be judged by their relevance to the task or problem confronted, not by the prestige or power of those who contribute. There must be objectivity in evaluation and reformulation. Although democratic groups need authority roles for effective coordination of their problem-solving activities, they need to learn to judge authority roles in terms of their contribution, not in terms of their general prestige.

5. The engineering of change must be anti-individualistic yet provide for the establishment of appropriate areas of privacy and for the development of persons as creative units of influence in society. The norms and standards by which a person thinks and judges are learned in the process of acculturation. Human rights and duties are grounded in cultural institutions and ideologies and are not independent of social relationships. To guarantee human rights, they must be guaranteed by appropriate social, political, and economic controls of human behavior, not by opposition to them. The determination of proper boundaries of individual over collective judgment in change must be based on collective judgment. Rights of private judgment can be defensibly defined and enforced on a democratic basis only by the process of collaborative planning. Groups must be trained to develop standards of acceptance of individual differences out of which resources for groups and institutional improvement can be developed.

It is important to remember that all change is not planned change. Bennis, Benne, and Chin (1961:154-155) devised a typology of change processes as an effort toward distinguishing planned change from other interrelated forms. The variables of mutual goal setting, deliberativeness of change, and power ratio between the change-agent and the client-system have been indentified as differentiating factors in the change process. The typology is as follows:

planned change entails mutual goal setting by one or both parties, an equal power ratio, and deliberativeness (at least eventually) of both sides.

indoctrination involves mutual goal setting and is deliberate, but it involves an imbalanced power ratio. Many total institutions fall into this category.

coercive change characterized by nonmutual goal setting (or goals set by only one side), an imbalanced power ratio, and one-sided deliberativeness. The distinction between coercion and indoctrination is complex and elusive. According to Bennis, Benne, and Chin, coercive change leads to a goal of collaboration over a period of time, and indoctrination does not have this goal.

technocratic change distinguished from planned change by the nature of the goal setting. The use of technocratic means to bring about change relies solely on collecting and interpreting data. Primarily it follows an engineering model in which the client defines personal difficulties as being derived from inadequate knowledge, assuming this to be accidental or a matter of neglect on the client's part. The technocrat colludes in this assumption and merely makes reports of the findings.

interactional change characterized by mutual goal setting, a fairly equal power distribution, but no deliberativeness on either side of the relationship. Unconsciously either may be committed to changing the other in some direction. Such changes may be seen among friends and married couples.

socialization change has a direct relationship with the interactional. A most obvious example would be the parent-child or teacher-pupil relationship. The incidence of greater deliberativeness on the "adult" side of the relationship brings specific cases of socialization into the indoctrination category.

emulative change processes associated with formal organizations in which there is a clear-cut superior-subordinate relationship. Change is brought about through a form of identification with and emulation of power figures by the subordinate.

natural change changes brought about with no apparent deliberativeness or goal setting on the part of those involved. It is a residual category encompassing accidents, quirks of fate, changes as the result of earthquakes or floods, and all other factors and causes that our limited knowledge cannot comprehend.

Bennis, Benne, and Chin emphasized that these classifications are limited, arbitrary and are perhaps too crude or pure to provide linkage to empirical reality, but they do provide suggestions as to how planned change can be distinguished from other change processes.

According to Benne (1961), it is a management function in organization not only to recognize when change has occurred, but also to anticipate impending changes and to make deliberate effort to shape these changes according to some criteria.

A conceptual scheme for analysis of the process of change was proposed by Kurt Lewin. According to Lewin (1947, 1961), periods of social change and periods of relative social stability should be analyzed together as follows:

1. Change and constancy are relative concepts; group life is never without change, merely in the amount and type of change existing.
2. Any formula that states the conditions for change implies the conditions for no change as a limit, and the conditions for constancy can be analyzed only against a background of potential change.

It is important to distinguish between actual change, lack of change, and resistance to change. Lack of change would occur when the conditions under which a group lives happen to stay constant during a given period: no one leaves or joins the group, no major friction occurs, facilities for activities remain the same, and there is an unchanged level of production.

If, however, the production level of the group were maintained despite loss or gain of membership or change in facilities, then resistance to change of rate of production is present. Mere constancy of group conduct does not prove resistance to change, nor does much change prove little resistance. Only by relating the actual degree of constancy to the strength of the forces forward or away from the present state of affairs can one speak of resistance or stability of group life in a given situation.

Social management requires insight into desire for or resistance to *specific* change. Lewin presents a system of analysis that permits the representation of social forces in a specific group setting. A basic tool for this analysis of group life is the representation of the group as a social field. This means that the actual happening is viewed as occurring in, and being a result of, a totality of existing entities, such as the group, subgroups, members, and barriers. The relative position of the entities as a part of the social field represents the social structure of the group and its ecological setting. What happens within the field depends on the distribution of forces within the field.

A MODEL FOR PLANNED CHANGE

Our conceptual framework describes the important factors of the change process. The descriptions also provide the opportunity to integrate and to refine understanding of the past periods concerning classical and behavioral thoughts of administration, since both make contributions to the process of change.

Change, as previously discussed, implies a systematic process that can be broken down into subprocesses or steps. Our conceptual framework consists of the following five subprocesses: input, sensing, conceptual acts, physical acts, and evaluation (see Fig. 2-7).

Forces for change as inputs

The forces for change can be classified into two groups: external and internal forces. External forces work from without the organization and are beyond the control of the administrator. Internal forces operate inside the organization and are generally within the control of the administrator.

EXTERNAL FORCES

Community demands. New scientific knowledge and technology make demands for change, higher quality and quantity of medical and nursing services. Changes in public education and income have heightened awareness of change for improved quality of health services. Recognition of participative action in the planning for health care brought about change because the community health program involves people, their children, and their families, first as patients and second as the sources of support for the health services, either as taxpayers or as private citizens.

Technology. Change in the quantity and quality of professional resources demanded the adoption of more automated materials or processes. Computers have made high-

speed data processing and the solution to complex service problems possible. New scientific knowledge paved the way for new techniques in vascular surgery, heart surgery, and organ transplantation. Expansion of equipment and capital investment have made possible more forms of remote control by physicians and nurses in their ministrations.

Education. The national nursing organizations, National League for Nursing, American Nurses' Association, and state boards of registration and education provide a continuing mechanism of pressure for more synchronized and synthetized action on behalf of nursing. The National League for Nursing promotes concerted action by nursing as a professional field and as a social force.

Environment. The nursing service administrator must be "tuned in" to movements over which she has no control but which, in time, control her organization's fate. The 1950s and 1960s witnessed a distinct increase in social activity. The drive for social equality posed new issues for nursing administrators. The drive for improved health care also posed new issues with which she had not been previously confronted. Sophisticated mass communication created potentials for nursing service but also posed a threat to those administrators unable to understand what was going on. Finally, to add to the problem, the relationship between government and health care facilities became much more involved as new regulations were imposed. These pressures for change reflect the increasing complexity and interdependence constituting modern living. The traditional function of nursing administration is being questioned, and new objectives are being advanced. No doubt the events of the future will intensify environmental forces for change.

INTERNAL FORCES

The forces for change within the organization can be traced to process and people causes. Process forces include (1) breakdown in decision making, communications, and interactions, (2) interpersonal and interdepartmental conflicts that reflect breakdowns in the human interactional process, (3) low levels of morale and high levels of absenteeism and turnover, symptoms of problems that must be diagnosed and dealt with, and (4) the design of health care facilities, bringing about a demand for more flexibility in the original designs.

Sensing
SENSOR'S RESPONSIBILITY FOR CHANGE

The nursing service administrator must continually consider the necessity for change. If it were possible to design the optimum nursing service organization and if the health care environment in which the facility operates were stable and unchanging, there would be little pressure for organizational change. But neither is the case. Nursing service organizational change is a pressing problem for the modern administrator; and in recent years, a wealth of literature has appeared that focuses on the need for planned change. Some health care organizations have instituted staff units whose mission is organizational planning. The planning units are specific responses to the need for systematic, formalized procedures to anticipate and implement changes in the nursing service organization. A nursing administrator utilizes the change model (Fig. 2-7) and considers each of the steps within it, either explicitly or implicitly, to undertake a change program. The prospect for initiating successful change is enhanced when the administrator explicitly and formally goes through each successive step.

The well-equipped nursing administrator is one who recognizes the multiplicity of alternatives. She is not predisposed to one particular approach to the exclusion of all others, she agrees with O'Connell (1968) that no change technique or change strategy can be judged superior on a priori grounds, and she avoids the pitfalls of standing still. The sign of decay, as Greiner (1967:119-130) observed, is "managerial behavior that (a) is oriented more to the past than to the future, (b) recognizes the obligations of ritual more than the challenges of current problems, and (c) owes allegiance more to departmental goals than to overall organizational objectives." Thus the administration of change implies a flexible forward-looking stance for the nursing administrator. This attribute is essential for using our model for change.

The model presumes that forces for change continually act on nursing service, an assumption reflecting the dynamic character of the modern world. At the same time, it is the administrator's responsibility to sort out the information that she receives from other departments and the overall organizational control system, as well as from other sources such as the community, that reflects the magnitude of change forces. Carefully analyzed information is the basis for recognizing the need for change. But once the nursing service administrator recognizes that something is not functioning, she must diagnose the problem and identify relevant alternative change techniques. The change technique selected as constrained by limiting conditions, must be appropriate to the problem (see Fig. 2-4). One example of a limiting condition is the prevailing character of the informal organization. The work groups may support some of the change techniques but obstruct others. Further limiting conditions include leadership behavior, legal requirements, and economic conditions.

The realization that a change program can be undermined underscores the fact that the choice of change strategy is as important as the change technique itself. One well-known and documented behavioral phenomenon is that people tend to resist change or at least to be reluctant to undergo change. An appropriate strategy for implementing change is one that seeks to minimize resistance and maximize personnel commitment. Finally, the nursing service administrator must implement the change and monitor the change process and change results. Our model includes feedback to the implementation and the input phases. These feedback loops suggest that the change process itself must be monitored and evaluated. The mode of implementation may be faulty and lead to poor results, but responsive action could correct the situation. Moreover, the feedback loop to the initial step recognizes that no change is final. A new situation is created within which problems and issues will emerge; a new setting is created that will itself become subject to change. Our model suggests no final solution; rather, it emphasizes that the modern nursing service administrator operates in a dynamic setting wherein *the only certainty is change itself.*

The process by which the solution to one problem creates new problems is widely recognized. Blau and Scott (1962) referred to it as the "dialectic processes of change," and they illustrated the dilemma by a number of examples. They observed that assembly-line techniques increase production but that, at the same time, employee absenteeism and turnover increase. Assembly-line work is monotonous and routine; it alienates workers and creates discontent; morale declines and personal problems emerge. Thus, a whole new set of difficulties is created by the solution itself. This phenomenon must be taken into account as a nursing service administrator considers changes.

COLLECTION OF DATA TO MAKE A DIAGNOSIS: RECOGNITION OF THE NEED FOR CHANGE

Information is the basis on which nursing administrators are made aware of the magnitude of the change forces. Certainly the most important information comes from the health care organization's preliminary, concurrent, and feedback control data. Indeed, the process of change can be viewed as a part of the control function, specifically the corrective-action subfunction. Analysis of quantitative and qualitative nursing services, financial statements, quality control records, and budget and standard cost information are important data through which external and internal forces reveal themselves. Declining patient census and withheld community resources are tangible indications that the health care organization's position is deteriorating and that change may be required. These sources of feedback control information are highly developed in most organizations because of their crucial importance.

The need for change goes unrecognized in many organizations until some major catastrophe occurs. The personnel seek the recognition of their professional organization before administration finally recognizes the need for action. The need for change must be recognized by some means, and the exact nature of the problem must be diagnosed.

Our framework has four steps, exclusive of the forces for change that must be completed if change is to occur, but the model refers to the goals to be reached. In terms of objectives, the goals can be described by asking the following three questions:

1. What is the problem as distinct from the symptoms of the problem?

2. What must be changed to resolve the problem?

3. What outcomes in terms of the objectives are expected from the change, and how will such objectives be measured?

The answer to these questions can come from information ordinarily found in the organization, such as departmental reports and records. Or it may be necessary to generate ad hoc information through the creation of committees or task forces. Meetings between administrators and personnel provide a variety of points of view that can be sifted through by a smaller group. Technical nursing problems may be easily diagnosed, but more subtle human relations problems usually entail extensive analysis.

One approach to diagnosing a problem is the attitude survey. Attitude surveys can be administered to the entire work force or to a sample of the personnel. The survey permits the respondents to evaluate and rate (1) administration, (2) personnel policies, (3) working conditions, (4) equipment, and (5) other job-related items. The appropriate use of such surveys requires that the questionnaires be completed anonymously so employees can express their views freely and without threat, whether real or fancied. The objective of the survey is to pinpoint the problem or problems as perceived by the members of the organization. Subsequent discussions of the survey results at all levels of the organization can add additional insight into the nature of the problem.

The approach that administration uses to diagnose the problem is a crucial part of the total strategy for change. The manner in which the problem is diagnosed has clear implications for the final success of the proposed change.

The diagnostic step must specify objectives for change. Given the diagnosis of the problem, it is necessary to define objectives to guide as well as to evaluate the outcome of the change. The objectives can be stated in terms of quantity and quality patient care, extension and expansion of nurs-

ing services, use of professional personnel, and satisfaction derived from nursing service.

Conceptual acts: strategy for development of planned change
CONCEPTUAL FRAMEWORK FOR PLANNED CHANGE

Any situation in which change is to be attempted is viewed as a dynamic balance of forces working against each other (Lewin 1947). One set of forces drives the situation toward the anticipated change (driving forces). Opposing forces tend to restrain movement from the anticipated change (restraining forces). When these two forces, toward and against change, are equal in strength, a level of *quasi-equilibrium* is occurring. This is a dynamic process in which the balance can be disturbed at any moment by altering either of the sets of forces involved. This balance of forces is shown as the level *L* in Fig. 7-1.

When discussing the means of bringing about a desired change, Lewin refers not to the goal to be reached but to a change from the present level of quasi-equilibrium to the desired one. This implies that planned change consists of transplanting the force field, in its entirety, to a new level of quasi-equilibrium. Two basic methods for changing the levels are proposed: adding forces in the desired direc-

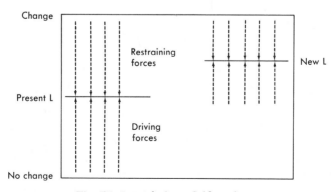

Fig. 7-1. Lewin's force field analysis.

tion or diminishing opposing forces. In both situations there may be change to a new equilibrium at a new level, but the secondary effect in each case would be quite different. Strauss and Sayles (1960) described the first method (raising pressure to overcome resistance) as being similar to slamming on the brakes of a car without taking the foot off the gas. It leads to tension and uncertainty and attempts to insulate the individual from pressure. The second method involves an attempt to discover and reduce forces of resistance to a particular change. It is comparable to allowing the car to slow to a halt without applying the brakes. It places the least strain on human relations.

Restraining forces are those related to resistance to change. According to Strauss and Sayles (1970), the most commonly recognized resistance to change is the resistance of employees to technological change, to automation, for example. Sometimes it is as violent at the managerial level as at a lower level. It may show itself in unexpected ways such as aggression, regression, scapegoating, fixation, and resignation, all of which may be traced to frustration from the inability to accept or to cope with change. One of the most obvious reasons for it may be economic. Will the change threaten jobs through displacement or inability to meet new skills demanded by change? Another reason may be inconveniences perceived by workers. Will they be required to learn new skills, work different hours, or move to a new location? They are threatened with the loss of the familiar.

Uncertainty due to lack of information about new goals will cause resistance through fear. Although factual information may be supplied, there is always the anxieties of the employees that arise from fears about how they will react in the new situation. This is exemplified by the fears of volunteers the night before induction into the service. With all the reassuring information they may have received from veterans, they still wonder how *they* will act.

Any threat to social relationships will meet with resistance. Even when physical change is not involved, the removal of a member from, or the introduction of a member into, an existing group tends to upset social relations. This may threaten leadership patterns and positions and hierarchical status of members. Individuals adjust their patterns of social relations to fit their own personality needs and in the formation of habits in job patterns. Any disruption of job patterns may threaten the balance between personality needs and job requirements.

Symbols raise special problems. They cannot be eliminated without threatening in someones mind the thing for which they stand. Small changes may symbolize big ones, particularly when employees are uncertain as to how extensive the program of change may be. With any shift, employees search for signs as to what may lie ahead. Treasured relationships and values may lie in a symbol. A threat to the symbol may be a threat to self.

A change substantially increases new orders to personnel. Many people resent taking orders at all. Levels of control from management may strengthen and reflect down the line, causing increased pressures and a feeling of decrease in autonomy and self-reliance among employees. It emphasizes their dependence on management.

Bennett (1961) challenged the assumption that all resistance is negative, asserting, rather, that it can serve useful functions in the change process; for example:

1. Resistance can force the leader to clarify more sharply the purpose of the change and the results to be achieved.
2. Resistance can disclose inadequate communications within the group.
3. Resistance often provides clues for the prevention of the possibility of unexpected consequences. It will force the leader into more careful examination of possible consequences.
4. Resistance can disclose the inadequacy of problem-solving and decision-making pro-

cesses so that the leader can determine whether or not relevant involvement of persons and groups in the change effort has been secured.

Driving forces are found in the desire for improved performance, decision to expand, effort to fully use potential, and built-in evaluation of objectives in the light of new demands (Lewin 1947).

DETERMINING REQUIRED CHANGES AND STRATEGY FOR PLANNED CHANGE

To determine required changes that must be dealt with before a change can occur, one should ask the following questions:
1. Which restraining forces can be reduced with the least effort?
2. Which driving forces can be increased?

A criteria in selecting forces to be modified may be as follows:
1. What forces, if modified, will be most likely to result in changing the level of the present condition in the desired direction?
2. What forces can be modified most easily or most quickly?
Careful analysis will prevent the many ineffective attempts at "shotgun" change.

Not only change but permanency of change should be the objective of any planning for change. According to Lewin (1947), implementation of a successful change involves the following three steps:

1. Unfreezing (if necessary) the present level of group habits
2. Moving to a new level
3. Freezing the group at a new level

It is also essential to recognize the limiting conditions that should be taken into consideration in planning the strategy for change in the implementation of the preceding three steps.

Recognition of limiting conditions: restraining forces on the administrative level. The selection of the change technique is based on diagnosis of the problem, but the choice is tempered by certain conditions that exist at the time. Filley and House (1969) identified three sources of influence

on the outcome of management development programs that can be generalized to cover the entire range of organizational change efforts, whether structural, behavioral, or technological. They are the leadership climate, formal organization, and organizational culture.

Leadership climate refers to the nature of the work environment that results from the leadership style and administrative practices of supervisors. Any change program that does not have the support and commitment of management has a slim chance of success. Administration must be at least neutral toward the change. The style of leadership itself may be subject to change; for example, sensitivity and system education are direct attempts to move administration toward certain styles—open, supportive, and group centered. But, it must be recognized that the participants may be unable to adopt such styles if they are not compatible with the style of their superior.

The formal organization must also be compatible with the proposed change. This includes the effects on the environment that result from the *philosophy* and *policies* of top management, as well as *legal precedent, organizational structure,* and the *system of control.* Of course, each of these sources of impact may itself be the focus of the change effort; the important point is that a change in one must be compatible with all others. For example, a change in technology that will eliminate employees contradicts a policy of guaranteed employment.

The organizational culture refers to the impact on the environment resulting from *group norms, values,* and *informal activities.* The impact of traditional behavior, sanctioned by group norms but not formally acknowledged, was first documented in the Hawthorne studies. A proposed change in work methods or the installation of an automated device can run counter to the expectations and attitudes of the work group. If such is the case, the change strategist must anticipate the resulting resistance.

The implementation of change that does not consider the constraints imposed by prevailing conditions within the present organization may amplify the problem that initiated the change process. Even if change is implemented, the groundwork for subsequent problems is made more fertile than what could ordinarily be expected. Taken together, these conditions constitute the climate for change and can be positive or negative.

Strategy for moving to a new level: desired goal. The selection of a strategy for implementing the change technique has consequences in the final outcome. Greiner (1967) emphasized reported changes and related various change strategies to the relative success of the change itself. He identified three approaches that are located along a power continuum with unilateral authority at one extreme and delegated authority at the other extreme. In the middle of the continuum are approaches that he termed shared authority.

Unilateral approaches can take the form of an edict from top management that describes the change and the responsibilities of subordinates in implementing the change. The formal communication may be a memorandum or policy statement. It is, in any form, a one-way, top-down communication. Shared approaches involve lower-level groups in the process of either (1) defining the problem and alternative solutions or (2) defining solutions only after higher level management has defined the problem. In either case, the process engages the talents and insights of all members of the organization at all levels. Finally, delegated approaches relinquish complete authority to subordinate groups. Through free wheeling discussions, the group is responsible for the analysis of the problem and proposed solutions. According to Greiner, the relatively more successful instances of organizational change are those

that tend toward the shared position of the continuum. Why is this the case?

As has been observed, most instances of organizational changes are accompanied by resistance from those who are involved in the change. The actual form of resistance may range in extreme from passive resignation to deliberate sabotage. The objective of the strategy is to at least minimize resistance and at most maximize cooperation and support. The manner in which the change is managed from beginning to end is a key determinant of the reaction of people to change.

The strategy that emphasizes shared authority has the strongest likelihood of minimizing resistance to change because it takes into account the "American culture pattern of equivalence between self-reliance and self-respect." Change imposed from the top, unilateral authority, runs the danger of creating resistance even though the proposed change may benefit the participants in every conceivable way by any objective standards. As has been recognized by the behavioral school of thought, an important means for overcoming resistance to change is to involve those who will be affected by the change in the decision to make the change.

The process of shared authority is composed of six phases. According to Greiner, these six phases accompany each instance of reported successful change.

1. Pressure and arousal
2. Intervention and reorientation
3. Diagnosis and recognition
4. Intervention and commitment
5. Experimentation and search
6. Reinforcement and acceptance

The strategy for implementing change, as described previously, involves supervisors and all personnel in the entire process. But it should be recognized that there is no guarantee that the strategy will work in all organizations. Indeed, some very basic preconditions must exist before employees can meaningfully participate in the change process. An intuitively obvious factor is that personnel must want to become involved. For any number of reasons, they may reject the invitation. They may have other more pressing needs, getting on with their own work, for example. Or, they may view the invitation to participate as a subtle attempt by administrators to manipulate them toward a solution already predetermined. If the leadership climate or organizational culture has created an atmosphere of mistrust and insincerity, any attempt to involve personnel will be viewed by them in cynical terms.

Stabilizing and freezing the new situation at the new level so that it will be maintained. Lewin (1947) introduced the idea of "social habit" as an inner resistance to change despite the application of forces at the level of social process. To overcome this inner resistance, an additional force may be required, sufficient to unfreeze the habit or the custom. Such a habit may be the values or standards of an individual's particular group in which the change is to occur. Of what value are these standards to the individual? Experience has shown that as long as group standards remain unchanged, the further the individual is expected to deviate from group standards, the more that individual will resist change. If the group standard is unfrozen, the resistance caused by the relationship between the individual and the group is eliminated. Most individuals stay close to the standards of the group to which they belong or wish to belong. In this way, the group level itself becomes a positive value or valence corresponding to the central force field, with these forces keeping the individual in line with the standards of the group.

It follows then that resistance to change should diminish if one diminishes the strength of the value of the group standard or changes the level of social value as perceived by the individual. This is one of the reasons for the effectiveness of collaboration by the group in planning for change or of *group-carried* changes. Studies have shown that it is easier to change individuals formed into a group than the individual performing alone.

If the change is to be frozen at a new level, there must be an awareness of the dynamic nature of the force field. According to Bennett (1961), when change occurs through the reduction of restraining forces and is accomplished by increased collaboration in the problem-solving process by those concerned with change, it is easier to stabilize, or freeze, at a new level.

As stated, group-carried change is more effective than change by an individual. When change involves people, action must be focused on helping them develop behaviors needed in the new environment created by the change. When the climate permits and maintains freedom for persons affected by change, their imaginations will be released to assist in the change effort. Through participation, human resources are developed more effectively toward accomplishing and maintaining the new performance.

Physical act: implementation of planned change

The implementation of the proposed change has two dimensions: timing and scope. The matter of timing is strategic and depends on a number of factors, particularly the organization's operating cycle and the groundwork that has preceded the change. Certainly, if a change is of considerable magnitude, it is desirable that it not compete with ordinary nursing service operations. Thus, the change might well be implemented during a less pressured period. On the other hand, if the problem is critical to good nursing service, then immediate implementation is in order. The scope of the change depends on the strategy. The change may be implemented throughout the department, clinical unit by clinical unit or department by department. The strategy of successful changes, according to Greiner (1967), makes use of a phased approach, which limits the scope but provides feedback for each subsequent implementation.

ALTERNATIVE CHANGE TECHNIQUES

The choice of the particular change technique depends on the nature of the problem diagnosed. The nursing service administration must determine which alternative is most likely to produce the desired outcome, whether it be improvement in the knowledge, attitudes, skills, or job performance of the organization's personnel or in material resources. As noted, diagnosis of the problem includes specification of the output that administration desires from the change. Donnelly, Gibson, and Ivancevich (1971) defined and classified these techniques according to the major focus of the technique, namely, to change the organizational structure, people, behavior, or technology. This classification of approaches to organizational change in no way implies a distinct division among the three types. On the contrary, the interrelationships among structure, behavior (people), and technology must be acknowledged and anticipated. Had nursing service administrators been asked a few years ago to advise on human problems in nursing service, their approach would have been limited to what is now called a *component* approach. Their thinking would have been directed at the components in the system— in this case, the people involved. They would have explored such answers as incentive schemes, human relations training, selection procedures, and possibly some time and motion studies. Their efforts would have been limited to attempts to change the components to fit in with the system as designed, no matter how poor the design might be.

But now nursing service administrators concern themselves with the *information* that must be *processed* by the system. Their concern is centered on the functions that have to be performed by the system and how these functions might best be performed. They concern themselves especially with how the system is designed to handle conditions of information overload.

An important contribution of the behavioral school is the documentation of the impact of organizational structure on attitudes and behavior. Overspecialization and narrow spaces of control can lead to low levels of morale and ultimately to low levels of service to people or low productivity. At the same time, the technology, distribution, and information processing effect may determine the structural characteristics as well as attitudes and sentiments of the health care organization.

Structural change. Changes in the structure of the organization ordinarily follow changes in strategy. Logically, the organizing function follows the planning function, since the structure is a means for achieving the goals established through planning. Structural change in the context of organizational change refers to administrative action that attempts to improve task performance by altering the formal structure of task and authority relationships. At the same time, one must recognize that the structure creates human and social relationships that gradually can become ends for the members of the organization. The relationships, when they have been defined and made legitimate by administration, introduce an element of stability. Personnel of the organization may resist efforts to disrupt these relationships.

Structural changes affect some aspect of the formal task and authority definitions. The design of an organization involves the definition and specification of job content and scope, the grouping of jobs into departments, the determination of the size of groups reporting to a single supervisor or coordinator, and the provision for staff assistance. Within this framework, the communication, decision-making, and human interaction processes occur. One can see, then, that changes in the nature of jobs, bases for departmentation, and line staff relationships are the foci of structural change.

Changes in the nature of jobs include any revision in the prescribed ways for performing assigned tasks. The origins of such changes are the implementation of new methods and new equipment. Work simplification and job enlargement are two examples of methods changes. Work simplification narrows job content and scope, whereas job enlargement widens them. Scientific management introduced significant changes in the way work is done through the use of motion and time studies. These methods tend to create highly specialized jobs. Functional nursing is an example of specialization by task; it narrows the scope and content of the job. Job enlargement, however, moves in the opposite direction, toward despecialization. Team nursing is an example of specialization by skill; it contributes to job enlargement.

Behavioral change. This type of change refers to efforts to redirect and improve employee attitudes, skills, and knowledge bases. The objective is to enhance the capacity of the individual to perform an assigned task in coordination with others. The early efforts to engage in behavioral change date back to scientific management and its methods of work improvement and employee training. These attempts were primarily directed at improving employee skills and knowedge bases. The employee counseling programs that grew out of the Hawthorne studies were (and remain) primarily directed at improving employee attitudes.

The educational programs for administrators have typically emphasized supervisory relationships. It is an attempt to provide supervisors with basic technical and human relations skills. Since supervisors are primarily concerned with directing the work of others, the content of these traditional programs emphasizes techniques for dealing with people problems, for example, how to deal with the troublemaker and the complainer. Emphasis today has shifted from traditional programs to programs including conceptual material encompassing communications, leadership styles, organizational relationships, and job relationships of those who are in different channels of authority but who must cooperate to get the work done. In contemporary management two prominent behavioral change approaches are the Strength Development Inventory Test by Porter (1973), which attempts to make the participants more aware of themselves and their relationships to others, and *The Human Organization* by Likert (1967), which relates people change and structural change. According to Likert, an organization can be described in terms of the following eight operating characteristics: leadership, motivation, communication, interaction, decision making, goal setting, control, and performance. The nature of each of these characteristics can be located on a continuum through the use of a questionnaire that members of the organization (usually supervisors) complete. Sensitivity training is another change technique that operates on the assumption that the causes of poor task performance are the emotional problems of people who must collectively achieve a goal. If these problems can be removed, a major impediment to task performance is consequently eliminated.

The traditional literature of administration has much more to say about the relationships between a superior and subordinates than about the supervisor to supervisor or department head to other department heads.

Technological change. This category of change includes any application of new ways to transform resources into the product or service. In the usual sense of the word, technology means new machines, such as lathes, presses, and computers. But the concept should be expanded to include new techniques with or without new machines. From this perspective, the methods of work improvement in scientific management can be considered technological breakthroughs.

The changes in organizational efficiency brought about by a new machine are calculable in purely economic and engineering terms. Whether the machine is a good investment is a matter of estimating its future profitability in relation to its present cost. These calculations are an important part of the administrative control function. Here, however, we are interested in the impact of the new machine on the structure of the organization. As some scholars have observed, technology is a key determinant of structure. They tentatively conclude that organizations with simple and stable technology can adapt more easily to a structure that tends toward bureaucratic organization, whereas organizations with complex and dynamic technology tend toward the more open and flexible system structure. Thus it would appear that the adoption of new technology involves a concurrent decision to adapt the organizational structure to that technology. Whether or not an inexorable and deterministic relationship between technology and structure exists, the fact remains that the introduction of technological innovation has far-reaching effects within the organization, as exemplified by nursing service organizations.

To catalog the impact of technological change on structure and behavior, Floyd C. Mann (1962) analyzed a number of actual cases and concluded that the adoption of new machines in the factory involves: major changes in the division of labor and the content of jobs; changes in social relations among workers; improved working conditions; the need for different supervisory skills; changes in career patterns, promotion procedures, and job security; generally higher wages; generally higher prestige for those who work; and around-the-clock operations. The degree and extent of these observed changes in structure and behavior depend on the magnitude of the technological change.

Evaluation: monitoring the process and results by use of feedback system

The provision of feedback information is termed the monitoring phase. From our model one sees that information is fed back into the implementation phase. It is also fed back into the input forces phase because the change itself establishes a new situation that will create problems. The monitoring phase has two problems to overcome: the acquisition of data that measure the desired objectives and the determination of the expected trend of improvement over time. The acquisition of information that measures the sought-after objectives is the relatively easier problem to solve, although it certainly does not lend itself to naive solutions. As we have come to understand, the stimulus for change might be the determination of performance criteria that administration traces to either structural, behavioral, or technological causes. The criteria may be any number of objective indicators, including decline in quality of nursing service and in number of people served, absenteeism and personnel turnover, and increase in in-service costs. The major source in feedback for those variables is the organization's usual information system. But, if the change includes the expectation that employee attitudes and morale must be improved, the usual sources of information are limited, if not invalid. As Likert (1967) has shown, it is quite possible for a change to induce increased service at the expense of declining personnel attitudes and motivation. Thus, if the administrator relies on the assumption that service and personal morale are directly related, the change may be incorrectly judged successful when improved service and cost reports come to attention.

To avoid the danger of overreliance on service data, the administrator can generate

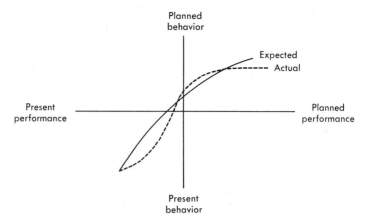

Fig. 7-2. Expected and actual pattern of results. (Modified from O'Connell, J. J.: Managing organizational innovation, Homewood, Ill., 1968, Richard D. Irwin, Inc., p. 156.)

ad hoc information that measures employee attitude and morale. The benchmark for evaluation would be available if an attitude survey had been used in the diagnostic phase. The definition of acceptable improvement is difficult when evaluating behavioral data, since the matter of "how much more positive" should be the attitude of employees is quite different than the matter of "how much more productive" they should be. Nevertheless, if a complete analysis of results is to be undertaken, behavioral measurements must be combined with service measurements.

The second problem of the monitoring phase is the determination of the trend of improvement over time. The trend itself has three dimensions: the first indication of improvement, the magnitude of improvement, and the duration of the improvement. A well-devised change strategy should include an analysis of what pattern can be expected. The actual pattern can then be compared to the expected.

Ideally, the pattern would consist of an index that measures the performance and behavioral variables. Fig. 7-2 illustrates a model that describes the necessary information for such an index. The solid line is the expected pattern through time. It shows a movement into acceptable behavior before a movement into acceptable

performance. The expected pattern may, of course, assume any configuration. The broken line is the plot of actual change through time. It reflects not only what is happening, but also the impact of corrective action that administration takes to keep the change program on course. If the expected pattern is valid, as originally conceived, the administrator's objective is to minimize the oscillations around the planned results.

In general, the monitoring phase is a specific application of administrative control. Before it can be effective, administration must provide for a measurement of the objective, information to compare actual results with planned results, and action to correct any deviations.

Change has become a pervasive fact of the modern world; it is therefore appropriate and logical to cast nursing service administration in a framework that emphasizes change. At this time, management of change does not imply random and unplanned responses to a changing environment. On the contrary, we have stressed the need for a systematic analysis of all facets of the proposed change program.

We think there is a critical need for planning, organizing, directing, and controlling the change process, as borne out by literature reporting change in various organizations. We emphasize that the manner in which the change is implemented bears heavily on the ultimate outcome. In fact, a change technique may fail because of ineffective implementation. We also stress the necessity for evaluating techniques and strategies in the context of the particular organization.

REFERENCES

Benne, K.: Democratic ethics and human engineering. In Bennis, W., Benne, K., and Chin, R., editors: The planning of change, New York, 1961, Holt, Rinehart, & Winston, Inc.

Bennett, T. R., II: The leader looks at change. In Schmidt, W. H., and Ayers, R., editors: Looking into nursing leadership series, Washington, D. C., 1966, Leadership Resources, Inc.

Bennis, W., Benne, K., and Chin, R.: The planning of change, New York, 1961, Holt, Rinehart & Winston, Inc.

Blau, P. M., and Scott, R.: Formal organizations, San Francisco, 1962, Chandler Pub. Co.

Commager, H.: The American mind, New Haven, 1960, Yale University Press.

Donnelly, J. H., Jr., Gibson, J. L., and Ivancevich, J. M.: Fundamentals of management, Dallas, Tex., 1971, Business Publications, Inc.

Filley, A. C., and House, R. J.: Managerial process and organizational behavior, New York, 1969, Scott, Foresman & Co.

Greiner, L. E.: Patterns of organization change, Harvard Business Review, **45:**119-130, May-June 1967.

Lewin, K.: Frontiers in group dynamics: concept, method, and reality in social science: social equilibria and social change, Hum. Relations **1:**1, June 1947.

Lewin, K.: Quasi-social equilibria and the problem of permanent change. In Bennis, W., Benne, K., and Chin, R., editors: The planning of change, New York, 1962, Holt, Rinehart & Winston, Inc.

Likert, R.: The human organization, New York, 1967, McGraw-Hill Book Co.

Mann, F. C.: Studying and creating change. In Bennis, W., Benne, K., and Chin, R., editors: The planning of change, New York, 1962, Holt, Rinehart & Winston, Inc.

O'Connell, J. J.: Managing organizational innovation, Homewood, Ill., 1968, Richard D. Irwin, Inc., pp. 10, 142-145.

Porter, E. H.: Strength, development, inventory, Pacific Palisades, Calif., 1973, Personal Strength Assessment Service.

Strauss, G., and Sayles, L.: Personnel: the human problems of management, Englewood Cliffs, N. J., 1960, Prentice-Hall, Inc., p. 61.

Strauss, G., and Sayles, L.: The human problems of adjustment, Englewood Cliffs, N. J., 1970, Prentice-Hall, Inc.

ADDITIONAL READINGS

Chin, R.: The utility of system models and developmental models for practitioners. In Bennis, W., Benne, K., and Chin, R., editors: The planning of change, New York, 1961, Holt, Rinehart & Winston, Inc.

Georgopoulos, B. S., and Mann, F. C.: The community general hospital, Ann Arbor, 1962, Survey Research Center and Department of Psychology, The University of Michigan.

Mann, F. C.: Psychological and organizational impacts. In Dunlop, J. T., editor: Automation and technological change, Englewood Cliffs, N. J., 1962, Prentice-Hall, Inc., pp. 50-55.

Reinkemeyer, A. M.: Nursing need: commitment to an ideology of change, Nurs. Forum **9**(4): 341-355, 1970.

Tannenbaum, R.: The introduction of change in industrial organizations, reprint from general management series No. 186, New York, 1957, American Management Association, Inc.

Tannenbaum, R.: When it's time for a change, reprint from General management series, New York, 1957, American Management Association, Inc.

Walker, D. J.: Our changing world—its challenge to nursing, Nurs. Forum **9**(4):328-339, 1970.

Chapter 8

INDIVIDUAL-TO-GROUP INTERFACE PROBLEMS

The health care institution is a complex social system whose most important input (patients and staff) is people and whose principal outputs (patient care and health) are personal service and information to people. Most of its work is done directly by human means; its major objectives—to direct individualized aid and professional attention to people who need or request it, to conduct research and training in the interest of such aid, and to supply high quality of service to the community—are all social in nature.

The health care organization is a problem-solving system whose principal components are purposive human beings who have the ability to act, interact, and communicate at will, to think and feel in both conscious and unconscious ways, to reason and solve problems, and to make decisions that may be rational or nonrational, correct or incorrect, self-oriented or altruistic, and organizationally relevant or irrelevant.

The organization is also a "living" system consisting of the orchestrated actions and interactions of numerous professionals and nonprofessionals in interrelated roles carrying out an extensive variety of specialized and interdependent tasks and functions. Their combined and converging work performances enable the organization to deal with particular problems and pursue specific objectives within its particular environment (Georgopoulos 1972).

Both the health care institution and its members are problem-solving systems. The major organizational problems that the hos-

pital deals with manifest themselves not only at the collective level, but also at the individual and individual-to-group interface levels. The behavior of individual members in particular roles affects problem-solving performance at the collective level. And conversely, each of the major collective problems discussed is reflected in the behavior of individual members in the organization and in organization-member relationships. This chapter is devoted primarily to organization-member relationships.

The conceptual framework utilized at this interface recognizes the complexity of individuals and the factors that influence their motivation to contribute to organizational goals. This conceptual scheme is built on research findings that indicate that an individual can usefully be conceived of as a system of biological needs, psychological motives, values, and perceptions (Schein 1965; Seiler 1967; Lawrence and Lorsch 1969). The individual's behavior is also determined partly by the specification and expectations of the job, ability or inability to relate to others, past life experiences, motivations, and personality characteristics. Behavior is influenced not only by the work environment, but also by life off the job. Even though individual behavior by and large conforms to that of society's expectations and cultural norms, the individual still remains highly individualistic in self-beliefs, motivations, hopes, and goals.

In essence, therefore, the objective of

organizational development at this interface is to obtain a fit between individual needs and the behavior required of the individual to accomplish organizational goals.

Different studies classify organizational and individual problems differently, but all have certain aspects in common. For example, according to Georgopoulos (1972), interdepartmental, intradepartmental, and individual level problems can be classified in seven categories: adaptation, allocation, coordination, integration, tension and role strain, output, and maintenance. Bennis (1969) classified them in six categories: integration, social influence, collaboration, adaptation, identity, and revitalization. Lawrence and Lorsch (1969) classified them in three: organization-environment, group-to-group, and individual-and-organization. Watson (1958) classified them in the areas of setting objectives, planning strategy, organizing, and controlling. Our survey of 35 directors and supervisors of nursing who attended the Western Interstate Commission of Higher Education in Nursing (WICHEN) Workshop on Nursing Service Administration (October 1972) classified problems in the following five categories: patient care, staffing, role conflict, communication, and resistance to change.

After analyzing each category of problem classification with regard to the most efficient way of presenting, diagnosing, and planning intervention, we decided to integrate the five points of view. Since Georgopoulos's classification is inclusive of all other approaches, except those of Watson and since our own administrative theoretical framework is so similar to that of Watson, we present the problems utilizing Georgopoulos's seven classifications within our own theoretical framework. For example, the problem of lack of adaptation at the individual or organizational level may actually be due to problems of inadequate planning for good adaptation or to lack of organizing, directing, or controlling for good adaptation. An advantage of using this framework is that the administrative conceptual framework can be used as a diagnostic tool in identifying the problems. It also guides the practitioner in planning a course of action.

The seven problems classified within our theoretical framework cover the entire input-transformation-output work cycle of the system, at the collective level and at the individual level. Some problems are encountered primarily on the input side, some on the output side, and others at intervening points. Problems manifest themselves as concrete difficulties, that is, in relation to the behavior and activities of individual members in the organization and in terms of organization-member relations. It is important to examine problems at the individual level to understand member behaviors in the system. Only by taking into account the problem-solving performance of the organization and its members in relation to these problems is it possible to assess the effectiveness of the system satisfactorily.

A word of caution with regard to the solution of these problems at the individual level, the problems are complex and persistent and do not lend themselves to definite solutions. Resolving these problems calls for nonflagging effort by the organization, for the problems shift in urgency and are not uniformly recognized in every health care institution. They are, nevertheless, problems that always confront the organization and must be handled at both the individual and collective levels. Moreover, the complicated problems are so multifaceted and interrelated that even considered individually and sequentially they defy solution (Georgopoulos 1972).

THE PROBLEM-SOLVING PROCESS

A problem exists at the individual level when there is an unmet need, when initially set individual objectives are not met or fulfilled, or when there is a deficiency in meeting the standard.

The problem-solving process is often

synonymous with the scientific process. This discussion concerns the problem-solving process, utilizing our administrative theory as a guide in making diagnosis, in identifying the antecedent factors of the problems, and in planning and implementing intervention.

Collection of data

The first step of the process is to gather relevant data that are classified under *input* (see Fig. 2-1). These data may consist of (1) signs and symptoms of a particular problem in the form of complaints from patients, individual members of the nursing staff, the community, or others, (2) feedback information received from previous evaluation, and (3) supplementary information gathered through interviews and other testing measures.

Sensing

The second step is to filter the relevant information from the irrelevant, called sensing. The investigator should categorize and analyze the relevant data in light of the conceptual framework, trying to get an overall picture of the problem. (The investigator may be the nursing service administrator, supervisor, clinical nurse specialist, or an outside consultant. Any of these people or other qualified persons who are charged with investigating the problem can be referred to as the investigator.) A conceptual framework ought to provide the perspective to regard trouble spots (input) as symptoms rather than as problems to be tackled head on. For example, a physician does not treat high temperature and increased white blood count as separate ailments, but attempts to find the cause of both and to make an accurate diagnosis. The conceptual framework provides a systematic and meaningful way of discussing underlying problems that produce diverse symptoms of trouble. For example, some problems may overlap several areas. The investigator can also sense and analyze the data in light of the administrative composite process. For example, do the symptoms point to a failure on the part of an individual or the superior in setting objectives, in planning, in organizing, in directing, or in controlling? For the individual to adapt to the job situation, appropriately allocate resources, coordinate functions, perform the duties of the job description, or create an environment in which role strain is minimal, that individual has to plan, organize, direct, and control each of these functions. Examining and analyzing data in the light of this process enables the investigator to identify the causes of problems and to make a diagnosis, that is, to formulate a hypothesis—the third step of the problem-solving process.

Diagnosis utilizing the administrative composite process (ACP) framework

Identifying the cause of problems and making an accurate diagnosis require the development of valid, reliable, and sensitive tools to measure the degree of severity or acuteness of the behavior problem. The same tools should also measure the success or failure of the proposed intervention.

A conceptual framework can be used as a diagnostic tool to identify causes of problems and to make a diagnosis (Watson 1958). In this discussion we use the administrative composite processes (Ac and Ap) as diagnostic tools in tracing problems.

SETTING OBJECTIVES (Ac)

In tracing problems for setting objectives, one must look for the following elements:

1. Are the primary objectives of the individual's work or services, which are set up either by the superiors or the individual, stated in terms of the exact nature of the behavior that the individual purports to render?
2. Are the objectives specific enough to guide and direct the individual and the superior?
3. Do the objectives take into consideration the demands of the consumer, that is, the nurses and their families, the patients, and the community?
4. Are the objectives set up in terms flexible enough to allow for easy adaptation to change?

5. Do objectives allow for adoption of new trends? Most of the professions, health care institutions included, are undergoing rapid changes. Advances in technology and science impose new demands on the individual and the type of services rendered.
6. Are the objectives planned and organized consistent with the resources available to the individual for achieving them?
7. Are the objectives reviewed and revised regularly in relation to consumer demands, current trends, and the individual's own growth and development?

In tracing a failure and in making a diagnosis of a behavior problem at the individual level, an investigator may find that many of the symptoms uncovered may be due to a failure in the area of objectives, such as uncertainty about the individual nurse's position or about job expectation and demands. An investigator may have to do a good deal of interviewing and studying to trace failures to the level of objectives. It may not be readily apparent, especially since some supervisors pay only lip service to the importance of setting objectives. But if a careful investigation does reveal a failure in this area, then the investigator can assure the director as well as the individual nurse that appropriate intervention to cope with the problem will bring significant results, not only in one area but in many.

If the investigator cannot trace the individual's behavior problem to the area of objectives, even though the diagnostic approach has been used, there may be no problem, objectives may be clearly stated and in flexible terms, or the investigator may not have gathered relevant data to answer each of the questions. Whichever is the case does not matter. The investigator can either proceed to the next step, the planning strategy, or formulate new hypotheses in the area of objective setting.

PLANNING STRATEGY AS A DIAGNOSTIC TOOL *(Ac)*

An individual in an organization needs a plan to achieve personal objectives and those of the organization. The individual needs a plan based on personal capability and potential and also on the characteristics of the organization, the resources available, and the conditions of the work environment—a plan that promises a profitable advantage to the individual and to the organization. Strategy in planning is closely related to the individual's specific position or job expectation.

Good strategy means recognizing the activities most essential to success at a particular time. A supervising nurse may need to shift from one situation to another, depending on her personal growth within the organization and on the needs of the organization. For example, for a time the supervisor may concentrate her efforts on mastering the new equipment at her command. At other times she may spend her energy in study to keep up with the advances in technology. At still other times she may emphasize improvement of patient care that her team members are giving to their patients. She may set aside time to teach her subordinates how to take care of colostomy patients. Furthermore, in emergencies the supervisor must set up priorities and put her efforts into handling the crisis before attending to her routine work. Unless the individual can gauge what areas need special attention at a particular time, she may find that her neglect of a critical point has resulted in inability to function and in dissatisfaction with her work.

Scheduling and coordination of activities are additional aspects of planning. For example, what does the individual expect to produce (or perform) within a specific period of time? What can be learned during the next two weeks or months? Setting target dates enables the person to plan activities and ensures achievements of specific goals by that date with relative certainty. Regardless of the kind of planning, an individual must be aware of the importance of sequence as well as the initial timing of a program or activity that is to be undertaken.

Therefore, in tracing the problems to

the planning stage, the investigator or the individual should ask the following questions as a diagnostic tool:

1. Do the signs and symptoms stem from failure to develop strategy or from some other aspect of planning?
2. Do the plans fulfill some aspect of individual or organizational objectives?
3. Are the target dates set up in realistic terms?
4. Are the scheduling, sequencing, and coordination of activities and plans congruent and realistic? That is, are the priorities that are set up appropriate?
5. Are the entering behaviors of the individual nurses up to par so that they can proceed from there to undertake new tasks?

Planning may thus be a valuable diagnostic tool that can aid the individual and the investigator in analysis of the individual's behavioral problems as well as problems occurring on the unit.

If the investigator cannot trace the causes of a problem to the planning stage for the same reason that they could not be found in the area of objectives, even though the diagnostic approach has been used, the investigator should then proceed to the next step of the administrative process and formulate a new hypothesis in light of further data.

ORGANIZING AS A DIAGNOSTIC AID *(Ac)*

Accurate analysis of a problem at the organizing level is extremely intricate, yet it is an area wherein snap judgments are often made (Watson 1958). Perhaps the most important asset that the investigator needs is a systematic way of talking about the whole job situation, the organization, and how it effects the individual's behaviors. Therefore, there is a need to examine the organizational system in terms of many mutually interdependent elements such as job structure, authority system, communication, social groups, and the individual. As the investigator examines each variable or dimension and tries to relate it to the individual's behaviors, it must be kept in mind "not only trying to see every factor that influences the situation,

but even more than that, the relation of these factors to one another" (Metcalf and Urwick 1941:181).

Job structure. In surveying the job structure for trouble, the investigator should examine varying points of view: that of a staff nurse for feasibility of methods and procedures and that of a clinical nurse specialist for analysis of tasks from the standpoint of simplifying functions, for analysis of the type of care each category of patients requires and for determination of qualifications of the persons assigned to perform at that level. The staff nurse and clinical nurse specialist can testify to the extent to which the job structure and the position that they themselves are given take advantage of their specialization and educational preparation. Are nurses given the opportunity to practice what they have been taught? Are they being prepared through in-service educational programs to undertake tasks for which they have not been trained? To underestimate a person's potential and capability leads to boredom, dissatisfaction, and frustration. Similarly, to push nurses to perform tasks for which they have not been adequately trained leads to frustration too; it increases the chance of error in the course of performing the task, leads to poor and unsafe patient care, and ends up in loss of self-esteem.

The investigator also needs to pinpoint the decision-making level and examine it to see if revision of centralization or decentralization at specific points will improve the job structure. Friction between people may turn out to be at the root of a problem. Some problems, otherwise diagnosed as, say, communication or authority faults, upon analysis turn out to be flaws in job specification.

Authority system. The assignment of a job to someone carries with it the allocation of authority to fulfill its responsibilities. Many problems erupt because of uncertainty about the amount of authority and responsibility a position requires. Areas of authority and responsibility often overlap between adjacent positions, for example, between staff nurse and team leader and between head nurse and supervisor, thus causing friction over job responsibilities and accountabilities. Many problems crop up, though, in which cooperation and peacemaking efforts work better in solving the problem than greater precision in defining authority (Watson 1958).

In tracing trouble at the authority level, the investigator needs to recognize whether symptoms of trouble stem from inadequate and uncooperative relationships between superior and subordinate or from the job relationship between people who are in different channels of authority, but who must nonetheless work together in the same area. The study by Myers and Turnbull (1956) on line and staff relationships illustrated that power cannot be allocated according to the simple traditional formula whereby the staff always "advises" or "persuades" the person in line position. There are staff nurses who know more than the supervisor about specific patient problems, or about the operation of complicated machinery, or about reading EKGs, and so on. The staff person often ends up with the actual power to make certain decisions, regardless of what the organizational chart says. The line person (supervisor) and the staff person (nurse) are faced with a conflict between delegated power and earned power. Because of the staff nurse's expertise in the clinical area and depending on the back-up support received from colleagues, the staff nurse's decisions may override those of the supervisor. Furthermore, depending on the attitude of other people toward the supervisor and on the strength of team spirit behind the staff nurse, the staff nurse can be as powerful as the head of a small informal organization. The danger to be on the alert for is that the supervisor's role and power will be considerably weakened.

Communication system. Assignment of jobs and allocation of authority determine the formal channels of communication. The informal channels elaborate the formal network through which people interact, and adequacy depends primarily on the individual's behavior and capacity for communication (Watson 1958).

Since clarity of communication is not easily achieved, the investigator may find the source of some problems right there. Another cause of trouble may be inadequacy of the formal organization's communication network. Informal organizations are threaded with grapevines of communication because needs of the individual or group have gone unheeded, notably need for more accurate information; need for belonging to a group, identity and affiliation; need for power; and the basic needs of security and rewards. Some of these problems of unmet needs may have arisen out of failure of the formal organization's communication system to provide adequate and accurate information at the right time or out of too much information being communicated indiscriminately and at the wrong time.

Once the investigator identifies faulty communication as the source of the problem, the resolution requires immediate attention of the directive. The solution is not an easy one. Training in communication skills may help after a time but immediate gains are likely to be limited to improving communication on the informational level and to developing sensitivity toward the individual's unmet needs, demands, and suggestions. It is also possible that people in top management and middle management will recognize their responsibilities as a distinct function—to create a better environment for communication (Watson 1958).

Social system. The formal relationships within a health care institution constitute a structure around which informal activities develop. Individual members in the organization are also members of many interlocking smaller groups (informal organizations) bonded together by common interests. A change can dislodge the social relations within the smaller groups, sending repercussions throughout the formal organization.

In the smaller social groups, common experiences, attitudes, and beliefs are shared, thus functioning to serve a need. They support the individual and give him a sense of security and belonging. Group norms within these social groups are powerfully effective in controlling individual behaviors. These social groups can be facilitators of achievement of both organizational and individual goals and objectives if the members of a group develop strong identification with their work, hence with the organizational goal assigned to them. Problems arise in several ways: (1) when organizational goals are incongruent with individual goals or when the achievement of one is at the expense of the other, (2) when changes are imposed on members of a social group without planning in advance how to effect the change in a manner that leaves undisturbed the individual's sense of security, and (3) when the modifier (therapist or supervisor) ignores the group norm in modifying an individual's "undesirable" behavior.

If the investigator, after applying the diagnostic approach to exploring a problem at the organizing level and having taken into consideration the variables of job structure, authority system, communication system, and social group in making the diagnosis, still has been unable to trace the cause, it may be necessary to look into the directing and controlling processes.

DIRECTING AND CONTROLLING PROCESSES AS DIAGNOSTIC AIDS *(Ap)*

Given a clear set of objectives and a method of how to reach them and by whom, the team leader or nurse administrator must put them into action and establish a form of control and follow up, in other words, direct them.

Control is the function of checking on performance and measuring results against some standard. The standard, depending on what is being controlled, can be stated in terms of target dates for completion of certain tasks or in terms of efficiency measures, such as number of patient care plans written and revised daily, frequency and quality of team conferences, reduction in patient call lights, and completion of assignments at the end of an eight-hour work shift. The control process must contain an "alert system" within the work situation, whereby inefficiencies or delays are detected early enough to make modifications; since it is not possible for individual nurses or managers to anticipate all events, they must be prepared to modify plans quickly. Installation of alert systems in the form of short-term target dates, command control sheets (master sheet for all activities for every patient every day) to check patient care activities, or frequent formative evaluations of performance enable detection of possible errors and delays in patient care procedures, so that plans can be modified midstream and errors corrected without loss of time and effort. The accuracy and efficiency of the control process depends on the sensitivity of the alert system.

The control process will be ineffective if someone at any level is uncertain about objectivity or has failed to plan ahead. Control is the difficult task of finding and reorganizing information that is critical. Relying on a single apparatus, such as formal reports from below, is not the only answer (McLean 1957; Watson 1958).

If the job of selecting objectives, planning, organizing, directing, and controlling is done effectively a coordinated effort results. To achieve successful coordination, individuals at all levels must know what they are striving for, how to get it, who does what, and when it is due and must be able to detect quickly the need to modify plans and activities. Coordination, therefore, is a composite of interrelated functions that depends on skillful management for effectiveness (Watson 1958).

If the investigator has researched and

interpreted the data carefully, a clearer view of the causes of problems occurring at the individual level will emerge. If analysis shows that the symptoms stem largely from failure in certain administrative composite processes, the investigator will be able to gather the evidence showing how these failures have inversely affected the behaviors of individuals and their work performance and have produced waves of reactions throughout the organization.

Intervention

Having diagnosed the cause, the investigator is faced with planning intervention, the fourth step in the problem-solving process.

Here again, the investigator will find the administrative composite process useful in formulating a plan of action. For instance:

1. What objective should individuals strive for, given their knowledge and capabilities and the requirements of the job?
2. What strategy concerning "what," "how much," and "when" of the duties of their job situation must individuals engage in to ensure personal growth?
3. How much and what kind of training and education do individuals need to adapt to changes in their job situation?
4. What control measures should the individual apply to accommodate unforeseen and changing circumstances and to ensure that individual and organizational objectives make their target dates?
5. Do the individuals reevaluate all these functions periodically and especially when feedback information from self-evaluation and control processes shows discrepancies and deficiencies in attainment of personal and organizational objectives?

Effective problem solving depends on the investigator's or director's ability to establish orderly relationships among factors surrounding the individual within the organization. The investigator must consider both individual and organizational objectives, plan for attaining the objective, and organize, direct, and control the situation so that the ultimate goal is accomplished, all the while bearing in mind that all fac-

tors are interdependent. The effective use of the administrative composite process in making both a diagnosis and a plan of action leads to success.

Evaluation

The final step of the problem-solving process is evaluation of the intervention. If necessary, the investigator proposes additional changes. Then, if the diagnosis was correct and the planned intervention accurate, significant reduction in the severity of the problem should result. If the problem still persists, then, depending on the results (feedback) of evaluation, new hypotheses are formulated and the whole cycle of the problem-solving process starts over again.

MANIFESTATION OF PROBLEMS AT THE INDIVIDUAL LEVEL

The rationale behind illustrating each of the problem areas is similar to that of medicine, in which students study each disease entity in terms of signs and symptoms, causes, manifestations, means of diagnosis, treatment, and prognosis to serve as a model when confronted with a patient problem. The majority of problems at the individual level are behavioral ones that are not directly observable but are inferred from other observable or measurable behavioral means.

Adaptation

Adaptation refers to the ability of the individual to respond appropriately to changes induced by the environment, to respond promptly to innovations, and to obtain resources.

Ability to change is essential for good adaptation. Change is constant and universal, and individuals are continuously faced with the unchanging law that change will occur—within their environment, between them and their environment, among their relationships with others, and within themselves (Murphy 1971).

Exploration of the theory of adaptation in relation to contemporary society and its environment requires that consideration be given to the needs of individuals, to the resources within or available individuals in relation to their environment, and to the needs and resources of the environment itself (Murphy 1971).

Humans are biopsychosocial beings who are constantly interacting wtih their environment. To adapt to these constant changes, individuals use various mechanisms (biological, sociological, or psychological) to cope with the situation. Bringing about an adaptive state frees the individual to respond to other stimuli. The adaptation level is determined by the pooled effects of the following stimuli: (1) focal, which is the immediate problem facing the individual, (2) contextual or background, which include other stimuli present, and (3) residual, which includes beliefs, attitudes, and past experiences that are relevant to the present situation (Roy 1970).

The needs of individuals are based on the following four modes of adaptation, and any change in the environment poses a threat to one or more of them:

physiological needs the ability of individuals to maintain homeostasis in the systems of nutrition, activity, elimination, fluid and electrolytes, respiration, circulation, and regulation as they interact with their environment.

self-concept individuals' positive or negative assessment of themselves, which is influenced by feedback from the environment and from their own reactions to themselves and the environment. Components are:

> *physical self* the way individuals see themselves physically and accept what they see.
> *personal self* the individual's character and self worth.
> *interpersonal self* self in relation to a primary social group (family) or secondary social group.

role mastery individuals' ability to organize their prescribed behavior in a specific setting and enact it effectively in a complementary interaction process.

interdependence the self-concept of individuals and their role mastery interact with other persons in the environment in an interdependent way (Roy 1970, 1971).

The two main adaptive mechanisms in individuals are the regulator, which works through the autonomic nervous system, and the cognator, which identifies, stores, and relates stimuli so that the symbolic responses can be made. The cognator mechanism works consciously through thought and decisions and unconsciously through defense mechanisms. Cognator ineffectiveness signals adaptive failure (Roy 1970).

Analyzing each adaptation problem in terms of (1) significant residual stimuli (individual's past experiences and past coping mechanisms), (2) the behavioral response to a given focal stimulus, and (3) the ACP diagnostic tool can lead to specific interventions. A system of nursing intervention can thus be made available for the supervisor or administrator counselor to work out the adaptation problems she may face in counseling individual employees. As a control agent, the nurse-counselor or supervisor can manipulate the physical and conceptual environment and adjust the stimuli in the work situation to obtain a positive response from the individual employer (nurse) and can promote adaptation by bringing about change from within the system itself. If the counselor-supervisor has succeeded, the individual employer has moved forward to a new adaptive, healthy state.

Within a health care institution, individual employees are bombarded with sensory overload. Some of the stimuli that suddenly require immediate response disturb the individuals' equilibrium and prevent them from coping effectively with the new demand. Constraints (that is, stimuli or situations to adjust to) are imposed on the individual by unions, professional organizations, community, family, and the organization itself. A health care institution with the rules and regulations of its present organizational form cannot function effectively without a good deal of compliance by members if they are to adjust to the requirements of the work technology and the physical features of the work place. Members must comply with the formal prescriptions of their roles, work group norms and professional standards, and overall policies and authority dictates and adapt their behavior to meet the needs of the organization and their co-workers (Thompson 1961; Etzioni 1964). These types of compliance demanded of the individual by the organization result in regimentation of behavior. Similarly, members cannot satisfy important personal needs and goals that are met through work without subjecting themselves to such organizational regimentation and behavioral constraints. At the same time, however, if some of the important psychological needs of the participants, including the need for affiliation and primary relation, are not met by the organization, members may create an informal organization with which to offset some of the work requirements imposed by the formal system.

Furthermore, professionals, including physicians and nurses, have strong needs for personal independence, prefer maximum freedom and autonomy in their work, and are averse to regimentation to which organizational prescriptions tend to lead.

One can therefore see that the job of adaptation is very complex. The organization and its members must reconcile their goals. That is, there must be a reciprocal relationship between organizational goals and individual objectives in which achievement of one facilitates the achievement of the other's objectives. Therefore, the signs and symptoms of maladaptation on the part of the individual will depend on the type of individual objectives that have not been accomplished. For example, if one of the objectives is "the staff nurses will be up-to-date with current advances in technology with regard to their specialties," then signs and symptoms of maladaptation with regard to this objective included such symptoms as failure on the part of the nurses to implement the new technique (for example, colostomy irrigation or application of the colostomy bag), signs of resistance to implement new procedures,

and patients not receiving adequate care.

Let us suppose these problem symptoms are brought to the attention of the head nurse, or supervisor, who is then asked to help the nurse in trouble. How can the head nurse make an accurate diagnosis and plan an intervention? She is now faced with the problem-solving situation. If she can utilize the adaptation theory in conjunction with the diagnostic tool of the ACP, she should be able to accurately diagnose and plan an intervention.

The first step of the problem-solving process is collection of data, that is, the signs and symptoms of the trouble. She will want to collect more information with regard to the focal, contextual, and residual stimuli, since the adaptation level is determined by the pooled effect of these three stimuli.

After collecting the data, she submits it to sensing, that is, to a method of categorizing the relevant data into a logical framework that can lead to an accurate diagnosis. Furthermore, she needs to identify which mode of adaptation is most affected, that is, physiological, self-concept, role mastery, or interdependence. The data (signs and symptoms) should guide her in determining the affected mode of adaptation. So far, however, the head nurse has probably not yet identified the cause of the problem, but she has a hunch that the signs and symptoms focus on maladaptation. Now, she utilizes the ACP diagnostic tool in determining its cause, that is, is it due to lack of knowledge of the objectives? If the objective-setting aspect is correct diagnosed as the cause, then the head nurse may proceed to determine if the planning strategy is correct. If she finds that the objectives were not properly set and that they were not explained to the individual, she then makes the diagnosis of failure in setting objectives, causing lack of adaptation to keep up with current advances in technology. She plans an intervention to properly establish objectives, ensures that they are explained to the employee, and accordingly plans to implement the objectives. If the intervention is correct, then the behaviors indicative of good adaptation should increase. For example, the nurse will read current literature on new technology and will seek opportunities to learn new techniques and many other behaviors.

Let us assume that the objective-setting stage was correct in that the problem was not caused there, then the head nurse should utilize the diagnostic tool of the planning strategy to find out if the cause of maladaptation lies in the planning stage. If the answer is yes, then the head nurse can utilize the same administrative composite process in planning the intervention.

Therefore, by applying this theoretical framework to the problem-solving process, the head nurse should be able to properly diagnose the adaptation problems and plan a course of intervention that will enable the staff nurse to better adapt to the work situation. Also, if the intervention is successful, the conceptual environment will also be positively affected; for example, other team members will consult the head nurse, she will be more motivated to teach others and to learn from them. She will also be able to utilize the resources that are available in the physical environment to function more efficiently, effectively, and economically.

Of course, the way to determine if intervention has been successful is to evaluate changes that have occurred in the individual, to determine the proportion to which individual objectives and organizational objectives have been accomplished, and to measure the difference between previous levels of achievement and the achievement of objectives after the intervention.

Maintenance

Maintenance refers to the individual's ability to preserve self-identity, integrity, basic character, and viability in the face of changes that are constantly occurring in the environment and within the individual.

Maintenance also deals with the individual's ability always to be coherent and able to handle the problem of personal survival.

An individual's ability in physical, social, and psychological self-maintenance is intricately related to powers of adaptation and maintenance of personal equilibrium in face of constant change.

The organization calls on its members to perform their roles reliably and to achieve and maintain high levels of performance (Katz and Kahn 1966). At the same time, members are faced with the problem of maintaining and updating their professional skills and knowledge, even though some of these skills may remain underutilized because of the nature and definition of work roles in the system (Georgopoulos and Christman 1970).

For individuals to maintain their professional status quo and keep up with the advances in technology and knowledge base, they have to keep themselves renovated and revitalized. Bennis (1969) introduced the term *revitalization,* or self-renewal, to embrace all social mechanisms that stagnate and regenerate, as well as the process of this cycle. Individuals should have the ability to fulfill the following four elements of revitalization: (1) to learn from experience and use the relevant knowledge when needed, (2) to develop and improve their skill to learn, (3) to analyze their own performance to acquire and use feedback mechanisms on performance, to be self-analytical, and (4) to control their own destiny.

The signs and symptoms of failure in self-maintenance resemble those of maladaptation: weakening of self-identity, loss of self-esteem, inability to cope adequately with changes and demands of new technology, backwardness in thinking, inability to learn from past experiences, and inability to utilize feedback information for self-improvement.

The means of solving problems of maintenance on the individual level also resemble those of adaptation. The administrative conceptual framework can be utilized to diagnose a maintenance problem and to plan a method of intervention to solve it.

Output

Output is defined operationally as the individual's ability to operate at top efficiency in terms of the amount and kind of patient care, acceptability, and cost. It also involves the ability of all members at all levels to maximize efficient and reliable role performance. Output depends on the system giving all members the maximum opportunity to achieve goals and job satisfaction (Georgopoulos 1966, 1972).

The reason for stressing the solution of output problems at the individual level in a health care organization is that this determines the organization's social efficiency, which depends on its human assets and resources. Social efficiency entails personal goal attainment for all members from top to bottom; it includes meaningful participation in the decision-making process, identification with the organization, opportunities for expressive behavior, satisfaction of intrinsic motives, and psychological rewards (Georgopoulos 1972).

The issues and difficulties in the area of individual output include quality, quantity, cost, and reliability of individual and group performance, input-output ratio problems involving sociopsychological efficiency of the system, and effort-reward balance and related motivation-to-work difficulties.

Furthermore, between inputs and outputs are the critical processes of resource allocation and control, coordination of effort, social and psychological integration, and organizational strain and its management. All intervene to immeasurably modify the relationship between input variables and outcomes. An individual with excellent inputs (knowledge base, experience, and specialization) may yield very poor output because the sociopsychological processes are upsetting the outcomes for the system or are taking place in ways that detract from efficient performance.

Another essential factor with direct bearing on the level and quality of performances and overall output of the individual is satisfaction of personal motives. Motives are unfilled needs or desires. Individuals are motivated to work primarily by economic rewards. Consequently, the psychological contract between the individual and the organization is effort in exchange for money. Schein (1965) also pointed out, though, that this assumption fails to recognize other social needs of the individual. The need for belonging provides the basic motivation for work. In this situation the psychological contract between the individual and the organization is satisfaction of social needs in exchange for individual effort.

Other behavioral scientists, such as Argyris, Maslow, McGregor, and McClelland, have shown that work in organizations is losing much of its intrinsic value. Their research indicated that this loss of meaning is related not so much to individuals' social needs as to their inherent need to use their capacities and skills productively and maturely (see Lawrence and Lorsch 1969; Schein 1965). These scientists view individuals as *self-actualizing*. The assumptions are that needs of humans are arranged in a hierarchy ranging from food and safety survival to social needs, self-esteem, autonomy, achievement, and self-actualization. The psychological contract between the individual and the organization is safety, social contact, affiliation, self-esteem, autonomy, and achievement expressed in terms of self-actualization in exchange for individual effort. The conflict inherent in this situation is that, while individuals ultimately seek independence and self-actualization, the organizational context places them in positions of dependency and constraint that prevent them from satisfying these higher-order needs (Lawrence and Lorsch 1969).

McClelland (1961) categorized higher-order motives in a manner particularly useful for our purposes. He identified the three important motives as need for (1) achievement (need for competitive success measured against a personal standard of excellence), (2) affiliation (need for warm, friendly compassionate relationships with others), and (3) power (need to control or influence others). The levels of these motives vary by individual.

High achievers are often viewed as possessing the need for a sense of competence or mastery (White 1963), and research studies have corroborated this view of humans as problem solvers (Herzberg, Mausner, and Snyderman 1959; Myers 1964). For example, in their work at Texas Instruments, Myers and his colleagues found that organization members in diverse jobs at several levels were motivated by the challenge of an opportunity for accomplishment in their jobs. The intrinsic involvement in the work and the sense of accomplishment derived were more important motivators than other factors, such as social rewards, status, physical conditions, and even economic rewards. The work of Herzberg and Myers suggested basically that individuals, in their transactions with the organizational setting, are motivated by a desire to use their problem-solving abilities. Furthermore, an organization can stimulate high achievement in the individual employee by instituting a formalized procedure for setting goals jointly with the individual member, for measuring performance against goals, and for evaluating such performance. This recommendation is consistent with McClelland's conclusion that the need for achievement is stimulated by feedback about performance against established standards.

Factors that determine whether a person is high in achievement, affiliation, or power is dependent on the past learning process and the individual's perception concerning whether or not personal objectives will be accomplished. When someone is offered a job situation, personal history causes that individual to perceive certain aspects of the current situation as potentially satisfying and others as less so. Therefore, whether a person behaves as a high achiever or affiliator in a work situation depends on the strength of that person's inherent motives and on the extent to which that person perceives that they will be satisfied (Lawrence and Lorsch 1969).

Satisfaction at work is determined by the degree of professional autonomy and self-expression an individual has and by a minimum of constraints. Members must be able to participate in the decision-making process and to function free of formal requirements other than those dictated by the nature of their tasks, roles, work interdependence, accepted professional norms and standards, and the major problems of the system (Georgopoulos 1972). Effective professional practice in the health care institution requires that leaders and supervisors ensure a balance between organizational constraint and personal need for professional autonomy and self-expression. Neither the authoritarian nor the pure human relations approach works effectively in supervising nursing departments (Georgopoulos 1966). Emphasis on high task orientation and consideration for the personal needs and goals of the employee seem to work best.

To preserve the motivation of the employee, the organization must facilitate the role performance and personal goal attainment of its members by removing obstacles such as external interferences, unnecessary complexity and uncertainty, role overload, and avoidable conflict and frustrations that demean the personal dignity and personal worth of participants or jeopardize their integrity, stifling individual freedom or unduly limiting their participation in the affairs of the system.

In summary, where there is failure in meeting the individual's needs—be they the basic ones of food and shelter or the higher-order ones of affiliation, power, and achievement that lead to the individual's self-actualization—the individual's output in the form of work performance and satisfaction decreases, which in turn, adversely affects the fulfillment of organizational goals. Managers and supervisors can usually recognize symptoms of a problem. They can point to lack of effort or results or to absenteeism or turnover, and often their explanation is that the individuals involved have a character weakness: they lack motivation. But, as Lawrence and Lorsch (1969) pointed out, managers and supervisors who offer this explanation fail to see the fallacy, notably that if individuals are not motivated to accomplish organizational goals it means not that they lack motivation but that they are motivated to do something else, even work against those very organizational goals. For example, the study of Roesthlisberger and Dickson (1939) showed that the restricted output of a bank wiring room could not be cited as proof that the workers lacked motivation. On the contrary, the workers were highly motivated to develop elaborate mechanisms to restrict production output.

The means of solving output and motivational problems at the individual level is to follow the problem-solving process explained earlier. The investigator or the problem solver can utilize the theoretical framework on motivation in conjunction with our administrative conceptual framework of ACP to diagnose output problems. Several valid and reliable tools are available in the psychological literature to measure motivational levels in individuals. Two instruments are available to measure the characteristics of individuals: the Thematic Apperception Test (TAT), which measures basic motives of need for achievement, affiliation, and power, and the California Psychological Inventory (CPI), which measures other behavioral characteristics (leadership, maturity, drive, and flexibility). An instrument to measure organizational climate, such as that prepared by Litwin and Stringer (1968), is designed to elicit individuals' perceptions of the structure in which they work, along the dimensions of structure, responsibility, risk, standards, rewards, and support. Our ACP diagnostic tool also enables the investigator to trace the causes and the underlying reasons for failure in output and motivation. It helps to discover if problems exist at the objective-setting stage, at which initial goals should have been set and explained to employees, or if the failure occurred at the planning, organizing, or implementing (directing or controlling) stage. Once an accurate diagnosis is made, intervention is planned accordingly utilizing our administrative conceptual framework.

Allocation

Allocation at the individual level refers to the individual's ability to delegate and utilize knowledge, experitise, energy, and personnel (members in the team) in the most appropriate manner; to handle problems associated with distribution of rewards, authority, and information among the participants; to ensure participation by all concerned in the decision-making process; and to solve problems concerning work specialization and the allocation of tasks and functions among members (Georgopoulos 1966, 1972).

As they go about their work, members must determine how best to accomplish certain tasks or meet specific requirements and how to allocate their energy and time among their various tasks and functions. As a team leader, the staff nurse must evaluate the condition of each patient, determine the amount and type of care needed, judge the capabilities and expertise of the team members, and make the assignment accordingly, that is, allocate responsibilities, all the while keeping in mind the institutions policies, rules, and regulations.

The same principle of allocation applies to the head nurses, supervisors, and directors of nursing, on their respective levels. In addition to hiring personnel and delegating responsibility, allocation for these individuals also includes budgeting of finances and distribution of equipment. The basic principles and concepts underlying efficient allocation are to evaluate the existing resources and needs, to define the goal, and to arrive at a means of attaining it. All these conceptual acts require the establishment of appropriate and attainable objectives, skillful planning, efficient implementation, and a control system.

Failure to carry out these administrative conceptual processes will result in problems in allocation. Signs and symptoms of poor allocation depend on where the problem is located, that is, in the realm of finances or personnel. At the staff nurse level, patients may complain of poor nursing care given by a team member, team members may complain of physical fatigue owing to overload of patient assignments or to lack of satisfaction from work because tasks were assigned that they did not feel capable or prepared to do. Other signs and symptoms may be in the area of accountability and responsibility. If members are not adequately informed of their job description, their assignments, and other position-related delegation of responsibilities, there will be lack of accountability on their part and perhaps an overlap of job responsibilities or omission of tasks stemming from conflict in areas of responsibility.

Lack of appropriate allocation of funding may result either in overspending or insufficient funds for such items as personnel, equipment, and maintenance.

The investigator can utilize the ACP diagnostic tool to ascertain the problem and to identify its causes. Depending on the location and cause of the problem, the investigator can use the ACP to plan an intervention.

Integration

Integration at the individual level refers to the individual's ability to mesh personal needs with those of the organization. It also involves the development of shared norms, attitudes, values, and understandings, which serve to provide a common universe of discourse for the different groups and members and help socialize and bind the members into the system (Bennis 1969; Georgopoulos 1966).

In health care institutions, identification with the organization, superior-subordinate relationships, and good communication—all indicators of integration—vary. The higher the level in the power structure, the better the commitment, the relationships, and the communication. These mechanisms weaken as the level descends.

Organizational goals and individual objectives must be integrated mutually and cooperatively. The institution must view each participant not only as an individual with personal needs, expectations, and value, but also as a member of a specific group in the system. The satisfaction of the needs of all participants and the integration of separate goals of the members with the goals of the organization assume special significance as the aspirations and expectations of members, especially at the lower levels, change.

The nature of work in health care institutions, along with the high levels of professionalization and specialization among its members and accompanying functional interdependence for all involved, necessitates the development and maintenance of complementary expectations and mutual understanding among the participants about one another's roles, work problems, and needs. Member compliance with formal rules and requirements is not enough if members are to perform their roles effectively. Performance of roles requires adequate coordination and integration of work effort throughout the organization and particularly at points where diverse and specialized activities converge, for example, in patient care. Good integration and coordination are essential for work efficiency and good patient care. But, again, much of this required integration and coordination must be achieved directly by human means and through voluntary efforts and spontaneous adjustments by its members (Georgopoulos 1972).

Increased specialization is a major cause of lack of integration. It makes interaction more demanding for all involved, frequently leading to fragmentation of tasks and functions with the result that individuals have difficulty understanding where they fit in the total picture. A great many of the members find their work uninteresting and unrewarding; problems of professional allegiance, organizational identification, and competition and conflict arise. These disadvantages can be minimized in all parts of the system through elaborate coordination, effective communication, and member cooperativeness (Georgopoulos 1972).

Other signs and symptoms of inadequate integration are lack of member commitment, low morale, psychological disinterest, alienation from the system, turnover, tardiness, absenteeism, problems of deviance and compliance, and nonadaptive and maladaptive behaviors (Georgopoulos 1972). Here again, the investigator can utilize the ACP diagnostic tool in tracing the cause of the integration problem and, accordingly, can plan a course of intervention.

Depending on the cause of the lack of integration, the investigator can suggest that a more systematic and adequate organizational socialization of members be undertaken when they enter the system, better matching of people and jobs when hired, and better role redefinitions that accommodate expressive as well as instrumental needs and behavior. Personnel policies, rewards, and incentives need to be based on extrinsic and intrinsic motivation and reinforcement. Members should be given opportunities to participate in decision making. To the extent that they are implemented, these factors improve the social efficiency level of the system (Georgopoulos 1972).

Coordination

Coordination refers to the individual's ability to articulate, interrelate, and regulate the many diverse but related activities and roles of different members at all levels so that personal efforts and energies converge in the attainment of organizational objectives. Coordination includes planning, programming, setting priorities, scheduling work, establishing routines, and standardizing work flow. The problems of sequencing, timing, and synchronizing the numerous activities in the system are the most important coordination problems the individual and organization face (Georgopoulos 1972).

Since all activities cannot be preplanned, standardized, or routinized much of the daily coordination of work in an organization depends on the voluntary and spontaneous adjustments that participants make in relation to their work, to each other, and to the system. Unplanned coordination requires adequate communication, feedback, well-developed mutual expectations, and reciprocal understandings among members in related jobs. Its success also depends on the degree to which the work-relevant expectations, attitudes, motivations, and values of members in related jobs are congruent or complementary; the degree to which members can satisfy important personal needs and goals within rather than outside the system; and the extent to which participants, regardless of professional role and formal status, are willing to cooperate and promote organizationally relevant behavior on the basis of self-discipline, professional self-control, self-regulation of individualistic activity, and internalized altruistic motivation (Georgopoulos 1972).

Numerous factors contribute to lack of coordination, for example, the crucial issue of balance between clerical and coordinative functions in nursing. Adequate organizational coordination is a necessary condition for good patient care and work efficiency. Much of required coordination has to be effected by nurses because they are present at the patient's side 24 hours a day and they are the greatest in number. Nurses are asked to serve as the repository of residual functions in the system so that they can carry out functions that are not normally their own when others fail to provide patients with the necessary services, supplies, supportive functions, or information.

Another factor is increased specialization. As specialization increases, members are forced to function within a more complicated work situation, in which communication and information-processing requirements grow more demanding, coordination needs become more pressing, sources of strain become multiplied, interdisciplinary collaboration becomes more indispensable, and the work of the organization depends on the performance of members who differ more and more in attitude, goal, skill, and function (Georgopoulos 1966). Furthermore, the other key issue of authority versus specialized knowledge, or the problem of a good balance between legitimate authority for decision making and knowledge on which decisions must rest, results owing to specialization (Thompson 1961).

Signs and symptoms of lack of coordination other than those already mentioned can be classified as poor communication, that is, lack of and delayed information and lack of feedback; for example, members show signs of disorganization, patient activities and tests are delayed or omitted, and food trays are delayed after diagnostic tests that require fasting. Members are frustrated and complain of doing nonnursing jobs; there is either overlap in work done or omission of certain tasks; confusion is at its height.

The cause of the problem of lack of coordination can adequately be traced by the use of the ACP diagnostic tool, especially the tool that taps the organizing aspect of the administrative process. The investigator has to look at the job structure, authority system, communication system, and the social group. Once these areas are cleared of blame, the investigator can look at the implementation (directing and controlling) to find out if planned objectives are actually being carried out. Again, depending on the source of the problem, it may be possible to use command control sheets or master control sheets that log patient care activities for each eight-hour work shift; these can also act as an alert system and help coordinate activities.

Strain: role conflict

Strain refers to the individual's ability to minimize, manage, or resolve tensions and conflicts that arise within organizations, particularly friction and confrontation among highly interdependent groups and members and among participants of unequal status (Georgopoulos 1972).

In health care institutions, people with extremely different skills, abilities, backgrounds, needs, attitudes, orientations, and values are in frequent interaction within a work structure whose requirements for functional interdependence and close cooperation are unmatched when compared with other complex human organizations. In organizations in which division of labor and specialization of roles and functions are extensive, the sources of possible stress, strain, and misunderstanding are numerous. The fact that the system can contain and resolve conflicts and contradictions is more an indication of member adjustment, voluntary cooperation, and involvement than it is an outcome of formal authority sanctions, high professional standards, or monetary rewards to complying participants (Georgopoulos 1972).

The behavior of an individual within a social system is conceived of as "the product of motivational forces that derive in large part from the behavior of members of his role set, because the role set constantly brings influences to bear upon him which serves to regulate his behavior in accordance with role expectation they hold for him" (Kahn and co-workers 1964:35).

Getzels (1958) conceived of behavior as a function of both nomothetic and ideographic dimensions of a social system. The

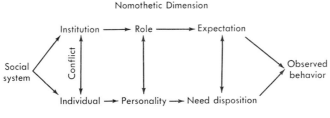

Fig. 8-1. Getzels' model of determinance of individual behavior and role conflict. (From Getzels, J. W.: Administration as a social process. In Halpin, A. W., editor: An administrative theory in education, Chicago, 1958, Midwest Administration Center, University of Chicago Press, p. 156. Copyright © University of Chicago.)

nomothetic dimension consists of institution, role, and expectations; the ideographic dimension consists of the individual and the individual's personality and need disposition. *Institution* designates agencies established to carry out organizational functions for the health care institution as a whole. *Roles* are the behavior expectations (such as duties, functions, and responsibilities) of the positions, offices, and statuses within an institution. Roles are defined in terms of expectation, and they are complementary.

Getzels presented his conception of the determination of the individual's behavior diagrammatically (Fig. 8-1). In the diagram each term on the two axes is the analytic unit for the term following it. For example, in the nomothetic dimension, institution is defined as a set of roles, and roles as a set of expectations. A behavior is derived simultaneously from the ideographic and nomothetic dimensions. The equation for this relation is $B = f(R \times P)$, where B is observed behavior, R is an institutional role, and P is the personality of the particular role incumbent.

According to Getzels (1958), in organizations there are three types of conflicts to be found that affect individual behaviors: (1) role-personality conflict, (2) role-conflict, and (3) personality conflict. These three types of conflict represent incongruence in the nomothetic dimension, in the ideographic dimension, or in the interaction between the two. Within the frame-

work of the theory, it can be generalized that such incongruence is symptomatic of administrative failure and leads to individual and organizational loss in productivity.

Role-personality conflict occurs as a result of the discrepancies between the pattern of expectations attached to a given role and the pattern of need dispositions characteristic of the incumbent of the role. An example is the situation in which a supervisor with an altruistic-nurturing personality (measured according the Strength Development Inventory [SDI] scale of Elias Porter [1973]) is asked to order, direct, reprimand, or fire a person, actions that require an assertive-directive personality (measured again by the SDI scale). Role-personality conflict results if the supervisor assumes this role uncomfortably and feels psychological pain and stress. According to Porter, there are three basic categories of personality or *relationship orientations*: altruistic-nurturing, *Blue* people; assertive-directive, *Red* people; and analytic-autonomizing, *Green* people. They differ from one another as follows:

sense of personal integrity Blue people view it as based on being genuinely helpful to others; Red, as being successful and gaining leadership over others; Green, as being self-sufficient, self-reliant, and independent.

derive personal satisfaction Blue, through success in fulfilling others' needs; Red, from success in directing accomplishments; Green, through success in managing resources.

basic approach to others Blue usually gets things

done for others; Red, through others; Green, independently of others.

view of cause of success Blue, a function of the exercise of concern for welfare of others; Red, the exercise of power and control; Green, the exercise of judicious foresight.

methods of exerting influence and leadership Blue, through reconciling differences and promoting goodwill and harmony; Red, by challenging, arguing, persuading, directing, and competing; Green, through establishing order, planning ahead, analyzing, and reserving judgment.

criteria for dispensing of rewards and incentives Blue, rewards should go to those people who are most helpful; Red, to the strongest person; Green, to the most analytic or judicious person.

judgment of others Blue judges others in terms of their helpfulness or selfishness or friendliness or aggressiveness; Red, in terms of strength and weaknesses (that is, who is strong versus who is weak) or winners or losers; Green, in terms of who is bright versus who is stupid or right versus wrong.

greatest source of satisfaction Blue people want to be thanked for things they have done for others, like to be needed, wanted, and liked; Red, from being challenged, followed, and being a winner; Green, from being respected for logic, perseverance, and fairness.

source of discomfort and threat Blue people experience threat and discomfort from anger and indifference and want to protect themselves from acting in an angry and selfish manner; Red, from seeing others show indifference toward them and withdraw their loyalty—they want to protect themselves from acting in a soft or gullible manner; Green, from others invading personal rights or from being over-helpful to them—they want to protect themselves from acting in a dependent and emotional manner.

view of self Blue person views self as needing to be more aggressive and hard-headed; Red, as needing to be more considerate of others and more planful; Green, as needing to be more sensitive and more self-assertive.

Each of these personality types has strengths that can be viewed by the other types as weaknesses. For example, altruistic-nurturing, Blue, individuals' typical support of others can be viewed as submissiveness, their loyalty as slavish, their trust of others as gullibility, their adaptability as spinelessness, their modesty as self-effacement, and their optimism as impracticability.

Assertive-directive, Red, individuals' ambitiousness can be viewed by others as ruthlessness, their competitiveness as combativeness, their self-confidence as arrogance, their persuasiveness as pushiness, their organizing capability as controlling, and their forcefulness as dictatorial.

The analytic-autonomizing, Green, individuals' cautiousness can be viewed by others as being suspicious, their analytical trait as nit-picking, their thoroughness as obsessive, their being methodical as rigidity, their being principled as purist, and their fairness as being unfeeling.

Everyone of us is a combination of all these three personality orientations, never simply one or the other. For example, if individuals are more Blue and Green than Red, they are the cautious-supporting type. If they are more Blue and Red than Green, they are the assertive-nurturing type. If they are more Red and Green than Blue, they are the judicious-competing type. If, however, they are equal parts of Red, Green, and Blue, they are the type of persons whose behaviors are very difficult to predict. Under conditions of conflict, an individual's actions may swerve more to one side than the other, depending on personality orientation. Porter's SDI scale (1973) is a valid and reliable diagnostic tool for assessing the strengths an individual uses in relating to others under two kinds of conditions: when relationships are proceeding smoothly and when they are not.

In role-personality conflict situations, persons placed in positions (nomothetic dimension) that require them to behave differently and inconsistently with their own repertoire of behavior (ideographic dimension) will experience dissatisfaction with what they are doing, will avoid the conflict-producing situation, will perform poorly in the duties prescribed by their position and role, and will avoid responsibilities.

As Getzels has pointed out, these signals of incongruence between nomothetic and ideographic dimensions are symptomatic of failure in the administrative process. On careful analysis, the investigator may trace the cause of the problem to failure in the areas of objectives, planning strategy, or the job structure aspect of organizing. Lawrence and Lorsch (1969), in planning a resolution to role-personality conflict problems, found it useful first to identify the behaviors required to perform a particular set of tasks effectively and then to determine the individual characteristics most often associated with them. For example, Lawrence and Lorsch (1967), in attempting to achieve more effective performance on the part of the *integrators* in an organization, made an analysis of the task and an examination of the personality characteristics of more or less effective performance on this job. It was learned from this two-pronged analysis that a relatively high need for affiliation, along with moderately high achievement, was associated with effectiveness.

Role conflict occurs when a role incumbent is required to conform simultaneously to a number of expectations that are mutually exclusive, inconsistent, or contradictory, so that adjustment to one set of requirements makes adjustment to the other very difficult. An example is the unresolved issue of balance between the performance by nurses of clinical and coordinative functions. The more coordinative functions nurses assume, the less time and energy they have to devote to patient care functions. As nursing accelerates specialization it will no longer be willing or able to carry out its coordinating activities and still discharge its professional responsibilities to patients and the organization (Georgopoulos 1972).

Another example of role conflict leading to role strain is in the area of commitment to the profession versus the organization. Professionals and specialists, nurses included, are usually more committed to their profession than to the specific organization. They have expert knowledge and technical competence to perform their roles autonomously, and conflicts arise because many decisions affecting them and their work are made by administrative people who have formal organizational authority and who may have good knowledge of the organization but very limited technical expertise. This situation leads to conflict and raises the issue of authority and the question of the proper balance between power and knowledge (Georgopoulos 1966).

The most common role conflicts occur within and between roles. This happens at the individual level when the manner in which persons think they are expected to behave (role perception) is different from the way others really expect them to behave (role expectation); for example, a supervisor may think the director wants most problems to be referred to her for consideration during meetings, whereas the director really thinks the meetings are too cluttered and wishes that the supervisor herself would make more decisions. Or it happens when two reference groups have conflicting expectations of a role incumbent; for example, the nurses' association may expect the director to press for higher salaries and less working hours per week, whereas the hospital board may expect the director to keep hospital costs down. Role conflict may occur among members within a reference group concerning their expectations for a role. For example, some nurses may expect their director or supervisor to initiate programs, but others may simply want her to stay out of their way and be ready to supply them with missing equipment and linen. Conflict can occur on the individual level over the relative saliency accorded two or more concurrent roles at a given point in time. This is the plight of nurses who at 3:30 PM may be torn between giving further help and care to patients and going home, so as to be there when their children return from school.

The signs and symptoms of role conflict are similar to those of role-personality conflict. There is confusion of roles, creating strain and unhappiness. Attitudes toward role and job are adversely affected, and one person's unhappiness infects coworkers, leading to dissatisfaction all around.

Here again, these signs and symptoms can be traced to failure in the ACP. Once the diagnosis is made, corrective action can be taken. In addition, Georgopoulos (1972) suggested that conflicts resulting from organizational constraints and regimentation can be minimized as members learn to accept and function interdependently, respecting not only their own needs but also those of others. The fact is inescapable that members within an organization must work interdependently, because the performance of each is always contingent on that of others.

Georgopoulos (1972) pointed out that a system-wide effort in the hospital can bring about effective role performance if a balance between primary and secondary relations is achieved by minimizing organizational requirements and constraints and by maximizing opportunity for professional autonomy and self-expression. Yet these efforts must be consistent with the patterns of functional interdependence that characterize work in the system. It is basically the responsibility of organizational leadership to achieve and maintain the balance. Balance is predicated on the conditions that members accept their interdependence and behave accordingly and that the distribution of influence and rewards in the system is acceptable to all.

Personality conflict occurs as a result of opposing-need dispositions within the personality of the role incumbents themselves. *Need-disposition* is refined by Parsons and Shets (1951) as the tendency to orient and act with respect to objects in a certain manner and to expect in return certain consequences. The conjoined word need-disposition "itself has a double connotation; for one, the tendency to fulfill a requirement

of the organism to accomplish an end state; for the other, the inclination to do something with an object that was designed to accomplish that end state" (Parsons and Shets 1951:114-115).

Personality conflict is illustrated by a comment from Charlie Brown, the "Peanut's" character, "I love mankind; it's people I can't stand." An example in the hospital is the supervisor who wants to please the director but dislikes doing certain tasks requested by the director. Such a conflict results in strain, discomfort, and conflict within the person. The cause of these problems can be found in the job structure aspect of organizing or failure in other aspects of administrative process. Once the cause is found, actions can be taken to remedy it or reduce the conflict.

A degree of conflict within organizations is inevitable, healthy, and productive of change, resulting in creative transformations that improve the structure and functioning of the organization. Lonsdale (1964) suggested that people who, because of their intolerance of ambiguity, attempt to resolve all conflict or to cover it up miss the fact that some amount of social disorganization makes for stimulating relationships and positive changes. But the question is, how much? There is no pat answer. Only further research of the antecedents and consequences of role and other types of conflicts can begin to answer this question.

Meanwhile, wasteful and pointless role conflict and strain can be reduced by analyzing and studying roles and communicating about them more objectively. Participants can observe role behavior of others and learn from this observation. They can read, study, and talk about roles and their meaning. They can role play and evaluate their own role behavior. To employ role theory in conjunction with the ACP provides a means for conceptualizing problems of individual performance within the organization in a way that yields keener insights and a deeper rational view of organizational behavior than heretofore possible.

CONCLUSION

The problems that occur at the individual-to-group interface level in a health care institution beg the question of how balanced or satisfactory the solutions can be. At this stage in the development of organization research, considerably more theoretical and empirical work is required. Hopefully, what has been achieved in the preceding discussion is a conceptual framework with which to start attacking problems that exist at the individual level. Although it may not solve every problem, the conceptual framework, if correctly used, should reduce the severity of the problem to manageable form.

REFERENCES

Bennis, W. G.: Organization development: its nature, origin, and prospects, Menlo Park, Calif., 1969, Addison-Wesley Pub. Co., Inc.

Etzioni, A.: Modern organizations, Englewood Cliffs, N. J., 1964, Prentice Hall, Inc.

Georgopoulos, B. S.: The hospital system and nursing: some basic problems and issues, Nurs. Forum 5(3):8-35, 1966.

Georgopoulos, B. S.: The hospital as an organization and problem-solving system. In Georgopoulos, B. S., editor: Organization research on health institutions, Ann Arbor, Mich., 1972, Institute for Social Research, pp. 9-48.

Georgopoulos, B. S., and Christman, L.: The clinical nurse specialist: a role model, Am. J. Nurs. **70**:1030-1039, 1970.

Getzels, J. W.: Administration as a social process. In Halpin, A. W., editor: Administrative theory in education, Chicago, 1958, Midwest Administration Center, University of Chicago Press, pp. 150-165.

Herzberg, F. J., Mausner, B., and Snyderman, B.: The motivation to work, New York, 1959, John Wiley & Sons, Inc.

Kahn, R., Wolfe, D. M., Quinn, R. P., and Snoek, J. D.: Organizational stress, New York, 1964, John Wiley & Sons, Inc.

Katz, D., and Kahn, R. L.: The social psychology of organization, New York, 1966, John Wiley & Sons, Inc.

Lawrence, P. R., and Lorsch, J. W.: New management job: the integrator, Harvard Business Review, **45**(6):142-151, November-December 1967.

Lawrence, P. R., and Lorsch, J. W.: Developing organizations: diagnosis and action, Menlo Park, Calif., 1969, Addison-Wesley Pub. Co., Inc.

Litwin, G. H., and Stringer, R. A., Jr.: Motivation and organizational climate, Boston, 1968, Division of Research, Harvard Business School.

Lonsdale, R. C.: Maintaining the organization in dynamic equilibrium. In Griffith, D. E., editor: Behavioral science and educational administration, in National Society for Study of Education, Chicago, 1964, University of Chicago Press, pp. 142-177.

McClelland, D.: The achieving society, New York, 1961, D. Van Nostrand Co.

McLean, J. G.: Better reports for better control, Harvard Business Review, **35**(3):95-104, May-June 1957.

Metcalf, H. C., and Urwick, L., editors: Dynamic administration: the collected papers of Mary Parker Follet, New York, 1941, Harper & Brothers.

Murphy, J.: Theoretical issues in professional nursing, New York, 1971, Appleton-Century-Crofts.

Myers, C. A., and Turnbull, J. C.: Line and staff in industrial relations, Harvard Business Review, **34**(4):113-124, July-August 1956.

Myers, M. S.: Who are your motivated workers? Harvard Business Review, **42**(1):73-88, January-February 1964.

Parsons, T., and Shets, E. A.: Personality as a system of action. In Parsons, T., and Shets, E., editors: Toward a general theory of action, Cambridge, Mass., 1951, Harvard University Press.

Porter, E.: Strength development inventory, rev. ed., Pacific Palisades, Calif., 1973, Personal Strengths Assessment Service.

Roethlisberger, F. J., and Dickson, W. J.: Management and the worker, Cambridge, Mass., 1939, Harvard University Press.

Roy, C.: Adaptation: a conceptual framework for nursing, Nurs. Outlook, **18**(3):42-45, March 1970.

Roy, C.: Adaptation: a basis for nursing practice, Nurs. Outlook, **19**(4):254-257, April 1971.

Schein, E. H.: Organizational psychology, Englewood Cliffs, N. J. 1965, Prentice-Hall, Inc.

Seiler, J. A.: A systems approach to organizational behavior, Homewood, Ill., 1967, Richard D. Irwin, Inc., pp. 51-81.

Thompson, V.: Modern organization, New York, 1961, Alfred A. Knopf, Inc.

Watson, E. T.: Diagnosis of management problems, Harvard Business Review, **36**(1):69-76, January-February 1958.

White, R.: Ego and reality in psychoanalytic

theory, Psychol. Issues, Monograph no. 11 3(3):24-43, 1963.

ADDITIONAL READINGS

Georgopoulos, B. S., and Matyko, A.: The American general hospital as a complex social system, Health Serv. Res. 2:76-112, 1967.

Murray, H. A., and Kluckhohn, C.: Outline of a conception of personality. In Kluckhohm, C., and Murray, H. A., editors: Personality in nature, society, and culture, New York, 1953, Alfred A. Knopf Co.

Sarbin, T. R.: Role theory. In Lindzey, G., editor: Handbook of social psychology. I. Theory and method, Reading, Mass., 1954, Addison-Wesley Pub. Co., Inc.

Searles, R. E.: The relation between communication and social integration in the community hospital, doctoral dissertation, Ann Arbor, 1961, University of Michigan.

Chapter 9

PROBLEM OF INTERDEPARTMENTAL RELATIONSHIPS: THE PROBLEM-SOLVING PROCESS

Anything that interferes with goal attainment is a problem and is a symptom of the need for change. In nursing service, any problem that affects the quality of patient care is a serious one, and the problem of interdepartmental relationships, which has plagued nursing from its inception, is especially so. The problem is escalating because of an increase in knowledge and because of rapid specialization, which have led to patient care contributions by many scientific specialists from different departments. What is the cause of poor interdepartmental relationships, and what can be done about this problem? Certainly, recognizing or diagnosing the problem is paramount, and deciding what action to take, once the problem is diagnosed, is close behind.

How can the nursing service executive put administrative theory to work in solving problems of interdepartmental relations? What does the literature have to say that will help in solving them?

The administrative theory within the systems framework (see Fig. 2-1) can be very useful. The specific concept for making a diagnosis of a problem involves all the processes of administration, namely, setting objectives, planning, organizing, directing, and controlling. The approach is not new; it constitutes the framework of analysis in much of the current literature on problems of administration. But often theories are presented without an adequate demonstration of how they can be put to work.

Our model, which distinguishes the administrative functions from the environment in which administration occurs, becomes a tool for problem solving. No other author, with the exception of Watson (1958), has used the administrative processes as a diagnostic measure, and Watson tried to give more and new meaning to the concept.

Furthermore, to be serviceable to nursing service administrators, a theory must enable them to understand the problems of an existing situation, provide assistance when a course of action is needed, and be flexible enough to be employed in the variety of situations that nursing service administrators encounter. The purpose here is to show that the composite process or the administrative processes provide a framework that satisfies these conditions.

Using this approach, we will follow a nursing service administrator—who must view an institution's situation from the top administrative level, use conceptual skills, and see the institution's problems as a whole—step by step through the job of examining the basic functions of administration and then of making a diagnosis of the problem or problems encountered.

INPUTS

The health care facility is seen as an open system; that is, it is a developing and innovative system. It receives inputs or information from the external environment (community, patients, and families) and from the internal environment (medical and nursing staffs, patients, and administrators). The following are examples of inputs from these areas.

From the community: the nursing service administrator obtains information requesting (1) more outpatient or clinic services, (2) more health instruction by nurses to patients before the patients leave the hospital, (3) better communication between physicians and nurses, (4) less waiting time for inpatients in treatment areas, and (5) reduction in cost of services.

From the nursing staff: (1) some departments are uncooperative in that they set their own time for patient treatment without considering the nursing department; (2) other departments feel "superior" because of their research work and added grant funds; (3) physicians interfere with requests of administration that the nurses work within stated policies; (4) nursing supervisors are blamed for too many things for which they are not responsible; (5) staff nurses feel they are too far removed from doing meaningful, high-quality work; and (6) the departments are too far apart in their thinking regarding the purpose of the organization.

From the medical staff: (1) lack of meaningful and productive communication with nurses, (2) diagnostic tests not done promptly, (3) requests for more nurses in all areas, and (4) requests made by administration regarding policy interferes with their authority as experts at treating patients under their care.

From hospial administration: (1) How can costs be cut in the nursing department? (2) What is the cost of a continuing education program for the department, and what is its contribution to patient care?

From patient: inadequate nursing care. For example, one female patient complained that there had been "too long a wait" in the admitting department, even though the physician had assured the patient that all the necessary provisions for admission had been made. The long wait that ensued resulted in a parking ticket to her husband. But her greatest complaint was that, despite the fact that her physician had told her there would be specific orders left with the nurse so that she would be prepared for home care, she was not taught by the nurse how to take care of herself after her return home. This caused her and her family much anguish. The dietitian had seen her only once, which seemed inadequate because after arriving home she realized that she did not understand the dietary instructions. During the morning of her last day the physiotherapy department wanted her early for treatment and told her to be "ready" in the morning. The therapist arrived just as her breakfast was being served. Her choice seemed to be either to miss the breakfast or miss the treatment; she decided to miss the breakfast. The patient wondered how much doctors and nurses communicated since she was told one thing by the physician concerning her treatment and another thing by the nurse. With such high costs, she had to go home as soon as possible. "Everybody is so busy including the nurses," she complained, "that nobody has time to really listen to what the patients are saying." Fig. 9-1 illustrates a representative day in the life of a patient.

From the nursing service administrators: Recognition of great strain within the nursing department is revealed on the faces of the nursing staff. According to the research study conducted by Arndt and Laegar (1970 *a* and *b*), nursing service administrators understand the meaning of a diversified role set and that they are in a boundary position. From their own observations, they know that there is lack of cohesion at the staff nurse level; the supervisors coordinate the work, but instead of permitting the staff nurses to

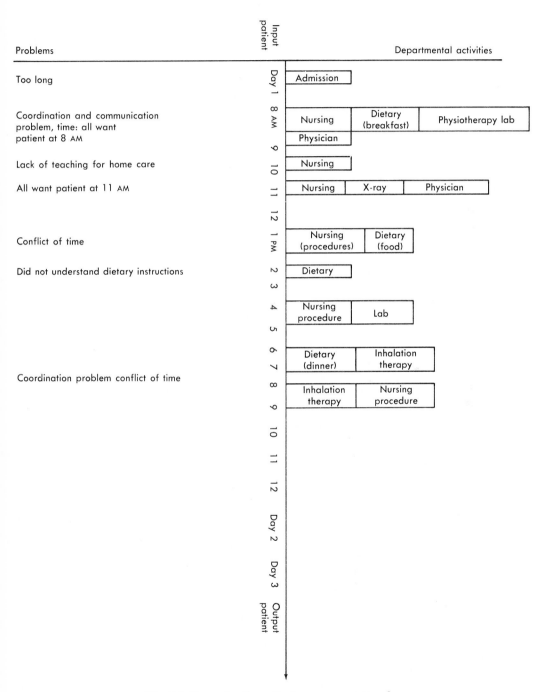

Fig. 9-1. Processing the patient: a representative day.

make their own decisions, the nursing service administrators interfere by doing so themselves.

SENSING AND ANALYSIS

After spending considerable time on analysis of the input received and her observations, the nursing service administrator attempts to draw up a statement of the department's problems: she finds the number of patients served by nursing declining, low staff morale, rising costs, and related difficulties. Her previous thinking has been along clinical unit lines, and she tends to think about the department head position in the same way—as a collection of people performing patient care activities, nursing services—about the cost involved, and other clinical unit responsibilities. Unfortunately, she finds that in dealing with departmental level problems she cannot make these problems fit specific clinical unit categories; the problems have a way of cutting across departmental boundaries.

It is difficult for her to decide whether the major problems represent inadequate nursing service, insufficient staffing, a limited budget, or personnel unprepared for the job; and it does not help to lump these problems together into budget, nursing service, and supervision. To tackle just the inefficiencies within each clinical unit or department is like stamping out minor fires without quenching the main blaze, but the nursing service administrator has trouble viewing the administrator's job in any way other than as a collection of department responsibilities. If there are inefficiencies within the departments, how else should the difficulties be eliminated except by tackling them one by one?

It is at this point that a theoretical framework can provide a logical system of inquiry. Using the systems approach, the nursing service administrator can first of all establish the fact that departmental activities are interrelated. The impact of a force, such as a change in procedure, in one department affects the entire organization's operation and is likely to produce ripples of reaction in other departments. Many of the trouble spots in various departments are probably related to one another. The first step is for the nursing administrator to regard those trouble spots as symptoms (not as individual, self-contained problems) and to try to get an overall picture, in other words, make a fundamental diagnosis.

Secondly, to get an overall view, the nursing service administrator needs some meaningful way of talking about the underlying problems that have produced diverse symptoms of trouble. At higher levels of administration, problems tend to overlap departmental boundaries, and the departmental tags such as nursing service, research, and medicine often do not fit. The composite process provides a better way of generalizing about these underlying issues. It not only offers a logical system of inquiry but also may suggest some additional analysis that the nursing service administrator may have overlooked when examining the basic data. Do the symptoms point to some failure of administration in setting objectives, in planning, in organizing, or in directing or controlling? Examining the symptoms in light of these processes may be very revealing for the nursing service administrator.

DIAGNOSIS UTILIZING THE CONCEPTUAL AND PHYSICAL ACTS (ACP) FRAMEWORK
Setting objectives

Although objectives are often discussed in broad terms, such as goals of the institution and responsibility to community and personnel, a narrower definition would be more helpful. The approach can be improved by pegging objectives to the specific part of the community's health care that the institution will offer. An institution's objectives can go beyond the service itself to the kind of demand involved, for example, more patient care in the form of home care.

What makes the matter of objectives so important is that most health care organizations are undergoing rapid and constant change. The fact that nursing care and nursing service change so rapidly tends to divert the administrator's eye from what is going on. Yet, it is easy to overlook trends threatening the existing patient care and services that are inconsistent with resources and goals. Consequently, unless administration regularly reviews its nursing situation and organizational objectives, it is likely to be too late in sizing up a new trend.

TRACING FAILURE

In diagnosing the health care facility's problems, the administrator may find many of the symptoms can be traced to a failure in the area of objectives, for example, uncertainty about the nursing service department's position within the health care system, the attempt to embark on programs without adequate resources, or a failure to adjust to changes in the external environment. An objective that often stands out by its absence is that the department of nursing is not present at the policy-making level. It is here that goals are set, decisions made, and direction given; it is the formative stage in which cooperation, coordination, and integration begin among department heads. The administrator also finds that an overall organizational goal or objective is missing. Otherwise, the review of her department's objectives, in general, shows them to be adequate, as are those from her clinical units as set up by her supervisors and head nurses, including individualized care and health teaching.

The nursing service administrator may have had to do a good deal of interviewing and study to turn up such a failure in policy planning formulation. It is not likely to be readily apparent, especially since administrators usually give lip service to the importance of setting objectives, even if they rarely do much specific work concerning them. But, if a careful investigation reveals a failure in this area, the nursing service administrator can give top administrators every assurance that intelligent efforts to cope with the problem will bring significant results—results that may show up not just in one department but in many.

It may well be asked, What is the important difference between the diagnostic approach and a more superficial attack on symptoms? If one starts with, We need better supervisors, we need more staffing, and we need to cut costs; the chances are that there will be plenty of evidence to support the case. A failure to set objectives is likely to result in identical conclusions. Consequently, the investigation will end prematurely, and efforts to set things straight, however drastic, will fall short. This is often observed among nursing services dominated by functional thinking, and it is no wonder that specialists and some consultants can almost always discover "what is wrong" in an ailing organization simply by applying their specialized knowledge.

But, when the diagnostic approach has been taken, the nursing service administrator may not trace the problem to objectives or, if so, only partly. This means that the other processes of administration must be examined.

Planning strategy

The need for a particular health care service in the community is the starting point for planning a strategy that can give the organization and nursing service a good advantage. Administration needs a plan for that service based on the characteristics and needs of the community, the resources of the organization, and the conditions of the economic environment—a plan that promises a good service. Planning strategy is, of course, closely related to the needs of the community.

An effective strategy involves recognition of activities that are most essential to the health needs of the community at a particular time. Health care efforts may shift emphasis at different stages of growth, and development as a social service has to adapt to external and internal environments according to demand. In one period, research may command special attention, whereas, in another, home care or some other activity may be more important. Unless administrators can gauge the areas that need special attention at particular times, they may find that the neglect of a critical situation has resulted in a loss of quality service to the people of the community.

All this may seem obvious enough in principle, but it is not so easy to effect in practice. For example, strategy becomes embedded in organizational policy, and policies sometimes become very sacred, so sacred that succeeding administrators may hesitate to change a particular policy, either because it is difficult to argue with success or because of the belief that present trends are fads that will soon disappear.

SCHEDULING AND COORDINATION

Planning of still another kind is also required. What quantity and quality of nursing care can be planned in advance with some certainty? Which departments should work most closely together?

The planning function brings into clear focus problems that arise from viewing the job of administration as a collection of departmental activities without relation to a larger purpose, namely, quality patient care. The admitting department may want different hours and longer time notices for patient dismissals. The operating room department, if left to its own devices, may want to standardize procedures more than the nursing department can accept. There may be brisk competition between departments for available resources. All the major departments must take part in planning, but administration must resolve conflicting purposes in terms of what will contribute most to attaining the organization goal.

DIAGNOSTIC TOOL

For the nursing service administrator the use of the diagnostic tool means that, regardless of the kind of planning, an appreciation of the sequence as well as optimum timing of a program is important. She must ask herself if any of the symptoms stem from failure to develop strategy or from some other aspect of planning.

If the plan is carefully thought out, some of the departmental problems may be budgeted for or anticipated. There are forces that influence planning in balancing the needs of one clinical unit or department against another. The administrator may have purposely taken a calculated risk and decided that, in view of its limited resources, the cost of temporary inefficiency in one area will be more than offset by the long-run gains in another, for example a department of continued education and nursing research. The question is whether the cost is greater than anticipated; and, if so, whether the plan should be revised. The presence of planning is thus a valuable diagnostic tool that can aid the administrator in analysis of the organization's problems.

Having reviewed her planning, the administrator comes to the conclusion that although the plan did not allow for the department heads to plan together, this step does not contain the key to her problems. She has to go to the next step in the diagnosis—another one of the processes, namely, organization.

Organizing as a diagnostic aid

The organization of an institution presents problems of adaptation as the institution grows. For instance, new divisions of responsibility may become necessary if certain activities, such as research and intensive care units, are to receive adequate attention or if different relationships among departments are required to reduce the strain on overloaded supervisors. It may be necessary to make decisions at different levels since overcentralization produces a slow-moving organization. New and old staff activities need to be fitted into the organization in ways that contribute to the quality of work and decision making. The administrator must also devote attention to the task of continued education of personnel.

The job of adaptation is complicated by the social characteristics of an organization. Change upsets the existing customs and routines, and vested interests oppose reduction in authority or shrinkage in the scope of activities. Moving too fast, therefore, can result in demoralization.

Accurate analysis of an organizational problem is one of the most difficult jobs there is; yet this is also an area in which hasty judgments abound.

Perhaps the most important tool the nursing administrator needs, if she hopes to delve very deeply in her analysis, is a systematic vocabulary governing organization. There is the tendency to distinguish between an "organizational problem" and a "human relations problem"—a dichotomy that would be more useful in dealing with discrete and distinct items. Unfortunately, a structural difficulty is likely to be accompanied by disturbed personal relationships and other problems; to focus on only one of the two produces a distorted picture. There are so many dimensions to an organizational situation that it is simple to find what one wants to find, be it a problem of status, bureaucracy, or any of a number of other concepts applicable in part but not exclusively so.

The verbal short cuts used in discussing organization produce mistaken notions of agreement. Agreement at a fairly high level of abstraction may conceal fundamental differences in the way the details of a situation are analyzed. Hence, we need to make a stronger effort to examine and talk about organizational systems in terms of the many mutually interdependent elements involved, such as structure, social groups, and individuals.

The task is complicated by the need to focus on the separate elements and also to retain an understanding of the total situation. By that we mean, in the words of Mary Parker Follet (1942:91-92), "not only trying to see every factor that influences the situation, but even more than that, the relation of these factors to one another." We are forced to resort to an analytical framework before proceeding. An organizational system has five dimensions, each of which can be examined separately as long as their mutual interdependence is kept in mind.

JOB STRUCTURE

In surveying the job structure for problems, administrators need various points of view. The staff nurse can judge the feasibility of methods and procedures; the supervisor or head nurse can analyze tasks from the standpoint of simplification of operations; the nursing service administrator and her immediate associates are concerned with whether the position structure takes advantage of specialization and whether nursing know-how is economical, affords adequate control, gets attention when needed, and is coordinated with related activities. The administrator can also examine the levels at which decisions are made to see if further centralization or decentralization at specific points will improve the structure.

The investigation may reveal difficulties that have shown up as frictions between people. Similarly, the inquiry may show that troubles in communications or lines of authority are in part symptoms. The failure that might be superficially diagnosed as a communications failure, for example, may really be a communications and job structure failure.

AUTHORITY SYSTEM

Assigning a job carries with it the assignment of authority to fulfill its responsibilities. In the literature of management there are many proverbs about the definition, allocation, and recognition of authority, all of which are useful as general guides but which are limited in value when the main concern is building cooperative relationships. Many problems crop up on the fringes of departmental responsibility, where solutions seem to depend more on cooperative intent than on precision in defining authority.

The traditional literature of management has much more to say about the relationships between a superior and subordinates than about the job relationships of people who are in different channels of authority but who must nonetheless cooperate to get the work done. In checking to see if symptoms of trouble are due to organizational failures, the nursing service administrator will do well to look at both types of interaction. Some writers have assumed that cross relationships between persons in different channels of authority would be properly influenced when necessary by appeal to the superior in charge of all the activities in question. In practice, these full-dress hearings often fail to produce cooperative behavior and, to avoid undesirable consequences, should be used only in cases of last resort.

Sometimes the way in which tasks can best be performed does not coincide with the manner in which authority, according to traditional beliefs, is supposed to be distributed. A study of line and staff relationships has shown that they do not reduce to a simple formula according to which the expert always "advises" or "persuades." As an expert in some matters, the staff person often ends up with the actual power to make certain decisions, regardless of what the organizational chart indicates. The danger, which may or may not materialize but which certainly should be watched, is that the line supervisor's role as an administrator will be considerably weakened as a result.

COMMUNICATIONS SYSTEM

Assignment of jobs and allocation of authority establish certain formal channels of communication, around which can be developed a system of communication that in turn is important to the support of the authority relationships. The informal channels elaborate the network through which people interact; here, adequacy depends primarily on the individual's behavior and capacity for communication.

Real skill in communication is so difficult to achieve that the administrator will probably be able to trace some of the trouble to this source. The problem is what to do about it once she has brought the matter to the "top" administrator's attention. In the long run, education may help, but in the short run, the gains are likely to be limited to improving other aspects of the organizational system that indirectly affect communication. It is also possible that administration will recognize its responsibility, as a distinct function, to create a better environment for communication.

SOCIAL SYSTEM

The formal relationships within a health care facility compose a structure around which informal activities develop. The members of the organizational system are also members of many smaller, interlocking groups (informal organizations) held together by bonds of common interest. Changes of many kinds can disturb or upset social relations within these groups, with repercussion throughout wide areas of the organization.

Social systems reflect the desires of individuals to share with others their common experiences, attitudes, and beliefs and, as such, give an individual the support and security that add meaning to the world of work. On the other hand, group norms are also an effective measure of control over individual behavior. Social custom is, of course, not always amenable to administration's purposes, but neither is it always opposed. The members of a group may develop a strong identification with their work and hence with organizational goals assigned to them. The social system as an aid to integration is very important.

The individual

An administrator is accustomed to judging the adequacy of individuals in performing specific jobs but also finds it impossible to ignore their ability or inability to relate to others. It is important to realize that although people are sensitive to the norms of the group, they also retain many individual feelings. Their behavior is influenced not only by the work environment but also by their off-the-job life. Although there may be some grounds for accusing members of contemporary society of being conformists with respect to items such as dress, food, and choice of movies, they still remain highly individualistic in their self-beliefs, motivations, hopes, and goals.

Interdependent functions

Since the preceding five dimensions of an organizational system are mutually interdependent, changes in one area will produce effects in other areas. All areas are likely to be affected from time to time by planning, controlling, and operating decisions, as well as by professional organizations, community norms, economic trends, and other factors outside the institution. The sensitivity of the organizational system and the interdependence of its parts can be illustrated in many ways. The following is an example of what can happen:

> The nursing service administrator decided to add new nursing skills to the service in an effort to improve patient care. Knowledge and skills in nursing were demanded that the present supervisor did not possess, so a new nurse was hired in her place and given the title of clinical nurse specialist. For many years that nursing division had been quite stable, with nursing care routines undergoing little change. Certain groups of skilled nurses had attained advanced positions with respect to responsibilities, income, and assignment. The new nurse's position and relationships to the organization, however, were never made clear.

Instead of functioning as a clinical nurse specialist, she assumed more and more directing duties, made changes in the physical arrangement and equipment, broke up some customary working habits, and changed groups that had been tightly knit. Some of the more skilled nursing groups complained directly to hospital administration, bypassing the nursing service administrator, and they were given an increase in salaries. Nursing personnel with less advanced positions became so concerned over job security that their work declined in quality and quantity. The new clinical nurse specialist became absorbed in details and neglected to establish relationships with her staff; nursing administration, following organizational tradition, left the division to be administered by the clinical specialist. The decline in patient care performance resulted in a poor nursing reputation for that division.

If the nursing service administrator confines her analysis to two or three aspects of the organizational system, she may again end up attacking symptoms instead of causes. In the preceding example, any trouble in communication, status, or line of authority is bound to reflect, at least in part, the failure of individuals or the disruption of the social system.

But, suppose the nursing administrator, following the diagnostic approach, still has not been able to identify the problem plaguing the institution. She can carry her investigation further and look at the directing process.

Directing as a diagnostic aid

The nursing service administrator, having surrounded herself with qualified people, still needs to acquaint these people with the purpose, goals, and objectives of the organization and the means for accomplishing them, that is, the purpose of direction.

The planning and organization scheme has provided the nursing service administrator with a mechanism for the attainment of purpose; she must now put the mechanism to use. The first function of the administrator to set that mechanism in motion is to direct its implementation (Tannenbaum 1949). Direction is the formal use of authority to guide nursing personnel. It involves devising purposes of action, methods, and procedures to be followed in achieving goals. The decisions to be made in connection with direction must determine "what," "how," "when," and "where." Developing the purposes of action provides the "what" content of direction. The nursing service administrator and her staff must formulate purposes, goals, and objectives of the department, but they must do so within the overall organizational goals. Departmental objectives may be broken down into those of the division, the location, and the individual. The final test is to have a particular objective for every person; all objectives should be coordinated to produce successive cumulative results leading back to the general objective for the institution as a whole.

The devising of methods or procedures to be followed in achieving purposes provides the "how," "when," and "where" of direction. Here again the broad and general decisions are made by the nursing administrator in conjunction with her staff, and these decisions are made ever more specific by successive staffs down through the line.

Directive decisions, once made, serve as a basis for the guidance of action. Most directive decisions are made to guide personnel in actions that are repeated frequently and rarely, if ever, to guide actions that are performed but once. To avoid unnecessary duplication in decision making, administrators have developed numerous devices or tools known by terms such as budgets, policies, procedures, rules, schedules, and designs. These devices release for other purposes much valuable time that would otherwise have to be devoted to redeciding and are also used by administrators as criteria of action, since each implies a standard of performance to be attained.

Examining the symptoms of the problem in terms of the directing functions establishes the fact that the purpose of the organization is clearly defined on paper, but the definition of the purpose is inadequate and not well understood. Provision has not been made for individual goals nor has the purpose to be achieved in the individual nurse's activity been made clear. Also missing is an effective set of well-written policies that will give members of an organization the security they need when making effective decisions.

Having improved her focus by examining direction, the administrator should give thought to making the processes complete by learning from the process of control.

Controlling as a diagnostic aid

Even though the administrator may visualize what the objective should be, how it should be reached, and who is to do the job and may put the plans into action, she still has to establish a form of control and has to follow up to see that plans are carried out. The administrator cannot always anticipate events, so at times, plans must be modified very quickly. A scheme is needed to apprise administration of what is taking place at the patient care level to prevent service and care from getting out of kilter.

Control is the function of checking on performance and measuring results against a standard. The standard depends on what is being controlled and can be in terms of target dates for completion of certain jobs or efficiency measures of some kind, such as unit cost, quantity and quality of patient care, and direct labor costs. At the lower levels of organizational activity, the techniques of the cost accountant and supervisor are easily applicable if tasks became crystallized into routines and procedures. But, if top administration is uncertain about its objectives or has failed to plan ahead, control at lower levels may be undermined.

Control is difficult at best, as experienced administrators know. There are difficulties in knowing what information is critical and how to get it. Relying on a single technique, such as formal reports from below, is dangerous. The confident nursing service administrator who never goes near a supervisor's department may find her confidence misplaced, for serious problems develop when there is a lag between the outbreak of trouble and the time it is reflected in reports. The goal of being completely informed will probably never be universally attained, but the tendency for bad news to be filtered out as information travels upward is a factor to reckon with.

Coordination is often linked with control. If an effective job has been done in selecting objectives, planning, organizing, directing, and controlling, the net result will be a coordinated effort. To achieve a coordinated effort, administrators at all levels must know what they are to attain, how to attain, who is to do each job, and when modifications of plans and activities are needed. In other words, coordination is not a separate and distinct function of administration but is a composite of other functions that are highly interrelated and that depend on skillful administration for their individual effectiveness.

Statement of diagnosis

If the nursing service administrator has done a careful job of investigating and interpreting the findings, there will emerge a clearer view of the organization's underlying problems than could have been obtained by thinking only in terms of departmental categories. The administrator now has some "handles" to grab. If her analysis shows that the symptoms stem largely from failures in certain administrative processes, she will be able to muster the evidence to show how these failures have produced ripples or even waves of reaction throughout the institution and will be able to avoid such generalities as "the organization needs more supervisors," or "the organization's problem is lack of funds."

Once she focuses on the symptoms and can make a diagnosis, the nursing service administrator must ask herself, What should I do about it? Here, once again, she will find the concept of the process of the administration useful in formulating a plan of action.

The aim of this particular method of analysis is to gain a fuller appreciation of the underlying problems that plague nursing service administration, rather than to focus attention on the superficial "tagging" of a problem as one, say, of staffing or of control, although there are many such problems common to all organizations. The manner in which a particular organization is affected and the way in which treatment should be administered vary from case to case. The underlying problem was found to be that the failure to centralize authority caused parts of the organization to develop their own internal objectives separate from and inconsistent with the general purpose. For example, the health care facility has as its general objective the care of patients, but in the process of organization, many secondary objectives may develop; the health care facility may be used as a field of research or education. Although neither of these purposes is inconsistent with the general objectives, it is important that they not be pursued to the extent that the main objective, that is, patient care, suffers.

It was also found that another failure stemmed from the fact that the executive had not set an overall organizational goal to which all departments could aspire. Furthermore, it was found that the nursing service administrator had not been invited to participate when overall institutional policy and plans were formulated, and thus department heads were not encouraged to plan together. Planning, which is essentially the controlling of time, became all important. In organizing, the importance of the relationships among the factors of the position structure, the social system, the individual, the authority system, and communication were not recognized. The informal groups formed among the personnel seemed to hold the staff together. Satisfaction was derived from association with people on the job. Nursing personnel were not matched to the job. The staff nurse was not assigned full responsibility and accountability for patient care nor was she given a number of coordinating functions. Norms and standards limiting the work processes were not understood. Decisions were made mainly at the supervisory level. Tasks as set up were unrelated and communication was almost nonexistent. Control of the work processes was not well understood. Controls were divorced from the work situation and split up into subtasks; the cohesiveness between subtasks rested with the organization rather than with the responsible personnel.

The diagnosis of the underlying problem confronting the nursing service administrator in our example may be stated as centering on interdepartmental relationships or integration resulting in fragmented patient care or the inability of the system to integrate itself. This includes functions associated with integrating the individual into the organization, securing their cooperation and compliance, and integrating all parts of the social system so that the total organization can achieve a certain overall sociopsychological unity and coherence. Development of common organization values, shared norms, attitudes, and mutual understandings, which can serve to provide a common universe of discourse for the different groups and members and to socialize and bind the members securely into the system, are all important in this area.

Georgopoulos (1972) identified seven categories into which all problems, be they organizational, individual, or group, can be classified: lack of integration, strain, minimized organizational output, lack of coordination, misallocation of resources, inability to adapt well to the external environment, and difficulty in maintaining itself or preserving its identity and integrity as a problem-solving system in the face of changes that are constantly occurring in the environment. When one of the seven problems is identified as the core problem, the remaining six also crop up.

INTERVENTION

The question now confronting the administrator is, How do I resolve the problem? The answer is clear: Work toward (1) improvement of interdepartmental relationships and responsibilities, (2) improvement of intradepartmental relationships, and (3) improved understanding of the nursing department in relation to the health care facility as a whole.

The next question is, What outcomes (or objectives) are expected from the change, and how are these to be measured? The objectives are (1) to improve patient care, fragmentation specifically, (2) to establish a total team effort for maximum achievement of the dominating objective, and (3) to establish measures of outcome.

Techniques of change

The choice of the particular technique of change depends on the nature of the problem the administrator has diagnosed. The administrator must determine what is most likely to produce the desired outcome. Donnelly, Gibson, and Ivancevich (1971) classified problems according to the major focus of the technique needed to bring about desired outcome. They identified the following three problems: (1) behavior, (2) structure, and (3) technology. The classification in no way implies a distinct division among the three types. On the contrary, the interrelationships must be acknowledged and anticipated. The change technique, according to the major focus of our problem, is concerned with changes in behavior (knowledge, attitude, and skills) and in job structure (tasks to be performed and effect of new machinery on personnel).

However, it is not necessary for changes in behavior and structure to start from scratch. Much work has usually been done in any organization. A fair amount of human relations and public relations work has been started. Task analysis and job descriptions are already available. Process analysis and routing schemes are in operation. All these things are, in fact, typical products of an organization that Lewin (1947) would describe as "frozen" and in "isolation." Processes and relationships are analyzed, quantified, and schematized according to a rational model. People are fitted in. In this static organization the essential thing is the way in which relationships and processes are administered and the way in which people are fitted in. The approach taken determines whether these processes and relationships are handled as open systems, open for innovation and development, or as closed systems.

Principles of problem solving
HUMAN RESOURCES IN ORGANIZATIONS

Relationships between subsystems are primarily supported by people who grasp the complexities of reciprocal interdependency and base their cooperation on mutual confidence. By trusting one another, these people create the space for effective functioning. A condition required to make this work is a profound insight into the

nature of interdependent relations and the characteristics of interfunctional and interpersonal trust and candor. One of the first insights in this respect is the notion that trust and confidence cannot be organized or constructed but must develop on the basis of a continuous process of development of interpersonal relations. This applies to work groups, departments, and hierarchical levels within the organization and is equally valid for relations with patients, families, the press, and others outside the institution. If one could visualize these processes, the organizational blueprint of this phase would depict a network of interrelationships, the level of consciousness of the people involved, and the degree of confidence that one has created for the other.

CONCERNING THE PROCESS ORGANIZATION

In the planning that takes place for the process organization many interactions occur among the various participating groups in the health care field. Personnel, flow of services, information streams, and circulation of equipment and supplies are but a few. In fact, it is possible to look at a health care facility as an extremely complicated mixture of processes, ranging from

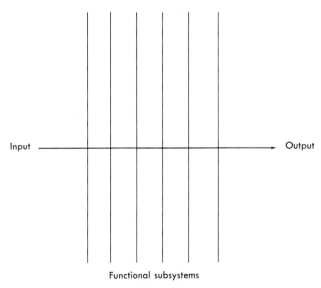

Input

Output

Functional subsystems

Fig. 9-2. Functional subsystem.

a one-time process to a cyclical one and from a short-term process to a long-term one, for example, handling correspondence at the administrator's desk (a one-day process) to administrative development (a long-term process lasting a year or more). It is customary now to see an organization and each of its constituent functions and departments as an *input-output system*, irrespective of whether the organizational unit is an educational department, an accounting department, or a clinic (Fig. 9-2).

It was already clear to the nursing service administrator in our example that it was not the vertical functional subsystems that are essential but rather the horizontal workflow passing the various departments and levels. An attempt was made by her staff to analyze these processes and to arrive at standard procedures. The standardization of procedures, however, evokes the "freezing" problem, whereby rules are applied automatically with little thought given to the actual problems themselves. Consequently, the problem of isolation may arise. In the development of organizational integration, it is of the utmost importance to help administrators and staffs to find a new approach to many of the standardized techniques, methods, and procedures. Cybernetics works with the principle of closed systems. The approach to organizational change should be the idea of open systems. The importance of an open system is clear when one recognizes that any organizational process is a subprocess of a larger process and, consequently, must be subservient to the larger process. For example, nursing is a subprocess of the total process of medical care, nursing is subservient to medicine, and medicine is only a subpart of a larger process beginning with the needs of the patients and ending with their satisfaction. Each process must be receptive to input from above and to change from within, technology changes and people changes; the whole process should remain dynamic to be effective. The essential lesson of experience in nursing service administration is that real change is accomplished only when people become self-reliant and function consciously within these processes. Only then is it appropriate to suggest that an organization move to an integrated system. A fundamental question therefore is, What conditions allow people and groups to act more self-reliantly and intelligently for the benefit of the greater unit of which they are part?

Intelligence may be defined as the ability to understand one's own work in the context of the larger whole. Insight and overall picture presume that one is able to lift oneself above the actual processes and actions. This requires keeping in mind the methods and ideas by which goals are accomplished, *policy thinking*. This is reflected in the style of action that is put into effect. For intelligent action one needs at least to understand the criteria by which solutions to problems are judged. Policy formulated at a high level and communicated down remains abstract. Policies come to life the moment that people are invited to check their invalidity while working. Consequently, people can really feel responsible for innovation in their work environment. In this way, it is possible to determine the limitations of certain policies, to discover shortcomings and gaps, and to improve and adapt these policies.

INTELLIGENT ACTION

Intelligent action is action that contributes to the whole. It allows people to regulate and maintain their own work within a framework of accepted limitations. This is only possible when administration accepts the idea of self-organization and self-control in the integration period. A necessary condition for this to happen is to make planning understood and visible —planning in the sense of norms in relation to quantity of output, quality, costs, and delivery schedules and short-term planning related to achievement. The crux of planning is for the participants to be so involved that self-organization takes place. This occurs particularly when the consequences of surpassing set norms and one's range of discretion become apparent. A good approach in this respect is *critical path planning,* leaving enough discretion for improvisation where needed. This method shows the interrelationships clearly.

Intelligent action for the benefit of the whole is closely related to motivation, to feel committed to relate one's work to that of others. This is possible when one is able to identify oneself with the goals, the meaning, and the social intentions of the job. In the beginning of a new organization, all this happens, to a certain extent, quite spontaneously. There is a direct emotional appeal because of the close contact among the administration, staff, and patients. Later on, planning obscures the goals. The organization is in danger of being removed from satisfying the needs of patients. Continuity and cost control become goals in themselves instead of conditions for serving patients in the best possible way. Where integration takes place, top administration regains its interest in determining the real needs of patients; community needs and motivation research try to make patient needs operational. The modern way to determining the needs of the organization and the process of managing by objectives go hand in hand to make progress in integration. Self-control can only be exercised when the goals of the organization become tangible in the minds of the staff. Self-control acts to motivate those who contribute to the achievement of organizational goals.

Constraints

The selection of the change technique is based on diagnosis of the problem, but the choice of change is tempered by certain conditions that exist at the time. Filley and House (1969) identified three sources of influence on the outcome of administrative development programs that can be generalized to cover the entire range of organizational change efforts, whether structural, behavioral, or technological. These sources of influence are leadership climate, formal organization, and organizational culture.

Leadership climate refers to the nature of the work environment, which results from the leadership style and administrative practices of superiors. Any change program that does not have the support and commitment of administration has a slim chance of success. Administrators must be at least neutral toward the change.

The formal organization must also be compatible with the proposed change. This includes the effects on the environment that result from the philosophy and policies of top administration, as well as legal precedent, organizational structure, and the system of control. Of course, each of these sources of impact may itself be the focus of the change effort; the important point is that a change in one must be compatible with all the others. For example, a change in technology that will eliminate personnel contradicts a policy of guaranteed employment.

Implementation of the proposed solution
LEVEL OF PHILOSOPHY

The first step in implementing the proposed solution is to be sure the top administrative force is educated in conceptual skills and, if they are not, to make a conscious effort to inculcate new ideas. A fundamental conceptual skill is the act of thinking in terms of development models. One needs to think in terms of processes and of ever-changing structures of different qualities and relationships.

TEAM BUILDING

The next step is building a cohesive administrative nursing service team, meaning to open up and discuss explicitly interrelations in the top team and to formulate goals and objectives for the organization and its policies. It is possible to start by working on the interpersonal relations and at a later stage to study objectives and policies. It is also possible to start with the study of objectives and policies and to evaluate the interaction and the social skills at the same time.

What applies to the top administrative team with respect to conceptual skills, interpersonal competence, and creative objectives and policies applies down the line step by step. Every associate or assistant administrator and her immediate colleagues (staff and line) form a ring. These rings should interlock for the sake of effective communication and development. When this process is set in motion, self-control and innovation become a reality. Usually, when there is an environment of trust and candor, the fruit of this process is the application of the *management by exception* philosophy, meaning that attention is focused exclusively on situations that are out of the ordinary and contrary to policy.

PROCESS ANALYSIS: HORIZONTAL LEVEL

Up to now the development steps in the vertical process have been highlighted. The lateral processes of change work straight through departments and organizational support. The nursing staff should become involved in change and innovation, should be assisted to understand their situation, and should learn to relate this to broader organizational goals and policies. Forming ad hoc horizontal groups often accomplishes this purpose. Bringing into the open the norms and standards that should regulate and limit these nursing care work processes is most important in this respect.

DEPARTMENTALIZATION AS INDEPENDENT UNITS

If the preceding steps have been successful, the organization will have become more accessible and tangible. The time has come to give greater independence to certain units of the organization. The overriding criterion for introducing the concept of independent unity is, of course, the overall objective of the organization. Functional units have secondary objectives. The greater the distance from the overall and real objectives, the less inspiring these secondary objectives are. It has been found that when an overall objective has to be transferred down the line more than three times, the motivation ceases. Independent units have genuine objectives, for example, their own service and cost responsibility. In practice, there are endless variations, for example, the relative autonomy given to research and legal units and the relative independence of the continuing education function of a large organization. Such units might also acquire the freedom to deliver their services to third parties. Alternatively, the parent organization is free to search the external environment for the best proposals. The principle of independent units is on a level higher than the subservient relationships, but the condition for serving that principle requires a higher degree of maturity of the parties involved. Moreover, the initiation of such working relationships promotes maturity, just as the subservient relationships suppress it.

The process we envisage may be described as a system of circles. The nursing service administrator determines whether the circles move upward or downward.

The nursing service administrator should initiate the principle of the independent unit by taking the following measures: (1) define the scope of action of policy decisions, that is, determine which policies are to be drawn up by central administration and which are to be left to the independent units, (2) promote nursing service assistant administrators throughout the department or organization, irrespective of units and independent units, and (3) adopt general policy principles that are supported by all the independent units in the organization.

STRUCTURING A SELF-MOTIVATING ORGANIZATION

The philosophy of a static organization excludes group building since jobs are perceived and organized as one-person tasks. When the task becomes too big, subtasks are created one level below. The relationship between these subtasks is determined at the level above, either by a staff department head or by a work-study group. Communication about work content becomes superfluous; consequently, communication is often negative and hostile to administration.

The full responsibility for coordination of nursing care rests with the supervisors, and their supervisory attention is directed downward. The same holds true for their own superiors, who are coordinating their work. Consequently, the static organization is autocratic and topheavy by nature. This organizational structure ravels, particularly at the lowest level, where there is really no essential cohesion, because the nurses are exempt from any responsibility for building groups; this discourages the feeling of belonging. The raveling process tends to penetrate the whole organization. The supervisors feel alienated and start organizing to establish their attitude toward higher administration.

In the integration process, it is mandatory to sew up the organization at the lowest level by forming horizontal groups that carry full responsibility and accountability for a number of coordinating functions. These functions are related to (1) the distribution of tasks within a work group, (2) elements of microplanning and self-control, (3) troubleshooting and preventive maintenance, (4) regulation of information flow, (5) rotation in the performance of particular jobs, and (6) introduction of policy and instruction of patient care tasks and innovations.

The sewing-up process has a multiplying effect. When larger responsibilities are delegated to the staff nurse level, the supervisors no longer need to be present continuously and can take the time to coordinate the various units and departments and to perform more important or equally important tasks.

Supervisors start to function as a link between staff departments and perform a highly integrating function. This means the supervisor's task has changed. She is making different decisions from those of staff nurse. In fact this process has spawned many staff departments. Our thesis is that where reorganization starts at the bottom, one or more administrative levels gradually disappear in consequence, and the role of staff departments alters in character. The supervisors' role will be to answer questions from below and give assistance rather than to pass instructions down.

DISCONNECTING PAYMENT FROM RESULTS

As noted, a serious symptom of the static organization is diminishing motivation among personnel. This leads to overemphasizing the importance of financial compensation. It is perfectly justifiable to say, Those who achieve more should earn more. However, the movement to pay according to results, which employed highly sophisticated scientific methods to measure performance and establish rates and created a psychological environment in which money interfered with cooperation and motivation among staffs and between staffs and supervisors, often transformed personnel into agitators who cared little about the content of their work. Integration development seeks to introduce an altogether new motivational environment. The introduction of clear and purposeful objectives, the encouragement of responsibility and accountability, and the restructuring of work processes require that compensation interferes as little as possible with actual performance and interpersonal relationships. Organizations concerned with health care have successfully moved from measured rates, via collective agreements, to fixed weekly and monthly salaries, all the while retaining the ability to set standards and control performance. The integration of staff is an important part of the integration process.

MAKING A DISTINCTION IN ADMINISTRATION AMONG RESOURCES, PROCESSES, RELATIONS, AND SUPPLY INFORMATION

An organization that proceeds along the lines outlined requires that a clear distinction be made among problems related to (1) the resources side of service, (2) work flow and process development, (3) human relations and all aspects of human resources that work to make service and the organization a success, and (4) the supply of information, quantitatively but also qualitatively.

Many organizations today start to look into their service process from the workflow (input-output) point of view, disregarding the myopic view that focuses on departments, functions, and components. It is quite possible for these organizations to adopt the organizational form of administration of resources and the administration of process development. In the area of human relations administration, this organizational form should be an integral part of administration itself and not primarily a task of staff departments and

Table 7. Objective indicators that measure degree of integration and improvement

Objective indicators	Pretest conditions	Intervention measures	Posttest conditions
1. Relationship improvement			
a. Conferences with physician daily and with other departments weekly	Insufficient or nonexistent	a. Careful scheduling of patient care activities between departments	a. Communication and decision making improved

b. Communication
    (1) Written
    (2) Verbal
    (3) Face-to-face
		b. To schedule daily and weekly conferences between department heads	b. Communication and decision making improved

c. Role determination
    (1) Determine patient's needs
    (2) How and by whom to be met
		c. Clarification of policies and procedures that affect interdepartmental activities	c. Roles determined

2. Patient care: rehabilitation			
a. Ability of patient and family to take responsibility of care at home such as care of wounds and care of diet	a. Unprepared	a. Improvements of nursing care procedures and instructions and appropriate teaching techniques	a. Patient and family better prepared for home care
b. Number of days of patient stay in hospital reduced	b. Too high	b. New equipment	b. Patient fewer days in health care facility
c. Writing and revising nursing care plans and recording patient progress	c. Missing	c. Implementation of care plans	c. Updated care plans
3. Team work: organization			
a. Coordination of care (1) Patient care activities (overlap)	(1) Too much overlap	(1) Integrated care for each patient	(1) Less overlap
(2) Delays in activities	(2) Too much delay	(2) Integrated program for each unit	(2) Fewer delays
(3) Number of errors	(3) Too many errors	(3) Integrate policy for health teaching	(3) Fewer errors

Room	Patient Name	Category	Admitted	Order received	History and physical completed	Nursing care plans completed	Respiratory therapy	Hematology	Chem	ISDT	Other	Routine	Special	Transport	Routine	Special	Miscellaneous procedure	Delay	Comments/Cause

(Column groups: Time — Admitted, Order received, History and physical completed, Nursing care plans completed; Laboratory — Hematology, Chem, ISDT, Other; X-ray — Routine, Special, Transport; Physical therapy — Routine, Special)

Fig. 9-3. Master control sheet for activities.

specialists. To achieve goal orientation, it is necessary to have a constant flow and judgment of information. The computer, with its data processing systems, plays an important role here. Only a flexible system built as a service organization instead of a power center can further the development of the organization.

EVALUATION

Measuring the outcome of objectives requires the acquisition of data measuring the desired objectives and the determination of the expected trend of improvement over time, the first being relatively easier to solve than the second, although neither lends itself to easy solution. The stimulus for change is deteriorating patient care—performance criteria that administrators traced to faulty interdepartmental relationships or lack of integration. The criteria may be any number of objective indicators, as shown in Table 7.

Fig. 9-3 charts the patient's activities and tells a nurse at a glance where the patient is at all times. This simple chart, which Porter termed Visibility Chart (1973), goes a long way in reducing error and in improving care.

The major source of feedback for these indicators is the organization's usual information system: care plans, reports on patient care conferences between nurses and physicians, minutes of conferences with other departments, and patients' records. With this in mind, it is meaningless to try to set standards in definite, measurable terms, even for the sake of making a more convincing or *scientific* evaluation. By so doing, the organization would allow evaluation to become an end in itself, rather than a means of obtaining better information on which to base judgments, and the results would be worthless for administrative purposes.

Fortunately, neither administration nor department heads demand or expect precision in such cases. Under such circumstances and until better methods are available, less specific and concrete standards can be accepted for administrative if not for research purposes. For example, in the case of human relations training, one can say that objectives will be achieved if most department heads believe that human relations training helped them to (1) understand and deal with other people and with their colleagues and (2) improve interdepartmental relationships.

This kind of standard can usually be improved, however, by identifying in advance the specific aspects of the interdepartmental relationships that education in human relations should help improve, for example, department heads' (1) willingness and ability to listen to each other, (2) attitudes and actions in explaining the "whys" of procedure changes to other department heads in advance of the change, and (3) confidence that colleagues will give fair consideration to ideas and suggestions. Standards, in whatever terms and with whatever degree of specificity expressed, are likely to represent (1) the expectations or requirements of administration, on the logical assumption that, for example, human relations education meets administrations' needs; (2) the expectations or requirements of department heads, on the logical assumption that unless human relations education also meets what department heads feel to be their needs it is not likely to be applied effectively by them in meeting administrations' needs; and (3) the recommendations or requirements of experts or authorities, on the logical assumption that organizations, programs, or activities that meet recognized requirements of good practice are generally more likely to succeed than those which do not.

Developing sources and methods of treating data

Having stated as specifically as possible what changes are expected to result from human relations conferences, it is possible to determine what kinds of data will indicate change, how and where to obtain this data, and how to treat it when it has been obtained.

Going back to human relations education for department heads, for example, it can be decided that any or all of these kinds of data will be accepted.

1. General impressions of department heads, colleagues, supervisors, and staff officials
2. Reports from any of these sources on actual incidents involving, or actions taken by, the department heads
3. Performance of department heads rated by supervisor
4. Observed behavior of department heads on the job
5. Scores on department heads' judgment tests
6. Records on absenteeism, suggestions, turnover, and grievances in the department heads' work groups
7. Results of attitude surveys among the department heads' employees and others

This kind of information is gathered from the same sources and in much the same ways described in the discussions on identifying these problems. The evidence sought, however, must now be pinpointed to the specific human relations objectives and standards established in advance.

The data gathered should be as complete as practical considerations permit, and it must include all reasonable, available indicators of success and lack of success.

Once the data has been gathered, the extent to which human relations or other objectives have been achieved can be judged by comparing the findings with the previously established standards. In addition

1. To obtain more accurate and precise estimates of the amount of change made, one must compare the same kinds of data for department heads *before and after* human relations education.
2. To help determine whether any changes found are due to human relations education or to something else, one must compare the same kinds of data for group education in human relations and reasonably comparable unprepared groups in the same environment, *matched controls*.
3. To help determine relative effectiveness of various educational methods, devices, timing, and instructors, one must compare the data

for *successive groups* of department heads exposed to the same educational content presented in different ways.

Pretesting the plan

After the evaluation plan has been developed, it should be pretested, approved, and put into effect. Since most of the operations involved in this process have already been discussed elsewhere in this book, they will be dealt with only briefly here.

The evaluation plan decided on should be tried out first on a small scale, to make sure that it is practical, that it obtains the kinds of data required, that this data can be treated as planned, and that it can be interpreted in meaningful terms.

Interview or questionnaire forms, for example, should be used on a trial basis with a representative population, and the evaluator should check carefully to see that the questions are clear, easily understood, and productive of the kinds of facts and opinions about which information is needed. The evaluator should also check to see how these responses can be reported and what kind of code, if any, may be required to classify and summarize them.

Collecting and analyzing data

The data collected must, of course, be relevant to the objectives of human relations education, and it must, as previously emphasized, include data on all the changes that human relations education was intended to produce. It should be as comprehensive as practical, drawn from sources that are representative, and systematically recorded. It must include all reported or discovered evidence, favorable and unfavorable, and should also include any available clues that will help relate cause and effect.

Information from available administrative reports and records should not be overlooked but should be used with caution; remember that information usually shows results without indicating cause.

Summary and classification of the data

should be very carefully done. If a coding system is used, different people should code an identical sample of the data independently and then compare results and resolve any discrepancies found.

Comparing findings with expectations

When the data have been collected and summarized in a reportable form, the findings can be appraised. There should be widespread and representative participation in this appraisal. It may be desirable to report the unappraised facts, possibly with some tentative suggestions about relationships and possible implications of these facts, to groups of those people most importantly concerned and let them make the appraisal by comparing the findings with the standards that had been set. This is the feedback process mentioned in analysis of data on change. All the observations made in that discussion are especially applicable to analysis of evaluation data, for as already suggested, change determination and evaluation are two sides of the same coin.

Planning and taking action on findings

Analysis and appraisal of evaluation findings discussed in the preceding manner not only indicate how well specific objectives are achieved, but also what changes are needed to make human relations education needs serve the needs of administration more effectively.

Ideally, the pattern should consist of an index that measures both the performance and behavioral variables. In general, the monitoring phase is a specific application of administrative control. Before the monitoring phase can be effective, administration must provide for a measurement of the objective information to compare actual results with planned results and must act to correct any deviations.

SUMMARY

Making a nursing service diagnosis of problems indicates the crucial need of the administrative processes as a diagnostic tool. We stress systematic analysis of all facets of the problem. Our analysis shows that the symptoms stems largely from failures in certain administrative processes, and the nursing administrator should be able to muster the evidence to signify how these failures have produced waves of reaction throughout the whole institution and should be able to avoid such generalities as, The nursing department needs better supervisors or better nurse practitioners. It further reveals the significant factor that a health care organization needs to be organized on an open systems basis and that functional thinking must be replaced by systems thinking.

REFERENCES

Arndt, C., and Laeger, E.: Role strain in a diversified role set: the director of nursing service. I. Nurs. Res. **19**(3):253-259, 1970*a*.

Arndt, C., and Laeger, E.: Role strain in a diversified role set: the director of nursing service. II. Sources of stress, Nurs. Res. **19**(3): 495-501, 1970*b*.

Donnelly, J. H., Jr., Gibson, J. L., and Ivancevich, J.: Fundamentals of management, Dallas, Tex., 1971, Business Publications, Inc.

Filley, A. C., and House, R. J.: Managerial process and organizational behavior, New York, 1969, Scott, Foresman & Co.

Follett, M. P.: Business as an integrating unit. In Metcalf, H. C., and Urwick, L., editors: Dynamic administration, New York, 1940, Harper & Row, Pubs.

Georgopoulos, B., editor: Organization research on health institutions, Ann Arbor, 1972, Institute for Social Research, The University of Michigan.

Lewin, K.: Group decision and social change. In Newcomb, T., and Hartley, E., editors: Readings in social psychology, New York, 1947, Holt, Rinehart & Winston, Inc.

Likert, R.: New patterns of management, New York, 1961, McGraw-Hill Book Co.

Porter, E.: Strength development inventory, Pacific Palisades, Calif., 1973, Rev. ed., Personal Strength Assessment Service.

Tannenbaum, R.: The manager concept: a rational synthesis, Los Angeles, 1949, The University of California at Los Angeles.

Watson, E. T.: Diagnosis of management problems, Harvard Business Review **36**(1):69-76, 1958.

ADDITIONAL READINGS

Bos, A. H.: Development principles of organizations. In Frank, H. E., editor: Organization structuring, New York, 1971, McGraw-Hill Book Co.

Etzioni, A.: Modern organizations, Englewood Cliffs, N. J., 1964, Prentice-Hall, Inc.

Follett, M. P.: Creative experience and dynamic administration, New York, 1924, David McKay Co., Inc.

Lewin, K.: Resolving social conflicts, New York, 1948, Harper & Row, Pubs.

Lewin, K.: Field theory in social science, New York, 1951, Harper & Row, Pubs.

Likert, R.: The human organization: its management and value, New York, 1967, McGraw-Hill Book Co.

Mullane, M. K.: Education for nursing service administration, Battle Creek, Mich., 1959, W. K. Kellogg Foundation.

Seckler-Hudson, C.: Organization and management: theory and practice, Washington, D. C., 1957, The American University Press.

Chapter 10

ALLOCATION OF HUMAN RESOURCES AND FUNDS

Unless adequate funds are appropriated to employ sufficient nursing personnel, the cause is lost in the beginning. This calls for a thorough interpretation of patient needs and for putting forth clear, emphatic arguments showing how the figures prove to be or represent essential requirements. A careful, convincing presentation of needs must be submitted to the administration yearly, in advance and according to the time specified by the administrative board.

In preparation of the nursing service budget, provision must be made not only for personnel requirements but also for adequate equipment and supplies. Also, if a record has been kept of the money expended during the current year for supplies and equipment, it will serve as a guide in proposing future requirements. Early planning and proposing of future requirements by the nursing service administrator will enable the purchasing agent to function more efficiently and produce a saving with no curtailment of necessary equipment. No hardship is greater than the lack of necessary tools, and this factor alone proves most detrimental to the medical and nursing personnel. The budget process is continuous, one fiscal period overlapping the other in different departments.

DEFINITION AND PURPOSE OF A BUDGET

Efficient operation of a health care facility can be achieved only by adopting a business viewpoint with regard to the institution's expenditures. The most important and effective technique is the preparation of a budget and a system of budgetary control. A separate budget should be made for each department with the responsibilities of each department clearly designated so that there is no overlapping of responsibility with consequent duplication of budgeting for one service or area.

A budget may be defined as a predetermined standard of performance in terms of the controllable costs for any given volume of service covering a specific period of time. The budget may be a variable one covering a series of volumes of services. It should be clearly recognized that the budget does not control costs but is a standard established by carefully considering past experience, standards for personnel and material, and the expected performance in terms of these experiences and standards. The budget for nursing service is the economic translation of that part of the aim of the institution that relates to nursing care of patients. The nursing service administrator is responsible for that part of the total budget of the institution that applies to nursing. The budget defines the limits of financial support for the nursing service department; therefore, it controls the scope and quality of the institution's programs.

The budget affects personnel policies that determine the quality and size of nursing personnel and, thus, the quality of patient care; it determines the amount and type of equipment, physical facilities, and other resources that will be available for nursing practice and research.

Goals and aspirations of the nursing service personnel are reflected in the budget. A budget that makes provision for quality of care, experimentation, and research helps to create a spirit of inquiry; on the other hand, a budget that is tight year after year stifles creativity of the personnel.

Budgeting involves the acquisition and expenditure of funds for nursing service, including the preparation of the budget and its control during the designated period. The effective allocation and control of expenditures has come to be a potent instrument of management efficiency. Budgeting methods are therefore a most important aspect of nursing service administration.

In general, the budget serves the purpose of bringing a system of communication into the area of policy making and operations so that the exchange of information on policies, programs, and finances is guaranteed. Furthermore, the budget, as an instrument of planning and managing the affairs of a health care facility, can and should provide the following:

1. The automatic, scheduled consideration and reconsideration of long-term ends of the health care facility
2. The basic information for a continuing examination of the relationship of the health care facility's budget to the economy and, in turn, encouragement of sound decisions with respect to these relationships
3. A comprehensive picture of the various programs and activities of the health care facility's departments and encouragement of a comparative evaluation of these matters in terms of their relative costs
4. A working basis for effective and continuing work relationships between administrators and the departments in the important matter of sharing responsibility for programs and policies of the health care facility

ADVANTAGES AND DISADVANTAGES OF THE BUDGET

Since the budget requires a complete program of activities planned in advance and an analysis of operations, it helps to clarify assignment of responsibility and authority and facilitates the tasks of supervision and administration. Moreover, the governing board of the health care facility and the administration, including nursing, are enabled to evaluate the nursing service position in the financial standing of the institution. The budget allows the nursing service administrator to criticize her own planning and at the same time provide a defense against unjustified attacks. It requires review of policies and accomplishments during the past year and the restatement of policies and plan of operation for the new fiscal year. It points out in what respects the estimates were good or poor. These facts, together with the reason for the differences, provide guides in preparing the budget for the next year. The budget guides nursing service administrators in what they can hope to accomplish within the next fiscal year with the funds or resources made available. Although a staffing plan is a budgetary control once it is in operation, the initial formulation of the plan needs to consider the financial resources available.

The budget thus gives direction, making it possible for the nursing service administrator to plan a program for the ensuing fiscal year with a reasonable amount of assurance that she will be able to carry out the program of her department. The annual budget also gives direction to institution-made projects. With the increase in institutional complexity and increased interest in expansion of services and in research, it is becoming necessary to make long-term budget plans and longer budget projections.

When the budget becomes a goal, that is, the end itself rather than the means to an end, it defeats its purpose. Institutional budgets must change to facilitate the attainment of new goals; this is the basis of the argument in favor of variable or flexible budgets that prevent the operation being locked in. Using the budget as a pressure device to force conformity results in problems in human relations. The trend is toward increased involvement of personnel in the preparatory stages of the budget (Argyris 1969). Overbudgeting, which occurs when budgets are so complete and detailed as to be cumbersome, is another pitfall to be avoided.

FACTORS DETERMINING NURSING SERVICE NEEDS

1. Types of patients admitted (such as medical, surgical, or pediatric), their lengths of stay, and the acuteness of their illnesses are fluctuating factors that must be taken into consideration.
2. Personnel policies, such as, salaries paid to various types of personnel, the length of the workweek and work period as well as flexibility in hours, the extent of vacation, statutory holidays, and sick leave are factors that can be monitored by the administration.
3. The size of the hospital and its bed occupancy: The large hospital requires more total personnel than does the small hospital to care for the same number of patients. This situation may be reversed in nursing, especially in very small hospitals where the factor of minimum coverage must be reckoned with (Block 1956).
4. The kind and amount of care to be given should be considered because they affect the number of hours of bedside care.
5. The proportion of nursing care provided by professional nurses to that provided by auxiliary personnel is important.
6. Amount and quality of supervision available and provided and the efficiency of job descriptions and job classifications should be taken into consideration.
7. The method of assignment of nursing personnel to patients (functional, case, or team method) should be taken into consideration.
8. The method of performing nursing procedures, whether simple or complex, and the method of record keeping and charting should also be considered.
9. Standards of nursing care should be kept in mind.
10. Physical layout of the hospital, the size and plan of the clinical units, the amount and kinds of labor-saving equipment and devices are all important factors.
11. Whether nonnursing functions such as messenger, dietary, and housekeeping are the responsibility of the nursing department must be considered.
12. Whether simple or complex reports are required by administrator is another factor.
13. Method of appointment of medical staff, size and activities of medical staff, kind and frequency of treatments and orders are all factors that determine nursing service needs.
14. Affiliation of the health care facility with a medical school or school of nursing, or both, is another important factor.

These factors indicate that each health care organization must be considered as a separate entity in planning for its nursing service needs.

DECISION MAKING IN THE BUDGET PROCESS

An analysis of the budget process shows clearly that from the initial steps in the formulation of the budget to the final step in its administration, decision making of a broad and significant character is involved. These decisions are made by many persons and many departments. Seckler-Hudson (1957) identified six areas wherein important decisions are made by one or many of those persons participating in the budget process. In some manner, and at some point or points, there will be (1) an analysis and comparative evaluation of the multitude of needs of the people who will be served within the jurisdiction of the budget, (2) choices made from among the many needs as to the programs and activities to be served by the nursing and other departments, (3) a decision on the creation of fiscal resources to meet the costs of the activities projected in the nursing service's budget, (4) a determination made concerning appropriations, apportionments, and allocations of funds among the many authorized activities and programs, (5) decisions made with respect to the administration of the plans and programs provided for in the budget, and (6) decisions made with respect to an accounting for performance and a justification of the budget.

A PLAN OF ORGANIZATION FOR BUDGET PREPARATION

There are certain prerequisites basic to preparing any budget and apply equally to that part of the budget for which nursing is responsible. First, a well-formulated budget organization with assignment of responsibility. The total, final budget, including the departmental components, should be prepared under the direction of one executive head, such as the treasurer, comptroller, business manager in the large organization, or the administrator in the small facility, who should be responsible for the administration and enforcement of the budget. Second, a budget committee should be formed. The coordinating committee (administrator, nursing service administrator, treasurer, and assistant administrator) might form the nucleus of the budget committee with representative departmental heads for discussion of items that related to their individual or interrelated departments. All department heads should be present when policies are being formulated.

INPUTS

The nursing service administrator receives and secures information or input on procedure for preparation of the budget in accordance with the financial management of the institution. Factors are (1) overall basis of financial management, whether free from debt, source of revenue, contemplated expansion or renovations, proposed increases or curtailment in any of the institution's various departments, (2) the economic, industrial, and health situation, locally and nationally, (3) effect on the institution's occupancy of additional facilities, and (4) accountability to the public through a board or a donor organization.

In addition, the nursing service administrator is furnished with the following procedure: (1) statement of the aims and objectives for the period in which the budget is being prepared; the administrative policy for future operations must be determined and stated; and (2) predesigned forms for submission of the budget information, including instructions with examples for using the forms; the kind of information the accounting office will supply; salary schedule for the department, including information regarding increases, new positions, and maximum and minimum quotation of salaries; policies affecting the budget, such as personnel policies, vacation, illness, health service, cost maintenance policies; contracts affecting personnel, such as Social Security, workmen's compensation insurance, and Blue Cross.

From the accounting department, the nursing service administrator receives an accounting classification with the income and expense items in the budget of each department following the account title as that used by the accounting department; essential statistics, including statistical and financial past performance; sound purchasing and inventory control and records; efficient admitting policy and records; and periodicity of budget: annual, biannual, or long-term plan. One of the fundamental prerequisites to good budgetary control and to the preparation of the budget is the ability to check actual performance with previous estimates.

The nursing service administrator may

also form a budget committee for her department. One of her major administrative responsibilities is to prepare the nursing service budget; this cannot be delegated to her assistants, although she should solicit the cooperation of her administrative and supervisory staff. The administrator cannot know all of the immediate and anticipated needs without their being made known to her by the members of the nursing service staff who are cognizant of these needs. Items to be requisitioned are introduced at meetings scheduled for budgetary deliberation, and attempts are made to justify these requests. Decisions are reached by the administrator in view of comprehensive needs. The discussion of the nursing service budget by the nursing administrator and her staff will help them understand the importance of controls. It will also impress upon those persons their responsibility for strict adherence to the budget specifications.

The nursing service administrator receives inputs from the nursing service budget committee. Some suggestions are received during the course of the year, but at a specific time the nursing service administrator formulates the budget. First, the personnel needs are stated. The number of personnel may be estimated on the basis of nursing service hours per patient per day on the clinical units and in special departments such as operating and delivery rooms, taking into consideration the personnel policies. Next, she ascertains what changes are contemplated, such as opening new facilities for patients and changes in other departments affecting the nursing service required, such as programs of education or research. Then, there is a review of the hours of nursing service per patient per day for the past budget year to determine (1) whether the amount of nursing care provided was comparable with what is considered safe nursing service. Figures for comparison should be available from the daily record of nursing service hours per patient per day and from the monthly

record prepared by the unit clerk and submitted to the nursing office; (2) whether the quality of nursing care met the estimated standards and whether this quality can be maintained by using more licensed vocational nurses by prearrangement of duties and responsibilities; and (3) whether certain dietary, messenger, or secretarial services for which nursing personnel are responsible could be more economically performed by other departments; facts and figures must form a part of this study.

Following this, the nursing service administrator recommends the salary scale for personnel. This scale should be considered well in advance. An organizational and classificational chart that briefly describes the responsibilities of each status of personnel in the department of nursing is essential. The committee must consider not only annual increases for tenure and salaries recommended by the recognized professional associations or the state or county, but also any contemplated changes in union agreements, if such exist, or in working conditions. Vacation, sick leave, and expected turnover should also be weighed. The nursing administrator is usually required to give considerable guidance in salary changes. Several devices in addition to the recommended salaries of professional organizations may be considered as tools to emphasize the need for good personnel policies as related to salary. These may include percentage turnover of personnel, for which figures can be secured from the personnel office. Finally, she requisitions equipment and supplies. Considerable assistance is gained from each member of the supervisory and head nurse staff who list their requirements.

SENSING

Many nursing service organizations have failed in their purpose because their administrators did not understand the importance of the environmental inputs and the structure and operation of the environment or did not have an appreciation of the environmental influences. For the nursing administrators, the input problem involves (1) the need to assess inputs, (2) consideration of the inputs that affect the budget and in turn the nursing program, and (3) the development of methods for effectively integrating these inputs with the budget to formulate the department's goals, objectives, and processes.

Among the various inputs from the environment with which the nursing service administrator must deal are the economic system or financial inputs, trends in cost, labor, industrial and health situations (locally and nationally), policies in operating areas, and their effect on the occupancy of health care facilities and personnel administration. To operate successfully, the nursing service administrator must understand these inputs together with their claims and predictions of the future on the organization. These inputs and their effects form a framework that must be considered when formulating a budget. With that assessment made, the nursing service administrator can proceed to establish objectives, make decisions, and plan with greater assurance than she could ever do in the vacuum that ignores environmental inputs.

PLANNING THE BUDGET

Choices from among the many needs will be made as to the programs and activities to be served by nursing service. The decision on programs and activities to be chosen for inclusion in the nursing service's budget involves the significant matter of determining relative values of many competing needs. The decision to include a program may determine the exclusion of another. Some financial resources are limited in relation to patient care demands; the decision makers must face the question as to whether the returns from the program included will be worth its cost in terms of programs excluded. According to Verne B. Lewis (1952:42):

Budget analysis, therefore, is basically a comparison of the relative merits of alternative uses of funds. . . . Budget decisions must be made on the basis of relative values.

There is no absolute standard of value. It is not enough to say that an expenditure for a particular purpose is desirable or worthwhile. The results must be more valuable than the results would be if the money were used for any other purpose. Lewis (1952:42) further stated:

Comparison of relative values to be obtained from alternative uses of funds is necessary because our resources are inadequate to do all the things we consider desirable and necessary. . . . The needs of people are many. Although the supply of resources has been greatly expanded in recent decades, the supply is still short in relation to demands. It would be nice if we had enough to go around, but we do not have. Some demands can be met only in part, some not at all.

Administrators have at their disposal only faulty tools to use in determining relative values of programs. They are always confronted with limited resources, with many competing programs, with department heads, and with sponsors urging that resources be spent for each of the particular programs. The administrator cannot meet all demands. But the question that must be decided somehow is, What choices are made from among the many competing interests for inclusion in the health care organization's program, and on what basis are these choices made?

The administrative concepts of the administrator's job are an excellent guide to budgeting. Utilizing the composite process in relation to the budget, the nursing service administrator may ask, What were the objectives for the past fiscal year? Have they been accomplished? How much of them has been accomplished? How well was the planning done? She has an excellent self-evaluation guide and a measuring stick as to how much has been accomplished according to the organization goals and individual objectives. What were the constraints? How much did they hinder the accomplishments? The nursing administrator finds the following administrative concepts useful in formulating a new plan of action:

1. What is to be accomplished during the next fiscal year in terms of resources and the requirements for care?
2. What kind of planning must nursing administration do to provide for increased nursing care, an intelligent strategy, and answers to the "what," "how much," and "where" of the service?
3. What kind of organizational structure, personnel, and training are required?
4. What kinds of controls should nursing service have if it is to be "fast on its feet" in adjusting to unforeseen and changing circumstances?
5. Does nursing service reappraise all these functions from time to time, particularly when control information shows unusual discrepancies?

Devising the budget
SETTING OBJECTIVES

The first step in devising her budget is for the nursing service administrator to identify the objectives, that is, the process of delineating in individual statements what is to be accomplished in the next fiscal period. The objectives may read: improve the care of patients through home-health teaching; improve nursing team and health team, dedicated to protection and well being of patients; improve conceptual and physical environment through improved relationships and working conditions; and improve quality assurance programs through feedback system.

PROGRAMMING

The second step is programming, the process of spelling out the means to be followed to reach each objective. Each detail must be carefully worked out so it is clear what elements are involved and in what amounts of time or size, so the financial forecast will be accurate. These two processes may be stated in another way: to formulate and adapt a plan of activities and programs for a stated time period, to relate program costs to re-

sources, to achieve the authorized plan according to a time schedule and at a cost within available resources, and to establish output measurements facilitating the effective attainment of the objective selected.

The planning of activities should fall within the framework of the policy of the health care facility in terms of which each specific program or activity is justifiable both to the administrator and to the board of directors or regents. In substance and detail, the planned program, budget materials, and justification should answer the following questions concerning each program in the budget: What are the ends to be served by the program? Why is this program being proposed? Can it be done better or more effectively by the nursing service than by any other department? How much do we propose to do during the next fiscal period? Is this a reasonable amount? What resources (personnel, equipment, and funds) will be needed to accomplish this? When do we anticipate completing the program? What feedback controls have been planned?

The details of programming for each objective may be spelled out under such specific headings as staffing, supportive services, administration, equipment and supplies, and evaluation (Dunn 1963). Each item is developed with justification of need, intended use, and anticipated cost, the last of which may be based on experience in the last fiscal period, with additions to accommodate increases in salary, personnel, or commodity needs.

The programming for each objective may also be spelled out under each of the following headings: structural development, behavioral development, and technological development.

Let us take the first objective, which states: improve the care of patients through home-health teaching. This objective may require an increase of 60 minutes out of each 24 hours of professional nursing time to be spent in direct patient care activities, namely, health teaching or preparing patient for home. The programming for this objective must spell out how these additional 60 minutes are to be gained.

From input and observation of accomplishments of the past year, the administrator may have found that the knowledge and skills of the professional nurse were not utilized to the fullest extent possible in patient care. Therefore, one solution might be to delegate 60 minutes worth of nonnursing activities, hitherto carried out by nurses, to some other group, such as transferring the transcribing of physician's orders to secretaries in the clinical unit or strengthening the nursing team and the health team through improved patient care conferences. This objective might also be accomplished by simplifying some outdated procedures through improving methods. Nursing service is concerned with programming for *each objective* and determining cost involved (four budgets): (1) personnel, based on staffing needs, (2) supportive services, (3) equipment and supplies, and (4) capital expenditures.

Personnel budget based on staffing needs
Categorization of patients and requirements of direct and indirect care in terms of quantity and quality staffing. There are a number of ways in which a nursing service administrator can analyze her personnel and staffing requirements for the next budget period. After all, the raison d'être of nursing service is to provide for patient care, and this takes personnel. The nursing service budget is concerned mainly with providing personnel for patient care. The method of accurate provision of personnel is a crucial factor. One method considered to be especially meaningful is to analyze nursing care requirements according to patient's need and to categorize patients that way.

Patient categorization according to nursing care needs is a change from the traditional method of simply counting the number of beds occupied. Requirements for nursing care are determined by criteria such as patient's physical restrictions, instructional requirements, nursing procedures, and emotional factors. Essentially, the degree of illness the patient is experiencing and how much care is required determine how many nursing personnel working hours are required. The point to be emphasized is that the amount of care required in a nursing unit is not determined merely by the number of patients in the unit; the aggregate load on the nursing staff is the statistically measured sum of the direct and indirect care needs of each patient. The essential requirement, then, is to arrive at a numerical figure representing hours by which to predict nursing load, a figure based on a realistic evaluation of patient needs rather than on patient census.

The nursing care that is administered to patients on physical restrictions (complete bed rest, partial bed rest, and the various stages of ambulation, for instance) can be studied and given a time value. Nursing procedure requirements are also given time values, for example, those that are continuous, those that take 20 or more minutes, and those that may take 10 to 20 minutes. Emotional factors can also be given a time value. For example, nurses spend time listening to a patient's fear of surgery, about a patient's family, and about anxieties. Health teaching needs also require a time factor. In this way the nursing care time requirements for patients in each category of illness can be estimated. This can then be broken down into the time requirements for each level of nursing care personnel on the basis of activities appropriately carried out by the professional nurse, the licensed vocational nurse, or by other nursing personnel. Simply multiplying the average number of patients in each illness category by the nursing care time they require gives the overall figure for nursing personnel needs. This can then be divided into the amounts of professional nursing, licensed vocational nursing, and auxiliary personnel time that will be needed.

By this operation, personnel requirements are determined and justified on the facts of patient care needs rather than on vague suppositions. That these are facts rather than guesses is supported by research studies carried out at Johns Hopkins University (Wolfe and Young 1965) and at the University of Illinois (Dunn 1963), which independently reported a marked similarity in the nursing care time requirement of respective categories of patients.

Determination of direct patient care requirements in terms of quantity. Wolfe and Young (1965) have in their extensive study been able to scientifically categorize patient care needs, determine the direct and indirect patient care requirements, and predict nursing loads. These researchers have classified patients into three categories, based on the patients' *degree of self-sufficiency.* The following categories list combinations of factors for categorization of patients:

Category I. *Self-care* patients are those who fulfill any of the following combinations: (1) ambulatory or up in chair, can feed self or may require cutting of food, and may bathe in bathroom or at bedside with help for back and extremities; (2) ambulatory with assistance, up in chair, and can bathe in bathroom or at bedside but may need help with extremities; and (3) same as 1 and 2, but, in addition, patient may have vision impairment, require oxygen therapy, or require intravenous feeding, but no two of these factors together.

Category II. *Partial* or *intermediate care* patients are those who fulfill the following combination of criteria: (1) Patient is ambulatory with help, can bathe self in bathroom or at bedside with assistance, requires complete assistance with feedings (except for intravenous feedings), has inadequate vision, and requires oxygen therapy (the last two conditions are optional and do not affect classification).

(2) Patient requires complete assistance to get up in chair and be bathed at bedside, can feed self or may require food cut or intravenous feeding, requires oxygen therapy, and has inadequate vision (the last two conditions are optional). (3) This patient is the same as 2, but this patient requires some assistance to get up in chair and be bathed at bedside. (4) This patient requires some assistance to get up in chair, can bathe self partially at bedside, and requires complete assistance with feeding. Inadequate vision and oxygen therapy are optional. (5) This patient requires bathing at bedside, can feed self, and may require cutting of food or intravenous feedings. Vision inadequacy and oxygen therapy are optional. (6) This patient requires special duty (private nurse) or continuous nursing assistance to the extent that special duty nurse must be relieved for meals.

Category III. *Intensive* or *total care* patients are those who have all the combinations not previously covered in category I or II. Includes any patient who may be otherwise classified under category I or II but who also requires suction therapy, is in isolation, is incontinent, has wound drainage necessitating change of bed linen, or suffers from marked emotional disturbance needing almost constant observation and requiring a single room.

The research findings of Wolfe and Young (1965) have indicated that category I patients, on an average, required 0.5 hour of direct patient care; category II patients required one hour of direct patient care; and category III patients required 2.5 hours of direct patient care. Based on these averages, a direct patient care index was derived that represented the total hours of direct care required on a nursing unit. This is expressed by the following formula:

$$I = 0.5N_1 + 1N_2 + 2.5N_3$$

I is the direct care index; N_1 is the number of patients in category I, requiring an average of 0.5 hour of direct care; N_2 is the number of patients in category II, requiring an average of one hour of direct care each; and N_3 is the number of patients in category III, requiring an average of 2.5 hours of direct care each.

Determination of direct patient care requirements in terms of quality. Having determined that quantity equals numbers in terms of hours of direct patient care requirements, one might ask, How does quality affect the budget? Quality may be defined as a measure of standards, and it is quality that determines quantity or the number of hours of care required. So, it is quality of care that controls the budget.

If the nursing service administrator has implemented a program for nursing care, then definite policies and procedures must exist. As a patient enters the health care facility an assessment is made of that patient's condition in relation to nursing care requirements based on (1) physical needs that determine nursing procedure require-

	AM		PM		Nite	
	Yes	No	Yes	No	Yes	No
I. Patient assessment to determine degree of self-sufficiency						
A. Biophysiological factors						
1. Procedures						
a) Suction						
b) O_2						
c) Diagnostic procedures						
2. Physical restrictions						
a) Complete bedrest (CBR)						
b) Binders to extremities						
c) Feeding						
d) Vision impairment						
e) Other						
B. Psychosocial factors						
1. Emotional needs						
a) Support necessary						
b) Explanation to reduce anxiety						
c) Listening						
d) Other						
2. Instructional needs						
a) Colostomy care						
b) Walking with crutches						
c) Home care						
d) Other						

Continued.

Fig. 10-1. Quality control observation sheet.

	AM		PM		Nite	
	Yes	No	Yes	No	Yes	No
II. Categorization of patients						
Have patients been correctly diagnosed and categorized?						
III. Planning and organizing						
A. Establishment of patient care objectives						
1. Have patient care plans been accurately made (written) regarding:						
a) Procedures						
b) Physical restrictions						
c) Emotional needs						
d) Instructional needs						
IV. Directing, controlling, and evaluating						
A. Have care plans been carried out appropriately rearding:						
1. Procedures						
2. Physical restrictions						
3. Emotional needs						
4. Instructional needs						
B. Have care plans been appropriately recorded regarding:						
1. Procedures						
2. Physical restrictions						
3. Emotional needs						
4. Instructional needs						
V. Overall evaluation—total						
Have corrective actions been taken?						

Fig. 10-1, cont'd. Quality control observation sheet.

ments and physical restrictions, (2) psychosocial and emotional factors, and (3) instructional needs. Assessment of the patient's nursing needs is a critical, continuous requirement and is the function of a professional nurse. Fig. 10-1 provides a guide for quality control assessment. The findings of the assessment process determine the patient's classification into either category I, II, or III. (There may be more than three *care classifications,* and which one of the three categories has the most seriously ill or the most complex nursing care requirements is an institutional matter of choice.)

Each category of patient care classification has requirements and established standards of care (also substandards and supportive evidence) and criteria for guidance, evaluation, and control. For each of the three categories described and inclusive factors, statistical evidence of the category of patients requiring nursing care influences the budget.

The standard set for each patient classification determines priority of care and is the beginning of the individualized patient care plan. The care plan is initiated at the time of assessment or on admittance of the patient and is coordinated with the physician's plan of care. The care plan is also a professional nurse's function, with regard to initiation, currency, accuracy, and special instructions.

The categorization of patients as to nursing care requirements is part of the care plan. Each category of care has standards set as to professional nurse's requirements; authority and responsibility are delegated, and accountability is established. For example, category III (seriously ill) patients may have to be cared for completely by professional nurses or by specialized professional nurses; category I patients also require professional nursing skills but not to so great an extent as category II or III. These patients may be cared for by newly graduated nurses, assisted by licensed vocational nurses and well-prepared nurse assistants. Provision must also be made for supervisory assistance and guidance to nurses. Classifying patients also classifies nurses as to competence required and thus influences the budget. For example, the more severely ill the patients admitted, the more professional nurses with specialized skill requirements needed.

Determination of indirect patient care in terms of quantity. Indirect patient care is defined as those activities conducted by professional and nonprofessional staffs away from the patient's bedside but on the patient's behalf and for the patient's welfare, for example, administrative duties, preparation of medication, paperwork (transcription of physician's orders and recording), communication, escorting and special errands, cleanup (other than those performed by housekeeping personnel), and travel (Wolfe and Young 1965). Mea-

sures of indirect care also depend to a large extent on the physical setup of the institution.

In a study at Johns Hopkins University, Wolfe and Young (1965) found that for a typical 30-bed medical nursing unit, the amount of time required for all activities classified as indirect care, rather than direct, remained constant at 20 hours for an eight-hour work shift. These 20 hours remained the same regardless of the number of patients in the clinical unit, their classification, or the number of nursing personnel assigned to the unit. It is significant to point out that the 20 hours of indirect care for the eight-hour work shift reported in the Johns Hopkins study included professional and nonprofessional personnel. On the other hand, the data verified that the amount of time required for direct patient care varied with the patient care index.

Therefore, findings from this study indicated that the total productive activity *(PA)* or the nursing load in hours was comprised of essentially two components: a constant one and one that depended on the classification of patients in a nursing unit. Therefore, one may say that the total nursing load or effort required of a typical medical or surgical unit for an eight-hour work period is $PA = I + 20$.

The 20-hour constant applies only at the Johns Hopkins Hospital and may prove invalid elsewhere, although research at the University of Illinois yielded the same results (Dunn 1963). These constants must be determined by observation and work-sampling studies in other institutions before expressions similar to these can be used with confidence. Although the approach is sound, the environmental context may differ from that in which these studies were conducted and may seriously influence the values of the coefficients to be used.

We feel strongly that indirect care should be measured quantitatively according to hours of time needed for communication with doctor and family and preparation of medications and qualitatively according to set standards. Indirect care influences the budget and the quantity and quality of nursing care that patients receive. For example, in nursing, communication with patients is emphasized. Much of this is done by the nurse during direct care hours with physicians and with families. But many nurses do not know what exactly to communicate. Nurses talk with patients and with their families and receive much valuable information, but they do not know how to successfully use the information in relation to health care. They communicate with some patients, physicians, and families but not with all patients because they lack the time. Nurses complain about too much committee work. Others complain that policies and procedures of the health care facility are not kept current, which is essential to patient care and need assessment. The indirect care area needs operation research concerning quantity and quality. Control measures need to be established. The observation sheet presented in Fig. 10-2 can be used to determine the indirect patient care index for each category of patient.

Indirect patient care needs	Categorization of patients		
	I	II	III
1. Preparation of medications			
2. Recording			
3. Communication			
Nurse—Physician			
Nurse—Patient and family			
Nurse—Team			
4. Escorting			
5. Physical environment			
Team arrangement			
Equipment			
Inventory			
6. Conceptual environment			
Conferences			
7. Writing of policies			
Planning			
8. Writing of procedures			
Planning			
9. Personal—Nonproductive			
Total number of different nursing personnel necessary for each category of patients.			

Fig. 10-2. Indirect patient care index: observation sheet.

Staffing formula

Let us put into operation the factors discussed by staffing a 50-bed clinical unit and accounting for both the direct and indirect care of patients.

Considering the average census to be 50 patients per clinical unit; the standard of care desired to be 4.7 hours per patient per day (4.7 hours was obtained by Abdellah and Levine and was reported as the *ideal* staffing pattern at the completion of their study in 1958); and the administrative and personnel policies, shown as administrative policies below, of the institution that determine the ratio of personnel to patients; we can now translate the following factors into a meaningful number of personnel for the clinical unit.

$$\frac{\text{Care needs of patients} \times \text{Days/year}}{\left(\text{Days/year} - \begin{array}{c}\text{Administrative}\\ \text{necessities}\end{array}\right) \times \begin{array}{c}\text{Daily hours/}\\ \text{employee}\end{array}} = \frac{\begin{array}{c}\text{Hours of}\\ \text{care/year}\end{array}}{\begin{array}{c}\text{Hours of care/}\\ \text{employee}\end{array}} = \begin{array}{c}\text{Number of}\\ \text{employees/unit}\end{array}$$

Care needs of patients = The number of patients/category on the unit ×
The standard of care/category or for the entire group

Days/year = 365

Daily hours/employee = 8

Administrative necessities =	Regular days off duty	104
	Holidays	9
	Vacation days	15
	Sick leave	12
	Leave of absence	3
	Continuing education	3
	Total	146 days/year

What shall be the percentage of professional to nonprofessional? The Abdellah and Levine study (1958) suggested a ratio of 55% professional nursing staff to 45% nonprofessional nursing staff. Thus

$$\begin{array}{c}\text{Number of}\\ \text{employees/}\\ \text{unit}\end{array} \times \begin{array}{c}\text{\% professional and}\\ \text{\% nonprofessional}\end{array} = \begin{array}{c}\text{Number of}\\ \text{personnel}\\ \text{in each}\\ \text{category}\end{array} \times \begin{array}{c}\text{\% distribution/}\\ \text{shift for}\\ \text{group}\end{array} = \begin{array}{c}\text{Number of}\\ \text{each category}\\ \text{on the unit}\\ \text{during each}\\ \text{shift}\end{array}$$

This formula is translated into meaningful figures for the ratio of 55% professional to 45% nonprofessional personnel with the same standard of care (4.7 hours) as follows:

$$\frac{50 \text{ patients} \times 4.7 \text{ hours} \times 365 \text{ days}}{365 \text{ days} - 146 \text{ days} \times 8 \text{ hours/day}} = \frac{85,775 \text{ hours of care/year}}{1752 \text{ hours/employee yearly}} = 49 \text{ employees}$$

(49 employees × 55% professional) × ⅜ = 10 professional (7–3 shift)
10 professional (3–11 shift)
7 professional (11–7 shift)

(49 employees × 45% nonprofessional) × ⅜ = 8 nonprofessional (7–3 shift)
8 nonprofessional (3–11 shift)
6 nonprofessional (11–7 shift)

This plan considers only the nursing personnel, excluding the clinical nursing specialists such as medical and surgical specialists. The administrative and supervisory personnel need to be added to the pattern also. A review of the pattern, using 4.7 hours of care as the standard of care, reveals the following numbers for the two levels of nursing personnel:

Level of personnel	55% to 45% ratio of 49 professional to nonprofessional nursing personnel
Registered professional nurses	27
Licensed vocational nurses	22

Indirect care must be determined by each health care organization. Some health care organizations have unit managers and more clinical secretaries. The auxiliary personnel contribute much to the indirect care. Therefore, each organization will have to determine how much time is actually spent by the nursing staff—professional and nonprofessional—on indirect care.

Calculation of indirect care index

The calculation of nursing personnel for indirect care utilizing (1) 20 hours of indirect care per eight-hour work shift as the standard and (2) the 55% to 45% ratio of professional to nonprofessional nursing personnel is as follows:

20 hours/8-hour shift × 3 shifts × 365 days/year = 21,900 hours of indirect care/year/30-bed unit

Using the medical unit in the Johns Hopkins study and applying the findings to the 50-bed clinical unit, we find that $21,900 \times \dfrac{50}{30} = 36,500$ hours of indirect care/year/50-bed unit. Each employee works 1752 hours/year, therefore $\dfrac{36,500}{1752} = 20.8$ or 21 (rounded number) employees are necessary to staff for the indirect patient care requirements for one 50-bed clinical unit for one year.

If we utilize the same ratio of 55% to 45% professional to nonprofessional nursing personnel (until each organization conducts its own study and determines the percentage of activities of indirect care conducted by professional and nonprofessional nursing personnel) the number of professional to nonprofessional nursing personnel would be

21 employees × 55% = 11.55 = 12 professional employees

Since the indirect care index is not dependent on the occupancy of beds, each eight-hour shift receives an equal number of employees.

$$\frac{12 \text{ professional employees}}{3 \text{ shifts}} = 4 \text{ professional employees for each shift}$$

21 employees × 45% nonprofessional = 9.45 = 9 (rounded off) nonprofessional employees

$$\frac{9 \text{ nonprofessional employees}}{3 \text{ shifts}} = 3 \text{ nonprofessional employees/shift}$$

When the overall staffing pattern is being calculated to account for both direct and indirect care, the administrative nursing personnel for the unit need to be included. Also to be taken into consideration are a unit manager available for 40 hours each week and three clinical clerks to staff two shifts with relief for their days off.

Therefore, after careful consideration and sensing of all the inputs and after the determination of direct and indirect patient care needs, qualitatively and quantitatively, the nursing service administrator is in a position to determine and allocate the professional, nonprofessional, and auxiliary nursing personnel to each clinical or service unit by utilizing the following computing methods of grouping: (1) by service units, (2) by classification of personnel, (3) personnel by hours of care, (4) by position, and (5) by ratio of professional to nonprofessional nursing personnel.

Correct and clear assessment of nursing care needs for patients is vital for interpretation and acquisition of nursing funds. The nursing service administrator needs to provide accurate and convincing figures and statistical data that reflect essential requirements of personnel. A careful, convincing presentation of needs must be submitted in advance to the chief administrator yearly and according to the time specified by the administrative board in order to secure adequate funding of the nursing department.

Support services, administrative expenses, specific equipment and supplies, and evaluation. Having determined the personnel requirements, the nursing service administrator must consider next the cost of the supporting services, administrative expenses, equipment and supplies, and the evaluation process.

The supporting services may be a teaching program for clinical secretaries to learn about transferring of physicians' orders or a consultation service to the health care team. The administrative expenses might include a new manual for the clinical clerks or the writing of new job descriptions. Another factor may be the introduction of new equipment, for example, a patient-to-nurse intercom system. The supplies and equipment needed would also relate to choice made to obtain the additional 60 minutes, but this might call for monitoring devices or electric beds or both. Evaluation is a systematic program to determine if the end result justified the means, each step carefully forecasting the program in total anticipated cost.

The objectives and the programs designed to meet the preceding items should be outlined in the budget and presented in the order of their priority. The more closely the objectives reflect the goals of the health care facility, the more helpful the administrator is likely to be when presenting the budget to the board of directors. It is more realistic to arrange these items in order of priority, because the administrative nurse can be certain of one thing, she will not receive all she asks for. But, once the nursing service administrator has been notified that a portion, or all, of her budget has been approved, she can take the next step, budget operation.

Besides the salary budget there are two more budgets with which the nursing service administrator is concerned, namely, equipment and supplies and capital expenditure budgets.

Equipment and supplies. The area of equipment and supplies is of concern to the nursing department. Improvement of nursing care to patients is often dependent on the physical facilities in the institution and on the quality and quantity of supplies and equipment. Therefore, nurses should be acquainted with the construction of the plant in which they work and with the materials they use. The nursing service administrator shares responsibility in overall planning for plant operation with other administrative personnel in the institution and for the effective use of supplies and

equipment within the nursing department. Her competency in these matters is reflected throughout the nursing department and contributes in large measure to economical and efficient management of the institution.

The nursing service administrator represents nursing in conferences and meetings with other department heads and explains needs and makes recommendations for nursing. She acts as a nursing consultant in any plan for new facilities, remodeling, or reallocating of space within the institution. Furthermore, the nursing service administrator directs and instructs members of the nursing department in evaluating and analyzing the relationships between the utility of plant, existent and obtainable, and nursing activities to be undertaken.

The ordering, accounting, and inventorying of supplies and equipment are coordinated with the overall system in the institution. There is close cooperation between the nursing department, administration, and the purchasing department in standardizing supplies and equipment. The nursing department assists in setting up a satisfactory index of articles in use and in the evaluation of safety, durability, appearance, utility, and cost of supplies and equipment in use and available. The nursing service administrator guides and instructs her assistants in analyzing needs so that she can be fully informed at administrative conferences, at which she shares in making decisions as to the kind and degree of responsibility for charge, maintenance, and availability of supplies and equipment. In the nursing department conferences, efficient and effective procedures and routines to be observed in use and care of supplies and equipment are formulated.

To assist the department heads, the accounting department should supply the description of each item listed in the budget including the amount of actual expense for the last complete year and the amount approved in the current budget. The department head should estimate the total amount of expense for each item for the current year and the coming year. This detail enlightens the department head and, more than any other, develops cooperation in administrative matters. To be at all accurate, the department head must review department procedures and usage of supplies and must avail herself of market knowledge to predict needs item by item for next year.

Capital expenditure budget. A list of items of capital expenditure required for new items of equipment and replacement of equipment for the coming year should be prepared. The form for the capital expenditures budget should have space for each of the items requested and should furnish (1) a complete description of the item, (2) the cost per item and the total cost, (3) space for recording the amount approved by the budget committee, and (4) space for supporting evidence of requirements.

Special budget forms, such as maintenance requests for painting, should be made out by each department head. Standardized accounting provides that the maintenance of building and general equipment be charged to the physical institution, whereas the maintenance of specialized equipment is charged to the department concerned. The budget for the physical institution will therefore provide for general repairs and items, and only items of a special nature will be provided for in the budget of individual departments.

Completed budget estimates can now be made for direct and indirect items of expense under the control of the nursing service administrator for the coming year. To develop cooperation and understanding between the department head and the administrator and to obtain preliminary approval for major changes or major items of equipment, the nursing service administrator should have the department budget reviewed by the chief administrator before its final completion and submission by the department head.

The actual arithmetic of budget compilation should not be done by the department head but should be left to the staff of the business office. Department heads should be encouraged to complete the totals in their work copy, which they retain, to acquaint them with the total cost of departmental operation. After such careful analysis and consideration, the budget will be established on a factual basis and will represent a well-organized plan for future operations. After all revisions are made, a master budget is prepared and submitted to the board of the health care facility for financial approval.

DIRECTING THE BUDGET: BUDGET OPERATION

In some manner, and at some point or points, decisions must be made with respect to the administration of the plans and programs provided for in the budget. That happens at the department level; it embraces all the many big and little decisions with respect to organizing for performance, scheduling, programming, and managing the operation of the department. It embraces determinations on matters of internal auditing of operations and fiscal matters, on performance reporting communicating upward in the department and to other parties concerned in the work, on records management, on work simplification and work measurement, and on the matter of performance standards. These many decisions grow by accretion into a formidable body of data, significant as a basis for decision making at higher levels of review. In a very real sense, the total budgetary process is measured in terms of the quality of the multitude of decisions that are made, and that must be made, within the operating department. If these decisions are unwise or basically unsound, many of them will never be corrected, for as the budgetary mechanism goes into full gear of operation, it waxes so large and complex as to defy meticulous supervision or policing. This fact raises several basic questions: Who shall direct and administer the budget? How shall this be done? What should be the preparation and background requirements of persons handling this work?

Control measures will vary according to the type of institution. Most tax-supported institutions tend to develop standards for such supplies and commodities as dressings, adhesives, and linens based on past experience. The non-tax-supported health care facility is more likely to use controls that relate more strictly to patient usage, for which patients can be charged, than to personnel usage. In either case, the nursing service administrator should get monthly reports of expenditures incurred by her department from the purchasing department, central service, or general stores. These should be broken down into the previously agreed upon categories from which the budget was prepared.

To emphasize the fact that budget activities are ongoing processes throughout the year, the nursing service administrator will then want to share financial statements with her department supervisors, head nurses, and staff nurses responsible for administering controls.

It is self-evident that the effective execution of a budget is entirely dependent on those people who use its elements of personnel or equipment. Therefore, through meetings such as staff conferences and in-service programs all nursing staff members should acquire a clear understanding of the budget. Coordination and cooperation with the purchasing departments must also be achieved for the effective operation of the budget.

CONTROLLING THE BUDGET: BUDGET REVIEW

Somehow and at some time decisions made with respect to an accounting for performance and a justification of the budget. If programs are authorized and funds for their administration are appropriated, the budgetary process has not been carried to its logical conclusion until there has been a satisfactory accounting of progress and performance and the use of resources, especially monetary funds. Each depart-

ment needs to be given some latitude in determining what techniques and methods to use in rendering an account of its performance to the chief administrator. As a minimum, though, each department should arrange for the following if possible:

1. Each department should install and use a work measurement system that is applicable to the peculiarities of the particular situation, including the establishment of performance standards. This system will serve as a basis for performance estimates and for supervision of program operations.
2. A continuous improvement of administrative reporting along functional lines should be maintained by each department. Those reports, if accurately kept, may serve as a basis for the department's later justification to the administrator, both with respect to its achievements and with further budgetary requests. The quality of the operating and financial reports determines, in large part, the effectiveness of communications within the department and with other concerned departments.
3. Each department should install and use a progressive record system maintained on a functional basis. These records and the organization's reports should supply the information required at higher levels of review in connection with proper decision making with respect to past performance and to future needs.
4. The continuous strengthening and improvement of accounting methods that are applicable to the peculiarities of the given program should be the concern of each department. Regardless of the variations in accounting systems, the results should yield adequate information concerning financial results of operations.
5. Each department should establish an adequate system of management analysis and a reliable system of internal auditing. Such a system should yield information concerning better ways of organizing in terms of program ends, more economical methods and techniques of operations, weak and strong spots in the use of equipment and funds, and more effective methods of presenting information to higher levels of budgetary review.

The variety of health care programs is great, and in the budget area of decision making no general detailed formula for accountability can be prescribed. It is preferable that the details be decentralized and that each department be held responsible for discovering and using the particular techniques suitable for a given program. Basically, the questions to be answered in this area are, Who shall be held accountable for results, to whom shall the account be made, and what are the appropriate facilities and methods to be used in connection with this accountability?

Comparison of estimates with actual expenditures. The key to a successful budget is the critical review of estimates in comparison with actual results. Reports should be prepared for each department on a monthly basis by the accounting office. This report should show the actual amount spent for each account classification in the current year and in the preceding year.

Variation in budgeted estimates. It is important that detailed comparisons be made rather than comparisons of overall results. The variation between budgetary and actual expenses in any one month is not a necessarily poor budgeting performance, as factors, such as time of vacations, vary the amount of graduate nurse personnel required. Monthly or quarterly figures should be used as a guide in judging the progress toward the entire figure. However, an investigation of variations must be made, and the cause of some variations should be analyzed to facilitate proper expense control.

Corrective action. When the important variations have been isolated, the nursing service administrator should take the corrective action necessary, or if this is impossible, she should state this in writing to the chief administrator. A budget supplements the nursing service administrator's experience and skill; it is not a substitute. It reveals any divergency early, so she may quickly and effectively control expenditures before the divergency becomes of any consequence. For example, a comparison of budgeted and actual expense items may reveal a substantial increase in salaries of general staff nurses for inpatient care. Also,

if fiscal management involves control methods, personnel participation, and a systematic approach, day by day, to items of expense, these can be compared to the estimates and allocations in the budget request.

In addition to the establishment of control methods and personnel participation, a third part of budget operation is the regular and routine comparison, item by item, of budgetary forecasts in contrast with actual expense. This leads to budget review in terms of a report. This review is a report summarizing the details of budget operation in relation to the stated objectives and should be carried out at stated intervals, perhaps at fiscal quarters. The review provides an opportunity to determine the status of stated goals and to readjust them, if needed, into more short-term objectives.

SUMMARY OF BUDGETARY PROCESS

The major stages of the budgetary process may be summarized as follows:

1. Formulation of the budget plan by the organization, departments, and chief administrator
2. Transmission of the budget plan by the chief administrator to the board of directors with the budget explanation, which provides unification between the administrative department head's program and the chief administrator's program on the one hand and the institutional policy and financial support on the other
3. Authorization of the budget plan by the board of directors through appropriation of funds; this is the final authorization representing a compromise between administration and department head's proposals
4. Administration of the budget plan by the chief administrator and department heads, economically, efficiently, and according to a time schedule
5. Accountability for performance and achievement of the budget plan by the chief administrator and department heads through a satisfactory reporting system and a further justification of future plans and activities

The formulation of the budget is one of

BUDGETING*

Functions of the nursing service administrator

Knowledge, skill, and appreciations

Secures information on procedure for preparation of the budget in accordance with the financial management of the institution

Budget definition: use of the budget as a planning device, tool of management, and means of evaluation of the program of the nursing service department

1. Overall basis of financial management: source of revenue, such as taxes, endowments, patients' fees, and special gifts
2. Accountability to the public: a board or a donor organization
3. Contracts affecting personnel: Social Security, workmen's compensation insurance, and Blue Cross
4. Basic system of budgeting and accounting in the institution: periodicity of budget, such as annual, biennial, seasonal, or long-term plan
5. System of accounting
6. Policies affecting the budget
7. Personnel policies: vacation, illness, health service, salary increments, cost maintenance, sabbatical leaves, and other prerequisites
8. Quality of equipment, supplies, and plant
9. Standard of nursing care
10. Educational program: in-service and staff education and conventions and other meetings for which expenses are paid
11. Criteria for a good budget: comprehensiveness, flexibility, reliability, and integrity
12. Types of appropriations: lump sums versus specific item, discretion, and diversion

Prepares the nursing service department budget

1. Gathers data for the budget

Review of previous and current budget experience; conference methods, receiving recommendations from assistants or nursing service budget committee; forecasting future needs: expansion, curtailment, or status quo; allowance for the unpredictable

2. Computes needs

Methods of computing: by grouping service units, classification of personnel or items, or personnel by hours of care or by positions; ratio of types of personnel, such as professional nurses to licensed vocational nurses or nursing assistants

3. Organizes budget
4. Presents budgets to administration for approval

Material by type or area of use, expendable or nonexpendable, depreciable or nondepreciable; organization of budget items in form and comprehensiveness

Submits justification of budget to administrator and, in turn, requests justification of administrator's decision

Basis of justification: objectives and standards of quality; contemplated expansions; other changes in personnel, procedures, and apparatus; departmental distribution of costs; methods of demonstration of mutual justification: graphic, statistical, and narrative; and the process of negotiation

*Adapted from Nursing Service Administration Seminar, University of Chicago, 1951, Edward Brothers, Inc., 1952.

BUDGETING—cont'd

Distributes appropriate information to members of the nursing department

Administers nursing department budget: controls expenditures

Periodically reviews the status of the budget

Uses budgetary data in staff appointments

Continually evaluates the program of nursing service in relation to adequacy of budget; analysis budget at end of period for use in preparing subsequent budgets; sets up inventory procedure to conform with that of institution

Information shared with assistants concerning operation of the budget

Correlation of expenditures with appropriations by specified periods

Priorities by time and urgency of need; preauditing: procedure for handling payroll

Adjusting personnel records to new budget

Dissemination of information to nursing units to promote efficiency and economy

---

the nursing service administrator's most important responsibilities and one which will have a direct bearing on the job satisfaction and nursing care responsibilities of her staff. Because of the necessity for justification, the programming for the budgetary objectives will be useful in directing the staff toward the achievement of specific goals, which, when reached, should increase the staff's sense of accomplishment. In addition, it is to the benefit of the patient and the health care organization to have a budget that is geared to early identified goals and accomplishment by well-outlined methods.

REFERENCES

Abdellah, F. G., and Levine, E.: Effect of nursing staff on satisfactions with nursing care, Hospital Monograph Series No. 4, Chicago, 1958, American Hospital Association.

Argyris, C.: The impact of budgets on people. In Litterer, J. A., editor: Organizations: structure and behavior, New York, 1969, John Wiley & Sons, Inc.

Block, L.: Budgeting for nursing service, progress in nursing service, New York, 1956, National League for Nursing.

Dunn, H. W.: The nursing budget, Am. J. Nurs. 63(11):M-12—M-16, 1963.

Lewis, V. B.: Toward a theory of budgeting, Public Admin. Rev. 4:42, Winter 1952.

Seckler-Hudson, C.: Organization and management: theory and practice, Washington, D. C., 1957, The American University Press.

Wolfe, H., and Young, J. P.: Staffing the nursing unit. Controlled variable staffing, Nurs. Res. 14(3):236-243, 1965a.

Wolfe, H., and Young, J. P.: Staffing the nursing unit. II. The multiple assignment technique, Nurs. Res. 14(4):299-304, 1965b.

ADDITIONAL READINGS

Budgeting procedures for hospitals, American Hospital association: Chicago, 1971, The Association.

Connor, R. J.: Effective use of nursing resources: a research report, Hospitals 35:30-39, May 1, 1961.

Houtz, D. T.: The unit manager in the hospital organization, Hosp. Prog. 1:73-78, February 1966.

Joint Commission on Accreditation of Hospitals: Accreditation manual for hospitals, Chicago, 1970, The Commission.

Sauer, J. E., Jr.: Cost containment—and quality assurance, too. I. Hospitals 46(1):64-70, 1972; II. Hospitals 46(2):78-93, 1972.

Vatter, W. J.: Operating budgets, Belmont, Calif., 1969, Wadsworth Pub. Co.

Young, E. G.: The nursing service budget, New York, 1957, National League For Nursing.

Chapter 11

THE NURSING ADMINISTRATOR: QUALIFICATIONS AND EDUCATIONAL PREPARATION

To effectively perform the duties and functions of an administrator for nursing services in a complex environment full of challenges and problems, a person must possess particular qualities and assume specific roles. The degree and the combination of these characteristics are dictated by the size, character, and type of health care institution to be administered. Administrators and educators agree on the basic attributes a person should possess to select, educate, and train nurses for the position of nurse administrator.

QUALIFICATION AND ROLE OF NURSE ADMINISTRATOR

The major attributes of a successful nurse administrator fall into the following three categories: (1) intellectual qualifications, the knowledge base relevant to administration of nursing services, (2) skills in the area of leadership, operation, and communication, and (3) personal characteristics, such as physical and psychological qualifications. Nursing administrators are successful to the extent that they utilize their talents effectively, make significant contributions to the health care organization, and receive personal satisfaction.

Intellectual qualifications

The intellectual qualifications of a nurse administrator focus on her ability to ac-quire and utilize knowledge. The determinants of the scope of intellectual abilities are (1) ability to comprehend and apply knowledge, which depends on technical competence, open-mindedness, sound personal judgment, and accurate sense of perspective, (2) ability to teach others, that is, knowledgeable in subject matter, a perpetual learner, active listener, and able to transmit knowledge clearly and motivate others, (3) ability to approach problems scientifically, that is, organize facts, give them proper weight, and place them in proper perspective, and (4) ability to develop a well-thought-out personal philosophy to guide and direct administrative actions and personal living.

MENTAL CAPACITY

To comprehend and apply knowledge of administrative principles, a nurse administrator must assume the role of the administrative composite process specialist, a system's specialist, and she must possess a broad base of knowledge in the Administrative Composite Process (ACP). The functions and activities of the nurse administrator as an ACP specialist within the sociotechnical system of the health care institution include (1) planning (policy formulation, setting of objectives, decision making, and planning programs of action), (2) organizing (principles, methods, and techniques of organization, such as division of work and assigning of tasks to appropriate individuals and nature of administrative responsibility, authority, and accountability), (3) directing: execution and coordination of the organized plan, and (4) evaluating and controlling: analysis, classification, and simplification of jobs, systems, methods, and procedures; qualitative and quantitative measurements of nursing activities; and ability to utilize statistics and accounting as means of administrative control.

An open sociotechnical system creates a difficult role for the nurse administrator, for administrative assignments do not have neat and clearly defined boundaries. Rather, the nurse administrator of today is placed in a network of mutually dependent relationships. The nurse administrator must successfully coalign people; apply institutional action, technology, and task environment; and formulate organizational design and structure appropriate to achieve a viable domain. One of the enduring objectives of the nurse administrator is to seek a moving equilibrium, since the parameters of the system (the divisions of labor and the controls) are evolving and changing. She deals with uncertainties and ambiguities and must adapt the organization to new and changing requirements.

Successful nurse administrators accept change as a byword and learn to deal with it in an organized, coherent, and positive fashion. The health care institution lives in a world of scientific advancement—medical, technological, and nursing—and must gear itself for constant change or perish of obsolescence. The health care institution must balance its set policies, standard operating procedures, and long-range planning, which are necessary to ensure stability and order, against its flexibility to alter policies and procedures that have become obsolete by changing circumstances. An essential intellectual attribute of a nurse administrator is the ability to heed signals indicating that

change is necessary. She should be emotionally constituted to follow the course of action that the signs indicate. The nurse administrator must also be able to read trends not only within her own field but also within the rest of society.

As an ACP specialist, the nurse administrator must also assume a leadership role. To function effectively and execute plans efficiently, she must know the elements and impact of leadership; accept the responsibilities and privileges of leadership; see the role of the leader as strategist, diplomat, and conciliator; and be aware of the social processes of adjustment, cooperation, and conflict in human behavior (American Council on Education 1954:37).

ABILITY TO TEACH OTHERS

As a teacher, the nurse administrator must be knowedgeable in the area of pedagogic theory and principle and be able to implement the principles of learning and instruction in actual staff development and teaching situations. As a teaching strategist, she must be able to identify teaching situations, understand the conditions and mediums of learning, be able to teach for transfer of learning, and master teaching methods and techniques in individual and group situations.

PROBLEM-SOLVING ABILITY

An essential intellectual qualification of a nurse administrator as ACP specialist is the ability to solve problems. A successful nurse executive must be able to identify problems clearly, have sensitivity to developing problems, spot symptoms of a gathering storm, and intervene during the early stages of development. If the nurse administrator is unable to anticipate problems, she will move from crisis to crisis, work will be interrupted repeatedly to put out a fire, and policies will be changed frequently in an attempt to meet the demands of each critical situation (Shaffer 1964). Therefore, development of an analytic mind, that is, the ability to think through a problem, obtain pertinent data, evaluate such data, and consider all direct and indirect factors, is of utmost importance.

The effective administrator also perceives her responsibility as being to help key staff think problems through by exercising their own judgment; she should extend every possible aid to them in arriving at a sound decision without giving them the answer. Furthermore, she provides the opportunity for staff to participate in the planning and decision making affecting patient care and the nursing department beyond the staff's specialty. Staff participation is essential for growth, and only the accountable nurse administrator can make this possible. When responsible nursing staff members are not brought into the discussion of problems early enough or if they have to push to be heard, they may assert themselves by dragging their feet, hardly the way to foster intellectual and professional growth in individuals or to take advantage of the rich opportunities at the corporate level for broadening experiences (Shaffer 1964).

DEVELOPMENT OF PERSONAL PHILOSOPHY

The final intellectual qualification of a nurse administrator is the need to have a well-thought-out guiding personal philosophy to direct administrative actions and personal living. If the individual is to have an effective and satisfying life as a nurse administrator in a health care institution, it is important that her personal philosophy in the following areas be in harmony with the institution's and with her position: (1) desire to serve and contribute to welfare of society, (2) respect for the dignity of human beings regardless of color, creed, race, and social or economic status, (3) awareness of spiritual needs and resources within herself and within others—attain understanding and not mere tolerance of others, and (4) leadership qualities necessary to administer the care of patients and to set a climate for clinical inquiry.

Skills

As a composite process specialist, the nurse administrator should have the special administrative skills of leadership, operation, and communication.

LEADERSHIP

Leadership exists when an individual meets organizational and individual needs and creates an environment and situation in which these needs can be satisfied. Research has shown that leaders are not born, but are cultivated; the specific training and education that leaders should have consists of increased sensitivity to diagnosing organizational, group, and individual needs and problems (Bennis 1960).

An important leadership skill that stems from the preceding principle is the ability to capitalize on what other members of the organization can bring to bear to satisfy existing needs of the staff. It is not possible for a single leader to fulfill all the needs of the group or organization because there are too many roles and functions that have to be performed efficiently and effectively. Implicit in this leadership skill is the nurse administrator's ability to understand and work with others.

Essential skills for a nurse administrator are the ability to motivate others to perform desirable behaviors and the ability to determine the means and the timing of dispensing rewards to staff members for accomplishing designated organizational and individual objectives.

The nurse administrator should be familiar with Thorndike's *Law of Effect* (1911), which points out that people tend to repeat behaviors that are rewarded and tend not to repeat behaviors that are not. This simple principle is frequently forgotten. As a rewarder and an agent who controls dispensing of rewards, the nurse administrator should know which rewards are in fact perceived as rewards, that is, which rewards have incentive value for the employee. This can be determined by ascertaining why staff members seek to work in their particular health care organization. An individual works in any organization to satisfy some personal need or needs. Needs of people are not simple. They are diversified, complicated, and at times unconscious. Individuals join an organization for a variety of reasons: some seek prestige and status; others, research opportunities or an opportunity for personal development; those with a strong social conscience want to help the sick and want to work with people; and still others work for financial reasons or for highly personal reasons. An astute, skillful, intuitive nurse administrator is aware of these factors and understands that needs vary among individuals and within the same individual at different times.

Another important aspect of motivation is for the nurse administrator to enable staff members to feel successful and to succeed by utilizing their talents effectively, thus making them feel that their contributions are significant to the health care organization, which in turn enables them to obtain personal satisfactions. Motivating people, therefore, requires (1) understanding of what each individual's satisfactions are, (2) recognition that most people want to do a good job and the right thing, and (3) encouragement of staff to use talents in making significant contributions.

The technique of *management by objectives* or *reality-centered leadership* is another important aspect of leadership skill that a nurse administrator should possess. Bennis (1960) referred to it as *problem-oriented leadership.* This entails establishing organizational and individual objectives, setting target dates for accomplishment of the objectives, and delegating tasks and responsibilities to appropriate people. Furthermore, when faced with problems or tough decisions of management, the administrator deals with them by exploring problems with the group, organizing the facts at hand, and involving people directly with the solu-

tion of the problem. She does so by communicating the problem, by insisting on involvement and participation, and by jointly working on the problem. This is management by objectives and not management by control.

Staff development and the ability to counsel are essential objectives of leadership. Developing staff does not entail teaching gimmicks, techniques, or giving pat answers to problems, but entails helping each staff member to become a more effective human being. These objectives are achieved by creating an environment in which self-development is encouraged and facilitated (Shaffer 1964:39).

The method of developing people deals essentially with the learning process. The concern of the nurse administrator is not only with problem solving, but also with teaching others how best to utilize their talents so that they themselves may become more effective problem solvers.

The nurse leader utilizes many teaching tools and strategies to produce learning, problem-solving ability, and actual experience or participation and to provide counseling or constructive criticism and climate for growth. Practice in actually solving problems produces learning. It is true that members learn from case studies, but attempting to solve problems successfully within their department has a special meaning for staff members. Within this framework of problem-solving strategy, the nurse leader has the following two responsibilities: (1) to ensure that the staff member has solved the problem satisfactorily and (2) to ensure that the subordinate is learning and growing through the experience (Shaffer 1964:40).

The use of constructive criticism to counsel employees implies the ability to counsel and point out the mistakes of employees without shattering their confidence. The criticism is focused on the error and not on the person, thus enabling employees to retain self-respect while facing mistakes realistically.

The professional growth of staff members in their daily performance on the job is the most important kind of growth, and nurturing it is an important aspect of the nurse administrator's position. The growth of individuals is either facilitated or retarded by the climate within which they work and that climate is set by the attitude and the behavior of the chief executive. The climate that enhances individual growth is characterized by (1) a clear-cut definition of responsibilities, (2) the feeling of freedom to perform tasks and make decisions that pertain to one's job and are within the policies established for the health care organization, and (3) the feeling that the staff members' ideas and opinions are welcome and that their efforts are appreciated (Shaffer 1964).

The ability to deal with individual differences and the ability to nurture creativity in individuals are essential leadership skills. Each individual feels unique in needs, talents, and aspirations and responds best to the leader who recognizes that and treats the individual so. The ability to handle individual differences efficiently and effectively entails (1) appreciation of the importance of a variety of talents to the success of the health care organization, (2) skill in recognizing and appraising diverse talents, and (3) versatility in blending talents harmoniously.

To encourage creativity, the nurse executive must have an attitude that embodies (1) genuine respect for the contributions of others, (2) willingness to accept their mistakes, and (3) humility to recognize that no one is perfect and that everyone has blind spots that can be effectively supplemented by the strengths of others (Shaffer 1964:38).

The nurse administrator who develops skill and versatility in dealing with individual differences has greater resources to draw on than the administrator who punishes disagreements and discourages creativeness.

OPERATION

The operational skills required are ability to make decisions, to delegate authority, and to organize and coordinate personnel and activities.

Decision making is the crux of an administrator's job, and a successful nurse leader soon learns how to make decisions. The operational skill of decision making requires the ability (1) to recognize when to stop gathering data and to pull the facts together to make a decision, (2) to act when it is time, (3) to plan and analyze data carefully, (4) to take risks, recognizing that risk is inherent in any major decisions, and (5) to utilize strategy, that is, (a) having an awareness that proper timing is often the key element in getting ideas accepted, (b) getting the proper support from influential people who can endorse and promote ideas at the proper level, and (c) recognizing the obstacles to new ideas and developing plans to overcome them.

Achieving results by utilizing others is the art of *delegation*. The nurse administrator can delegate formal authority but cannot delegate responsibility; ultimately, it is the administrator who is accountable for the conditions and operation of the nursing department within the health care organization. She can only hope that the person who accepts the authority also accepts the responsibility, or accountability, that goes with it. She delegates authority at two levels: performance level and decision-making level. The delegation of authority at the decision-making level is the highest expression of confidence and trust the nurse executive can bestow. At this level the nurse administrator assumes a new role, that of delegator of authority. She becomes the disseminator of information, enabling her assistants (subordinates) to make sound decisions. The nurse administrator's concern has shifted from deciding *what* the decision is to *is it the best* decision (Shaffer 1964).

Organization and coordination of the

activities of others constitute two more essential operational skills for the nurse administrator. The need for effective administration of nursing services has been widely asserted, especially as health care organizations grow in size and complexity, requiring more conscious planning and organization and rational control on the part of the nurse administrator in the face of mushrooming communications problems. As health care institutions expand, the position of the nurse administrator becomes one of a coordinator. She is expected to coordinate the activities within the organization's environment and between the health care organization and the community at large.

To do so efficiently, the nurse administrator has to demonstrate understanding of administrative and organizational processes, for it is through these processes that effective administrative behavior of coordination can be achieved (Arndt 1965).

COMMUNICATION

To delegate decision-making authority and get things done through others, the nurse administrator must know how to communicate with her staff. The art of effective communication entails the following:

1. Skill in articulating the objectives and long-range plans of the health care organization is necessary to communicate properly.

2. Ability to report, explain, and interpret the institution's policies in light of specific problems that her staff is dealing with is an important aspect of communication.

3. Awareness of the fact that nonverbal communication skills are important tools in administration. Attitudes and feelings communicate far more than words. The staff will learn to read the signs in facial expression, attitude, tone of voice, and gestures, which will either facilitate or inhibit channels of communications between herself and the staff.

4. Ability to listen and pay attention is an important aspect of communication. A nurse administrator must know how to listen in a way that encourages members of the staff to express their opinions and communicate and to learn from them in the process (Shaffer 1964).

Personal traits

The personal traits of the nurse administrator may be categorized as physical and psychological.

PHYSICAL QUALITIES

Good health is the first physical requirement. In addition, the top nurse executive must possess a high degree of endurance, capacity to withstand stress, strain, and pressure, ability to work long hours under difficult circumstances when required, and perserverance to pursue objectives. Finally, she should express vitality, which is a reflection of the fortitude and liveliness of the person. Vitality bespeaks forcefulness and personal attractiveness, strong elements in leadership quality (American Council on Education 1954:32).

PSYCHOLOGICAL QUALITIES

Psychological qualities are attributes of character (the sum total of an individual's mental habits, which are a result of learned behaviors) and personality (that aspect of character that is workable in influencing other people).

Character. The important attributes of character for a successful administrator are as follows:

1. Integrity in moral soundness. This refers to the nurse administrator's standard of conduct in relationships with other people who can be trusted with respect to honesty, loyalty, honor, reliability, and sincerity.

2. Self-discipline takes the form of self-understanding and self-control of attitudes and feelings. The nurse executive who takes the time to attempt to know and understand herself better minimizes the

risk of having emotional factors adversely affect her judgment. Self-understanding requires the willingness to face even unpleasant facts about one's self. Self-control of attitudes and feelings is the ability to look at one's own thinking, beliefs, and attitudes objectively and to recognize prejudices, biases, fears, and other feelings that distract one from sound reasoning and judgment.

3. Responsibility is willingness to accept accountability for one's own duties or acts and those of associates and staff members, as well as to accept social responsibility to the community, which requires understanding of and sensitivity to the social, cultural, economic, and political environment in which one must function.

Closely associated with the sense of social responsibility is the attribute of humanism that a nurse administrator should possess. This refers to her mode of thought and action, which is based on an abiding interest in and an affection for people and society in general.

4. Stability is a manner of living characterized by firmness and steadiness in conduct that does not waver with uncertainty or vacillate with indecision.

5. Industry is the ability to utilize talent and strength in accomplishing something worthwhile. This requires initiative, diligence, and perserverance.

Personality. Personality is a personal trait that is psychological in nature. It is the aspect of character that is workable in influencing other people.

1. Self-confidence, courage, and the ability to sell ideas to the administration, the governing board, and the public are essential personality characteristics. In addition, the nurse administrator should have intelligence, warmth, persuasiveness, and the ability to influence others. A nurse administrator who is persuasive has a keen sense of appropriateness and timing, can distinguish relevant from irrelevant facts in a given situation, and can marshal and present facts convincingly, attracting rather

than commanding assent. Furthermore, if she is to be a true leader, she must become involved in activities outside her profession. In addition to selling her own ideas to influential people, the nurse executive has to interpret to the public and to other professional groups changes that are occurring in nursing education, nursing practice, and the profession in general, for to fail to do so represents a disservice to her profession and to her own role as a director (Young 1969).

2. Personal magnetism and tact help determine a person's charisma and are derived from innate and acquired characteristics. The innate aspects of personal magnetism are the manifestations of emotion and temperament; the acquired or the learned aspects owe to good manners. Emotional balance and pleasant temperament are prerequisites, but only conscious effort and self-discipline develop them.

Closely associated with personal magnetism is tact, a sensitive mental awareness of what to say or do when dealing with others, so as to achieve a purpose and to avoid giving offense. It is a learned behavior that develops from self-control, self-discipline, and consideration for others when emotion and temper threatens to overcome judgment (American Council on Education 1954:34).

3. Cooperation is the ability to adjust to group decisions and to work in harmony with others and is the measure of the nurse administrator's capacity to link her will with the purpose of others.

4. Ability to inspire and motivate entails transmitting enthusiasm to others and exerting a positive influence on others. Personal magnetism, enthusiasm, and the ability to inspire others form a triad of attitudes in a balanced personality. For a nurse administrator to inspire others, she needs to be knowledgeable, perceptive, and able to communicate her ideas.

5. Determination and willingness to pay the price of success are also essential personality characteristics. The price the nurse

administrator has to pay is measured in time, responsibility, and ability to withstand loneliness. She is expected to go far beyond the 40-hour workweek and often will be taking work home. She is responsible for the welfare of hundreds of people who depend on her judgment. Loneliness of command is often one of the most difficult burdens a chief executive must bear. It may require that she discipline associates who are friends. She may be cut off from the grapevine. Often she is called on to make unpopular decisions, some that she cannot discuss with any of her associates (Shaffer 1964:44).

6. A sense of humor and a sense of perspective are essential to other personality characteristics. Humor helps to keep things in perspective and prevents undue brooding. The administrator with a sense of humor knows she may make errors and is able to laugh at herself and with others. Humor, when sensitively used, helps to dispel anxiety and allows for the "light touch" during some difficult situations. Sarcasm, which has its roots in the hostile realm, has no place in effective administration. The wise and just administrator is sensitive to the feelings of others and utilizes humor in moderation and for reason.

EDUCATIONAL PREPARATION OF THE NURSE ADMINISTRATOR

A nurse administrator of this caliber who is qualified to assume the requisite roles must be educationally well prepared. The education of the nurse administrator has raised issues of tremendous magnitude that have direct bearing on the demand and supply of nurse leaders and their preparation.

Salient educational and professional issues facing the field of administration of nursing services and the academic preparation of the nurse administrator

Some of the questions that are being asked concerning the position and the preparation of the nurse administrator are as follows: Do we really need nurse leaders? Should nursing schools prepare nurse administrators, or should other related disciplines prepare administrators for nursing services? Should the preparation for nursing service administration be at the level of the master's degree, or should it be on doctoral level? Does the nurse administrator need clinical specialization? If yes, does the specialization have to be in nursing?

The question, Do we really need nurse leaders? has received overwhelming affirmative support from scholars in the field of nursing education and nursing service administrations (Arndt 1965; Mullane 1959, Finer 1964; Miller 1971; Young 1969). Implicitly and explicitly, these scholars have all stated the nation's need for nurse leaders; we agree. Health care agencies rely heavily on the leadership of nurses educated for and responsible for creating and administering new patterns of organized nursing services. More recently, nursing educators and nursing research grant donors have ignored the fulfillment of this need. To emphasize clinical specialization at the expense of nursing administration research reduces the number of potentially capable nurse leaders in the field of nursing service administration, as experience has shown. The critical need for nursing leadership should be reflected in a reexamination of master's degree programs with a view toward providing the minimum educational preparation for the majority of nursing service administrators.

Graduate education needs to devote more attention and study to the issue of preparing nurse administrators who can create and maintain a nursing care system for delivery of optimum and individualized care to patients and a nursing education system that will educate and prepare creative, independent nurse practitioners at all levels of competence.

Another important issue lies in the area of educational preparation of the nurse administrator. Should graduate programs in nursing prepare nurse administrators? Or, should other related disciplines assume the responsibility for educating them? Should trained nonnurse administrators organize and direct nursing care services? Also, if schools of nursing assume the responsibility of educating nurse administrators, should the candidate be required to have a clinical specialization?

Before we can answer the question of whether a nurse should administer the nursing care services and, if so, what her educational preparation should be, we need to know whether or not an advanced clinical specialization in nursing is a requisite for the nurse administrator (Miller 1971).

It is our opinion that some advanced clinical specialization in a specified field is essential for the administration and the delivery of nursing care services. It enables the nurse administrator to be more sensitive in predicting or diagnosing problems existing at the patient care level and those facing the nurse practitioner. In so doing, she can plan, organize, direct, and control the delivery of nursing care services more efficiently, and she can create a physical and conceptual environment that is conducive to delivery of optimum patient care in which nurses are able to practice what they have been prepared for.

Which department of the university should assume the responsibility for educating nurse administrators? We feel it is the responsibility of schools of nursing to prepare nurse leaders to administer the delivery of nursing care services. Doctoral programs in nursing are now available in a number of universities. The programs emphasize research and the building and testing of nursing theory, the basis for nursing practice. Nurse administrators prepared in these programs will also need to acquire knowledge in administration through course work in other related departments, such as business administration and behavioral sciences. The interdisciplinary approach to educational preparation has the advantages of maintaining the student's identity with nursing as a discipline and fostering the concept that administrative and organizational skills are tools by which the primary goal of nursing service, that is, the delivery of direct nursing care services to patients, is achieved.

Another advantage of doctoral study in nursing is that it can relate the ongoing research in nursing administration more relevantly to nursing practice than can primary education acquired in another discipline (Miller 1971:42).

With respect to whether the educational preparation of the nurse administrator for university schools of nursing, for university hospitals and clinics, and for large and complex health care organizations be at the masters or doctoral level, Miller (1971), Young (1969), and McNerney (1960) were of the opinion that it must be at the doctoral level, and we concur. The sophistication required to collaborate effectively with other health professionals and planners requires in-depth education and training in research, nursing practice, and other related disciplines, which only preparation at the doctoral level can provide.

If research findings are to form the knowledge base for nursing practice, nursing service, and nursing education, the major university schools of nursing and nursing services should stress research focused on nursing care problems of patients, how best to organize nursing-care services, and how best to educate practitioners (Miller 1971:41).

There are several ways for the nurse administrator to pursue a doctoral level education, assuming first that there are some basic knowledge areas essential for a nurse administrator. Graduate level course work in nursing and related disciplines and research work in clinical nursing and nursing service should have the highest priority as a required area of study. Obviously the functions of the nurse administrator should be directed toward a better system of providing direct nursing care to patients in a diversity of settings. With the variety of highly educated professional nurses and technical nurses and nurse assistants that make up her staff, it is essential that the nurse administrator be a competent practitioner who can utilize the nursing skills and potentials of the staff to the fullest extent. Furthermore, she must be knowledgeable in the area of nursing practice and nursing research to interpret to other health professionals and the community the role that nursing plays in the delivery of a total health care system. For the nurse administrator to understand how complex organizations operate, thrive, change, or decline with the changing needs of society, she needs to have advanced knowledge in systems theory, organizational and administrative theory, social sciences, theories of learning and instruction, comprehensive health planning, economics of health, statistics, and humanities, in other words, the eclectic theory of the four schools of administrative thought: scientific management, behavioral science, social science, and scientific management.

Formal academic education of the nurse administrator

The purpose of the academic period is to select students of outstanding promise and to provide them the opportunity to gain knowledge and develop abilities, skills, attitudes, and understandings that will constitute a base for their growth into responsible and competent nurse administrators. If an individual is to meet the qualifications demanded for administration of nursing services, she must be endowed with specific attributes and must successfully complete an educational and training program extending over several months or years to develop the requisite knowledge base, skills, and capabilities.

A meaningful program of education for nursing administrators must provide the basis for education in the future. Given the certainty of change and the uncertainty of its direction, it is an unassailable proposition that in university education for nurs-

ing service administration the highest value must be placed on the development of acuity of the thought processes of students rather than on particularized subject matter or on present operating practices (Arndt 1965:9).

In a world in which the most prominent characteristic is change, the qualities of adaptation, flexibility, ingenuity, creative thinking, imagination, and exercise of judgment are the keys to effective functioning and the mastering of numerous problems generated by an increasingly complex society and health world. It is the fact of modern life and modern thought with which nursing service administration must come to terms (Arndt 1965).

AIMS AND OBJECTIVES OF ACADEMIC PROGRAM OF STUDY FOR ADMINISTRATION OF NURSING SERVICES AT THE DOCTORAL LEVEL

These goals are presented as guides in developing the present and future programs in nursing service administrations to meet current and future needs, realizing that constant experimentation is necessary within reasonable limits and that resources will vary in different universities. The suggested curriculum is a standard that can be used in the planning of present or future programs in nursing service administration.

The central purposes of graduate level education in the administration of nursing services is to enable the student to develop a base of fundamental knowledge and a disciplined mind capable and competent of researching problems in nursing administration, education, and practice and to become a competent practitioner in administration of nursing services. It is also the purpose of graduate level education to discipline the character of the nursing student for future growth and development in administration of nursing services, in civic responsibility, and in personal life.

Instruction is planned specifically to enable each student to acquire the following abilities:

1. To demonstrate a thorough, integrated fundamental knowledge of organization, management, and administration of nursing services.

Rather than imparting factual information to students, the aim is to inculcate a versatility of mind for the task of nursing administration and to orient them to their surroundings. The nurse administrator needs to have a firm grasp of fundamental knowledge, principles, methods, and techniques on which to rely in meeting the challenges of administration of nursing services, or she will be lost in a maze of facts and details.

2. To demonstrate competence in the orderly, analytical exploration, solution, and handling of problems in the area of administration of nursing services.

Competence in nursing service administration is dependent on the student's ability to analyze situations, to recognize and diagnose problems, to determine issues, to seek pertinent facts, and to exercise imagination in developing an alternative course of action to make decisions under pressure. Such conceptual skills are supported by the ability to understand the human factor, to utilize figures effectively, to draw on a fund of substantive knowledge, and to draw on another's specialized skills and knowledge.

3. To develop skill and knowledge for dealing effectively with other people, individually, in groups, and through written communication.

The ability to work effectively with others is perhaps the most crucial skill of all. Understanding human nature and the importance of individual motivation and group relationships is critical for the successful formulation and execution of policies. The student should be knowledgeable not only of the methods of directing others but also of the relative advantages and disadvantages of accomplishing tasks or organizational objectives through force of authority, that is, by coercive means, persuasion, and autonomous or group thinking. The student should also demonstrate ability in written and oral communication and participate in meetings of various forms.

4. To demonstrate understanding of the economic and social system in which the health care organization operates.

The general economic and social developments of society impinge on the control and behavior of individual social institutions. As administrative responsibility increases, attention to the relationships between the individual organization, the community, and the overall economy and their effect on the nursing department occupies an increasing portion of the nurse administrator's time. Graduate nursing students are encouraged and placed in a position to think of their particular administrative environment in the perspective of the broad social and economic foundation and its external impact on the institution, in the perspective of historical development and gradualness of change, and in the perspective of health care organization as one agency of society and of health and also as a field of endeavor dependent on group thinking, action, and sharing to achieve advancement.

5. To develop in the student an inquiring mind, independence of thought, and a maturity of character.

To improve on the heritage of their predecessors, future nurse administrators must be taught to explore, inquire, investigate, question, and think creatively. They must conduct scientific research and develop practical judgment. To achieve progress, they must emulate and excel, not imitate.

SOME TEACHING STRATEGIES AND AREAS OF EMPHASIS FOR GRADUATE EDUCATION IN NURSING SERVICE ADMINISTRATION

The essential areas of concern and some of the teaching strategies that need to be incorporated into the program planning and instruction of nurse administrators are as follows:

1. The need for in-depth teaching of principles of administrative theory and practice for nursing services utilizing analytical and quantitative procedures.

Graduate schools of nursing that prepare nurse administrators for responsible leadership positions in complex organizations and in the community at the doctoral level need to be aware of the necessity to teach and to engage the student in learning the dynamics and organizing principles of the field of administration for nursing services, rather than simply to convey a mass of facts about the field. Graduate schools of nursing should move in the direction of specialization in depth, which refers to a deepening of understanding or intensifying of skills and insights in the field of nursing service administrations (Duce 1966).

Methods of investigation, canons of interpretation, and conceptual systems that are conducive to the understanding and use of facts about nursing service administration are principles that must be flexible and open for investigation and revision as new facts dictate. The teaching of these principles enables the students to view the organization as a system composed of interdependent parts in which the whole is greater than the sum of its parts.

2. Utilization of technological advances.

New concepts and methods of instruction need to be introduced that allow programs to be tailored to meet the needs of the individual student. Some of these new concepts—notably, independent-study programs, cooperative participation in research, and group dynamics—have already been introduced. But graduate education in nursing has not recognized so well the role of technology as an instrument of research. If properly integrated into the teaching learning process, such techniques as programming, model building, and simulated administrative experiences can enhance the graduate student's educational development. Through computerized management games the simulated experiences provide students with a variety of vicarious learning experiences without the frustration and danger of too early a participation in actual administrative responsibilities. It is an excellent supplement to and often substitute for the case-study method, role-playing, and the more conventional graduate experiences.

3. The need for fertilization across disciplines and the need for off-campus education.

The graduate programs in nursing service administration need to draw more on the basic disciplines of the university for support, and these disciplines in turn will find new sources of insight from cooperation with nursing administrative studies. There is not only a great opportunity but also a valid need for meaningful cross-fertilization among university disciplines and fields of study on developing a new area of concentration such as administration for nursing services (American Council on Education 1954:90).

Graduate educational programs in nursing service administration are as much the responsibility of the institutions and nursing service departments that students are being educated to serve as they are of the graduate nursing schools. Therefore, graduate education needs to engage more and more in activities in cooperation with institutions off the campus. There cannot be a sharp line at which education ends and practice begins. The objectivity that scholarship requires and the involvement that practice demands are complementary rather than contradictory and must be developed together in education and continued in practice (Duce 1966). Graduate education should act as a dynamic link between formal education and full responsibility of administrative practice. This is possible only if there is an effective method of combining essential aspects of both in the educational programs. Therefore, administrators of nursing services and nursing educators need to work together in planning and implementing graduate nursing programs that prepare nurse administrators capable of meeting tomorrow's rather than yesterday's needs.

4. The need for research training in nursing service administration.

A necessary condition for any effective teaching program in nursing service administration is a vigorous, well-structured research framework in which the demands for creative capacities are paramount. Establishing a milieu in which meaningful research can be conducted is one of the primary responsibilities of a nursing service administration educational program. Integrating research methods and values into the student's development is the responsibility of the educational system. Whether the research is basic, applied, action, or any other is not so important as whether the student has acquired the knowledge and skills and developed the attitudes of openness, experimentation, and disciplined investigation.

Another major concern that has particular relevance to education for nurse administrators is the basis for developing content of educational programs. We agree with Miller (1971) that not until nursing education and nursing service are more closely related in university medical centers will there be instituted the kind of research that supplies the knowledge base for the form and content of nursing curriculums preparing practitioners for all levels of nursing, including administration.

PROPOSED CURRICULUM FOR GRADUATE LEVEL EDUCATION OF THE NURSE ADMINISTRATOR

Undergraduate educational preparation as prerequisite for admission to graduate level study. The nature and quality of the preparation that students bring with them from their undergraduate years are of paramount importance.

In addition to the basic nursing courses and clinical experiences that lead to the baccalaureate degree in nursing, each student should have a broad, general education in the liberal arts and sciences as a minimal requirement. Nursing administration involves the humanities, the arts, and the physical, biological, social, and nursing sciences. General education builds the foundation for advanced specialized studies. It aims to develop in all students the competence to exercise constructive critical judgment on and to achieve some understanding of the diverse and particular problems, materials, and methods they have encountered in the foundation courses.

Aims of undergraduate nursing education

1. First-level nurse practitioners should be capable of practicing professional nursing in any state or country.

2. Students should demonstrate competence in comprehension and expression in words.

3. Students should demonstrate knowledge and understanding of the human institution and the values with which the law deals. More specifically, the students should demonstrate understanding of (1) economic systems of societies, (2) political organizations of societies, (3) democratic processes, (4) social structure of societies, and (5) cultural heritage of Western and other societies.

4. Students should develop sound judgment and competence in problem-solving ability. This teaching process is necessary to develop the power to think clearly, carefully, and independently. Creative power in thinking requires a development of skills in (1) beginning research, (2) fact completeness, (3) fact differentiation, (4) fact marshaling, (5) deductive reasoning, (6) inductive reasoning, (7) reasoning by analogy, (8) critical analysis, and (9) constructive synthesis.

Graduate educational program in nursing service administration. The academic period of graduate study is one of synthesis and integration. It assumes that the candidate for the master's degree will have a background in basic courses of nursing service administration and that the candidate for the doctoral degree will emerge with advanced knowledge and skills in application of the principles of administration of nursing services and competence in conducting research and in effectively utilizing its results.

The chairman of the university graduate program in nursing service administration should assume the responsibility of selecting students whose work and performance in academic courses have been high in quality and broadly based so that the level of graduate courses and seminars proposed for this aspect of professional study can be pursued.

Throughout the graduate program, master's and doctoral, are five threads that form the curriculum on which nursing service administration courses are formulated. The continuum progresses from the simple to the complex.

Administrative composite processes. The first area of concentration deals with basic and advanced principles of nursing service administration. More specifically, it is concerned with teaching administrative conceptual acts, planning and policy formulation; organization and operation of nursing services; decision making; and problem solving. It also deals with physical acts of directing nursing services and with analysis, evaluation, and control to ensure that the planned objectives of the nursing service department have been successfully implemented and achieved.

Educational objectives. The educational objectives to be achieved by the student in the area of administrative composite processes are based on the student's ability to do the following:

1. Develop and demonstrate an understanding of the fundamental principles and processes of nursing service administration

2. Implement these principles and processes in reaching intelligent administrative decisions of performing effectively the duties of a chief executive of the nursing department

3. Demonstrate an understanding of the objectives of a health care institution and

become competent in formulating long-term and short-term plans for achieving them

4. Become competent in making decisions, appraising operating situations, determining what alternative actions are pertinent to a situation, and foreseeing the consequences of each alternative

5. Identify problems in organizational planning, organizing, directing, and controlling departmental duties and activities in different types of health-care organizations and to plan and implement a course of action in solving these problems

6. Conduct a scientific investigation of organizational and individual level problems that occur in the department of nursing

7. Develop competence in exercising a directing and coordinating influence among diversified groups, which will make for a well-integrated nursing service department

8. Demonstrate understanding and competence in the utilization of administrative tools with which to analyze, evaluate, and control the nursing department

To perform the preceding functions effectively, the student should demonstrate knowledge in the following areas:

a. Financial evaluation, that is, understanding and interpreting balance sheets, expense distribution, reserve investments, and establishment of rates and charges, for example

b. Budgetary control and cost analysis, that is, establishing a budget of operation for analysis and control

c. Statistical evaluation, that is, knowledge and understanding of the value and use of statistical data concerning the operation of the nursing department, for example, evaluation of the statistics regarding work performed and services rendered by the nursing department, standard of operating efficiency, comparison of standard of patient care, and knowledge of qualitative aspects of evaluation in addition to the quantitative analysis

9. Demonstrate knowledge and understanding of the effects of external (sociological, political, legal, or economic) constraints on the appropriate functioning of the organization as a whole and nursing department in particular, constraints that may have an inhibitory effect on the organization and its nursing department

10. Demonstrate knowledge and understanding of the internal activities of the nursing department and their direct and indirect relationships with the activities of other departments whose activities vary widely from those of nursing and be knowledgeable of the types of specific problems commonly found in other departments

The emphasis throughout the program should be on creative thinking and on the exercise of intelligent judgment in such matters as selecting and weighing administrative factors in given situations; interpreting qualitative and quantitative data and determining their applicability; evaluating the tangible and intangible variables that need to be taken into consideration in making administrative decisions; and developing sound and realistic standards of performance, delegation, communication, supervision, and evaluation as means of implementing administrative decisions.

Learning experiences. The type of learning experiences offered to students to achieve the preceding educational objectives varies from course to course, from one objective to the next, from one institution to another, and from teacher to teacher. The majority of objectives may be achieved, however, by supplying the following types of learning experiences, either separately or in combination:

1. Teach courses in small seminar groups (10 to 15 students) to permit frequent and thorough presentations, discussions, and analysis by each student of a large number of problems and situations involving the experience of many organizations and institutions, with special emphasis on health care institutions, such as hospitals, clinics, and nursing departments in each institution
2. Lectures

3. Case studies
4. Independent studies
5. Clinical observations
6. Simulated clinical experiences and computer assisted instruction
7. Field trips

Courses

Introduction to principles of administration

This course offers a study of the basic principles underlying the administrative process as it functions in various forms of organized society. It focuses on organization, structure, delegation of authority, decision making, rewards and sanctions, discipline, coordination, authority, and other characteristics of administration procedure. It also deals with the basic principles of administrative planning, organization, direction, and control and with application of these principles in various types of activities.

(Course can be offered in another department such as business administration or hospital administration and is required for master's and doctoral students.)

Nursing administration

Nursing administration is a study of the administrative composite processes in nursing and the critical examination of the theory and practice of administration processes and techniques. Subjects covered are organization as an open sociotechnical system and the nursing department a subsystem within it; explanation of the administrative composite processes in nursing and principles of policy formulation for the organization and its nursing department; organizational procedures; implementation of planned changes; and critical appraisal of the role, duties and responsibilities of trustees, administrators, and nurse administrators.

(Course is offered in department of nursing and is required for master's degree and doctoral students.)

Problems in administration of nursing services

This course offers the identification, interpretation, and critical analysis of problems faced by the nurse administrator and the development of skills in effective resolution of these problems. Subjects covered are analysis of problems that exist at the group-to-group, individual-to-group, and individual-to-individual interface levels. The specific problems to be examined are the problems of adaptation, maintenance, output, allocation, integration, coordination, and strain (role conflict).

(Course is offered by the department of nursing and is required for doctoral students and elective for master's degree students.)

Social and economic aspects of delivery of health care

This course is a survey of the social and economic forces and constraints affecting administration and financing of delivery of health care and their effect on provision of nursing care. The need for health care insurance, group hospitalization, socialized medicine, and the role of government in the provision of prepaid medical care are discussed, and the relevant issues are critically analyzed.

(Course is offered by the department of nursing and is required for doctoral students and elective for master's degree students.)

Managerial accounting

The functions of accounting with reference to administration of health care organizations are offered is this course. Emphasis is placed on the relation of accounting to budgetary control, internal check, and analysis of revenue and cost in terms of departmental units.

(Course can be taken in department of business administration or hospital administration and is elective for doctoral students.)

Quantitative controls in administration

This course is aimed at developing ability and skill in using the basic quantitative techniques (accounting, statistics, and budgeting). Emphasis is placed on planning a budget for an organization or a departmental unit and determining the role of quantitative data and techniques in administrative planning and production and financial or cost control.

(Course can be taken in department of business or hospital administration and is required for master's degree and doctoral students.)

Executive direction and control

Basic principles of leadership, authority, delegation of authority, responsibility, accountability, legal implications, and the role of executive control in each of these areas is offered in this course. The principles that underlie operating controls and the various control practices are covered.

(Course is offered in department of nursing and is required for master's and doctoral students.)

Business law

This course covers the nature and social functions of law, social control through law, and the law of business and health care organizations. The basic principles of the law of contracts and agency and negotiable instruments are discussed.

(Course is offered by department of business or hospital administration and is an elective course for master's degree and doctoral students.)

Conceptual environment. The second area of concentration deals with the principles of human relations skills within the health care organization and between the organization and the community.

Educational objectives. The educational objectives to be achieved by the student in the area of conceptual environment are based on the student's ability to do the following:

1. Demonstrate understanding of the theories and principles of human relations in administration and apply these principles by utilizing proper methods and techniques for achieving them

2. Demonstrate understanding and awareness of the importance of sound relations between the nursing department and its various communities (local, regional, and national) and demonstrate skill in bringing about a cooperative relationship by interpreting the goals of the health care institution and its nursing department to these communities and the needs and requests of these communities to the organization and its nursing department

3. Apply the theories and principles of group dynamics in group meetings and in group counseling situations

4. Demonstrate understanding of human behavior under normal situations and when individuals are in conflict

5. Clearly communicate the goals and objectives of the health care organization and its nursing department to the nursing staff

6. Demonstrate sensitivity in early detection and diagnosis of problems such as poor employee morale and employee discontent with work conditions

7. Demonstrate knowledge and awareness of the role of the informal organization within the formal organization and skill in utilizing the potential power of the informal organization to achieve the goals and objectives of the organization and its nursing department

8. Demonstrate skill in teaching strategies and apply the basic principles of

learning and instruction in actual staff teaching situations

9. Identify problems in any aspect of human relations and conduct a scientific investigation that leads to clarification and eventual resolution of the problem

Courses

Human relations in administration

This course offers a systematic study of the principles of human relations in administration, with emphasis on their application to the field of nursing. Special topics discussed and examined are formal and informal organizations, communication, participation, introduction of change, use of control systems, and development of understanding and cooperation.

(Course is offered by the department of nursing and is required for master's degree and doctoral students.)

Personnel administration

This course offers a systematic study of principles, methods, and techniques used in administering a sound personnel program—personnel practices and policies. Subjects studied are methods of development of optimum human relationships within the organization, recruiting and selecting the nursing work force, job analysis, job evaluation, management and supervisory training, training of nursing staff and technical employees, communication, transfer and promotion of employees, wage and salary administration, employer turnover and employee morals, and evaluating personnel work and personnel budgets.

(Course can be offered either by the nursing department or by business or hospital administration and is required for doctoral students and elective for master's students.)

Health care organization and the community

This course is a systematic study of the role of the health care organization and its nursing department in meeting the health needs of the community and their relationship with other agencies, such as medical, nursing, allied professions and their organizations at the local state and national level, insurance companies, unions, and other community organizations. Discussion of health care organization and its nursing department as an educational institution for the physician, nurse, and others is also included.

(Course is offered by the department of nursing and is elective for master's and doctoral students.)

Group behavior in health care institutions

The course focuses on the problems of social control, legitimization of authority, and processes of decision making in relation to organized social life in the complex settings in which nursing is practiced.

(Course is offered by nursing department and is elective for master's degree and doctoral students.)

Teaching strategies in nursing

The focus of this course is on the application of theories of learning and instruction to actual teaching situations (patients, students, or staff). Subjects covered are conditions of learning, models of instruction, variables influencing learning and instruction, and essential teaching strategies.

(Course is offered by the department of nursing and is required for doctoral students and elective for master's students.)

Physical environment. The third area of concentration is concerned with the different patterns and structures of health care organization. It specifically deals with people structure and physical structure of the organization. *People structure* refers to characteristics of the organizational chart, for example, tall versus short and line versus staff positions. Physical structure refers to the architectural design of the institution and the heating, lighting, and ventilation systems, which influence working conditions and delivery of patient care. In addition are discussed the purposes, functions, financing, and methods of operation of the major health care organizations, voluntary and public, that provide diagnostic, therapeutic, and preventive health services or engage in health education and research at the international, national, state, or local levels.

Educational objectives. The educational objectives to be achieved in the area of physical environment consists of the student's ability to do the following:

1. Demonstrate understanding of the basic principles underlying the necessity for different types of health care organizations (for example, consumer-sponsored, profit or nonprofit, and private or tax-supported) and their effect on the nursing department and the delivery of health care

2. Show evidence of understanding the basic principles and characteristics of dif-

ferent types of people structure, for example, organizational charts that are tall versus short and line versus staff, channels of authority, and communication

3. Identify problems of people structure inherent in each area that influences delivery of health care to patients and conduct a scientific investigation that leads to clarification of the problem and eventually to its resolution

4. Demonstrate understanding of the physical structure of the health care organization and its effect on working conditions, work efficiency, and safety factors

5. Participate in planning and improving the physical environment of the health care organization

6. Identify variables that affect the physical structure and the people structure of the organization, encouraging those that facilitate the operation of the system and inhibiting those that hinder its efficiency

Courses

Social structure of organization

This course covers the general principles underlying the development of the administrative organization of the whole institution and its nursing department. Specific subjects covered are type of ownership, purposes, characteristics, financing methods, and people structure, that is, organizational chart, line and staff positions, authority systems, and channels of communication. Presentation of case material that deals with relationships between staff nurse and staff nurse, staff and supervisor, supervisor and supervisor, and top and middle management is included in this course.

(Course is offered by the department of nursing and is required for master's degree and doctoral students.)

Physical structure of organization

This course deals with the general principles underlying the physical development of the organization and its nursing department. Specific topics covered are principles underlying the architectural design of the institution; physical factors affecting delivery of health care; and characteristics of each department that affect the physical structure of the institution, administration of the physical plant, maintenance, heat, light, power, ventilation, utilities, and procurement and storing of supplies.

(Course is offered either by the department of nursing or hospital administration and is required for doctoral students and elective for master's students.)

Research. The fourth area of concentration deals with the development of cognitive skills in the utilization and actual performance of scientific investigation. Research is threaded through the entire curriculum in all areas of studies.

Educational objectives. The educational objectives to be achieved in the area of research consist of the student's ability to do the following:

1. Demonstrate understanding of basic principles of research and of the problem-solving process

2. Demonstrate understanding of basic principles of statistics and demonstrate competence in handling data and in presenting results of analysis

3. Demonstrate competence in utilization of research findings

4. Demonstrate competence in identification of specific problems encountered in administration of nursing services

5. Test hypotheses and theories of administration for nursing services

6. Use statistical findings as evaluative tools

7. Conduct a scientific study leading to a master's thesis and a doctoral dissertation that fulfills the requirements of a scientific research

Courses

Introductory statistics

This course deals with fundamentals of research, language of research, statistical concepts, planning of research, interpretation of research outcomes. It includes an introduction to descriptive statistics, mean, median, mode, and variance; normal curve tests; and discussion of the concepts of validity and reliability.

(Course can be offered by another department and is required for master's degree and doctoral students.)

Experimental design: intermediate statistics

Covered in this course are *t* test correlation, regression analysis, analysis of variance, and randomized block and factorial designs. Internal and external threats to the validity of research conclusions are also discussed.

(Course can be offered by another department and is required for master's degree and doctoral students.)

Experimental design: advanced topics

This course deals with introduction to Latin square and fractional factorial design, analysis of variance and covariance, and multivariate analysis of variance.

(Course can be offered by another department and is required for doctoral students only.)

Research in nursing

This course deals with the examination of processes for exploration, experimentation, and validation of knowledge in nursing. Specific emphasis is given to the treatment of problems of inquiry in a clinical setting. This course may be taken in conjunction with writing a thesis.

(Course is offered by nursing department and is required for master's degree and doctoral students.)

Research on thesis

This course entails conducting a scientific study on a nursing problem; thesis is required.

Research on dissertation

This course entails conducting an extensive scientific study. Oral defense of the proposal, dissertation, and final defense of the dissertation are required for doctoral students.

Nursing specialization: clinical and administrative. The fifth area of concentration deals with the development of clinical nurse specialists and beginning specialists in administration of nursing services. It is essentially the aim of the master's degree program. At the doctoral level, concentration is directed toward the development of advanced knowledge and skill in administration of nursing services and competence in utilization and performance of scientific administrative research. This program of study is planned and conducted jointly by the university (through the program director and other faculty members) and the health care organization (through the nursing administrator and her staff). The period of internship or clinical experience in nursing service administration forges a link between formal education and learn-

ing on the job. It is a carefully planned and executed transition period, intended to help the student implement formal education by observing procedures and personally performing them in actual or simulated situations or both. The experience enables the student to acquire understanding, perspective, and confidence.

Educational objectives. The educational objectives and courses in the area of clinical specialization in medical, surgical, developmental, maternal-child health, and psychiatric nursing are set up by the program chairman of the specific subject. The objectives in the administrative aspect of nursing specialization consist of the student's ability to do the following:

1. Observe the application of theories and principles of administration in actual administration of nursing services

2. Observe the nurse administrator (preceptor) as she relates, communicates, and works with the governing board of the organization, the administrator, medical staff, various departments, nursing staff, unions, and community

3. Participate in making administrative decisions under the intimate guidance and coaching of a carefully selected nurse administrator as the preceptor

4. Work with other nursing staff in middle management and with other professionals in performing various duties

5. Perceive and understand the philosophy of the leaders in the field and also the preceptor's philosophy, motivations, ethics, and methods of dealing with people and with problems in the complex world of the health care organization, nursing department, and community by working closely with the preceptor

6. Demonstrate competence, precision, thoroughness, and skill in putting administrative decisions, policy changes, or new procedures into operation when given responsibility for these functions

7. Demonstrate willingness and skill in serving as liaison person between the health care organization and one or more

other agencies when asked or allowed to perform such duties

8. Demonstrate evidence of learning from experience and show improvement in skill and understanding of principles of administration

9. Identify administrative problems in clinical situations and conduct a scientific study that leads to the clarification of the problem and eventually to its resolution

10. Analyze critically problems and issues occurring in administration of nursing services

11. Educate and inform the preceptor *indirectly* on the current advances in knowledge and research findings in nursing service administration

Courses

Clinical specialization in nursing

The focus of this course is on the application, refinement, and extension of professional knowledge and skills in a clinical field of the student's choice. The course includes supervised practice in the clinical area of the student's choice.

(Course is offered by the department of nursing and is required for master's degree and doctoral students.)

Internship in nursing service administration

This course deals with directed learning in nursing service organizations and with critical appraisal of the issues and problems occurring in the field of administration of nursing services and appraisal of applicability of concepts of administrative theory.

(Course is offered by the department of nursing and is required for master's degree and doctoral students.)

SPECIFIC LEARNING EXPERIENCES FOR INTERNSHIP PROGRAM

The internship program consists of clinical experience for the student nurse administrator; it ranges on a continuum from observation and operational work experience to significant projects whose implementation or solution is primarily the responsibility of the student intern.

The internship period is designed for and tailored to the individual student, depending on needs but within an agreed framework of training. The chairman of the university program is expected to inform the preceptor about the student's educational background and experience and about the student's strengths and weak-

nesses so that the internship period supplements, challenges, and strengthens the previous experience of the student and does not merely utilize skills already developed.

The student nurse administrator is given responsibility for putting administrative decisions, policy changes, or new procedures into operation. The student should be given experience in administrative problems and problem solving in as many areas as possible.

The student intern is given the opportunity to attend as many meetings of working committees as possible in the hospital or in agencies with which the institution participates.

CONDITIONS FOR PRECEPTORSHIP

The conditions for preceptorship are similar to the education and training of hospital administrators proposed by the Commission on University Education in Hospital Administration (American Council on Education 1954).

The conditions essential for preceptorship for the education and training of nurse administrators are as follows:

1. The preceptor should be well qualified to discharge duties to the university and should be knowledgeable about the objectives of the entire program of study.

2. The internship program should be worked out in detail by the preceptor with the aid and approval of the chairperson of the program in the university so that the program can be coordinated with the work of the academic year and used as a basis for evaluation.

3. Adequate channels of communication should be established to ensure that the performance of the preceptor and of the student during the period of internship is equal to that of the academic period. A close relationship and a reporting system should be established between the preceptor and the university faculty. Each should visit the other's institution and hold conferences and attend combined faculty meetings.

4. Continuous evaluation of the preceptor and the student is necessary if they are to improve in their performance.

5. There should be a constant group of competent nurse administrators from which the university can draw its staff of preceptors. Preceptors who are familiar with the objectives, plans, and problems of the program make superior instructors, an essential element in making the internship period an integral part of the university program.

Throughout the program of study and internship, the university must have complete authority in establishing and maintaining standards of admission, instruction, internship training, and qualifications for degree.

SUMMARY

We are of the opinion that for a nurse administrator to effectively and optimally assume the role of a leader, conceptualizer, thinker, composite process specialist, problem solver, coordinator, integrator, a change agent, and many other roles, she has to be well prepared academically and experientially. The curriculum presented in this chapter is an attempt to prepare such a nurse administrator.

REFERENCES

American Council on Education: University education for administration in hospitals, a report of the commission on university education in hospital administration, Washington, D. C., 1954, The Council.

Arndt, C.: Some views on: teaching and research in nursing service administration, J. Nurs. Educ. 4(1):9-13, 1965.

Bennis, W. G.: Problem-oriented administration, Hosp. Admin. 5(1):49-70, 1960.

Duce, L. A.: Graduate education in administration—some recent developments, Hosp. Admin. 11(1):28-41, 1966.

Finer, H.: Administration and the nursing services, New York, 1964, Macmillan Pub. Co. Inc.

McNerney, W. J.: Formal education beyond the master's degree, Hosp. Admin. 5(1):71-88, 1960.

Miller, D. I.: Issues in graduate education: education of nurse administrators for complex settings, J. Nurs. Educ. 10(2):37-44, 1971.

Mullane, M. K.: Education for nursing service administration, Battle Creek, Mich., 1959, W. K. Kellogg Foundation.

Shaffer, R. O.: A measuring stick for the administrator, Hosp. Admin. 9(2):28-45, 1964.

Thorndike, E. L.: Animal intelligence, New York, 1911, Macmillan Pub. Co., Inc.

Young, L. S.: The modern nurse administrator, J. Nurs. Educ. 8(3):13-14, 1969.

ADDITIONAL READINGS

Gallagher, A. H.: Educational administration in nursing, New York, 1965, Macmillan Pub. Co., Inc.

King, I. M.: Toward a theory for nursing, New York, 1971, John Wiley & Sons, Inc.

Mercadante, L.: Education for service—the challenge, Nurs. Forum 8(2):151-159, 1969.

Ramey, I. G.: Meeting today's challenges to nursing service and education, Nurs. Forum 8(2):160-175, 1969.

Chapter 12

LEADERSHIP

Probably as much has been written about leadership as has been written about any other area of organizational behavior. Leadership is present in any group, almost by definition, whether it be composed of children, adults, or baboons. Our concern is with adults. We differentiate leadership from supervision. Supervision is concerned with acts issued from a formal or appointed position in the organization by someone with authority, the *legal* right to act. Legal, here, means issued officially by the organization. Leadership concerns acts issued from a formal or informal position in the organization by someone with power, the ability to act, which implies nothing about the legal right. What is leadership? Some behavioral theories and research findings have projected the impression that leadership is a synonym for managership. The realities of formal and informal organizational life indicate that this assumption is not correct. Leaders are found not only in the administrative hierarchy but also in informal work groups. We are concerned with the exercise of leadership by individuals in the formal administrative hierarchy. Applewhite, in *Organizational Behavior* (1965), listed many definitions of leadership, for example, (1) "the process by which an agent induces a subordinate to behave in a desired manner" (Bennis 1959:295), (2) "the process (act) of influencing the activities of an organized group in its efforts toward goal setting and goal achievement" (Stogdill 1950:4), (3) "(a) helping the group to find the machinery or means to a goal (syntality) already agreed upon and (b) helping the group to decide upon a goal (synergy) that is satisfactory in the sense that the group can stably pursue it" (Cattell 1951:176), (4) "leadership is an influence process the dynamics of which are a function of the personal characteristics of the leader and his followers and of the nature of the specific situations" (Richards 1966), and (5) "interpersonal influence, exercised in situation and directed, through the communication process, toward the attainment of a specified goal or goals" (Tannenbaum and Massarik 1957).

A review of the leadership definitions indicates that they are very similar. The common core running through these five definitions is that leadership is a process whereby one individual exerts influence over others in the group. The important implication of the influence-interaction feature is that leadership occurs only when there is interaction between individuals.

Concept of power: an influential theory

Attempts have been made to depict the basis on which an administrator may influence a person or a group of persons. One of the most concise but insightful approaches is offered by French and Raven (1960). These two researchers defined five bases of power as follows:

1. Coercive power. This power is based on fear. A person perceives that failure to comply with the wishes of the superior will lead to punishment.
2. Reward power. This is the opposite of coercive power. A person perceives that com-

pliance with the wishes of the superior will lead to positive rewards.

3. Legitimate power. This type of power is derived from the position of a manager in the organizational hierarchy. For example, the hospital administrator possesses more legitimate power than the assistant administrator, and the director of nursing service possesses more legitimate power than the supervisor.

4. Expert power. An individual with this type of power is one with some expertise or special skill or knowledge. The possession of one or more of these variables gains for the possessor the respect and compliance of peers and personnel.

5. Referent power. This power is based on a follower's identification with a leader. The leader is admired because of one or more personal traits, and the follower can be influenced because of this admiration.

These five bases offer a distinction between the power bases. These can be reclassified into two major categories: (1) power based primarily on organizational factors and (2) power based on individual factors.

Coercive, reward, and legitimate powers specified primarily by the individual's position in the organization. Supervisors in an organization are at a lower administrative level in the institution than nursing service administrators, and consequently their coercive, reward, and legitimate power bases are significantly less than those of nursing service administrators. Upper level administrators are allowed various institutional facilities and resources, whereas administrators at the lower levels cannot utilize them. Position also affects the use of power in regard to the discipline process. Supervisors can reprimand their personnel (coercive power), whereas nursing service administrators can reprimand supervisors.

The degree and scope of a nursing service administrator's referent and expert power bases are dictated primarily by individual characteristics. Some administrators possess specific qualities (for example, skills or attributes) that make them attractive to their personnel, although the administrators are working within an organizational system. Thus, the individual nursing service administrator controls the referent and expert power bases, and the organization controls the coercive, reward, and legitimate power bases.

Katz and Kahn (1966:302) added another concept to the fivefold power framework for studying leadership. They proposed an incremental influence category in the following manner: "we consider the essence of organizational leadership to be the influential increment over and above the mechanical compliance with routine directives of the organization."

The incremental influence factor could be described in the French and Raven approach as a combination of the referent and expert bases (Student 1968). The essence of the influence theory is that the organizational and individual characteristics of managers are related. Thus, the act of influencing or leading others depends on the organizational system itself and, among other things, on the perceptions that subordinates hold of their leaders.

The influence framework can be utilized to identify the functions that a leader is supposed to perform in an organization. Many distinct behavioral viewpoints of leadership functions are espoused by individuals studying leadership behavior. Three interpretations of what the leader should and must do in the organization have been classified as the psychological, sociological, and anthropological views.

Leadership job

The identification and clarification of the job that leaders are expected to perform in any organizational system is a controversial issue. It may be looked on from the standpoint of psychology, sociology and anthropology. The behavioral approach to leadership has not yet clearly explained the organizationally related functions of a leader.

From the psychological viewpoint the primary function of a leader is to develop effective motivation systems. The leader must be able to stimulate subordinates in such a manner that they contribute positively to organizational goals and are also able to satisfy various personal needs.

The Maslow need hierarchy (1965) could serve as a model for the leader in developing the most effective motivation system. The Maslow need hierarchy stressed two ideas: (1) only needs not yet satisfied can influence behavior, and (2) human needs are arranged in a hierarchy of importance. When one level has been satisfied, a higher level need emerges and demands satisfaction. The leader, by being familiar with the premise that "man does not live by bread alone" but is interested in psychological growth, can develop programs that achieve optimum contribution from his personnel. A program that focuses on the entire need spectrum—physiological, security, social, self-esteem, and self-actualization—is assumed to have a higher probability for motivating successfully than a partial program that focuses on some but not all needs.

In the psychological viewpoint, the French and Raven power theory is an integral part. To consider only organizationally controlled power sources, coercive, reward, and legitimate, leads to the development of incomplete and often misdirected motivational programs. The leader must also consider referent and expert power bases in developing motivation programs.

The sociological approach to leadership is seen as a facilitative activity. The leader is perceived as establishing goals and reconciling organizational conflict between followers and exerting influence by performing these activities. The establishment of goals provides the direction that followers often require. It guides followers to know what type of performance or attitude is expected of them. The goals also influence the interaction patterns that de-velop between followers. This leads to specific group characteristics, such as communication networks, cohesiveness, and status hierarchies. Conflict among followers can become so disruptive that nothing positive is contributed to the organization. When this occurs, a leader's influence must be exercised to minimize the disruptive conflict within or between groups.

The anthropological approach to leadership perceives the values and purposes of the people being led.

SELECTED LEADERSHIP THEORIES

Efforts by behavioralists, or behavior scientists, have indicated that there is interest among them to organize the numerous theories. Instead of creating more theories of leadership behavior, the focus is on systematically organizing and categorizing what is already available. There appear to be three broad leadership theory categories that have evolved from the recent stop-and-organize efforts. They are (1) the trait theories, (2) the personal-behavioral theories, and (3) the situational theories. Donnelly, Gibson, and Ivancevich (1972) illustrated that the trait and personal-behavioral approaches can be integrated to some degree to yield the situational approach. Some of the situational theories emerging have borrowed from the trait-theory approaches and from various personal-behavioral-theory approaches. Therefore, it is best to consider each of the approaches as having many similarities and some differences.

Trait theories

The focus on various personal traits of leaders as criteria describing or predicting success has been in effect for some time. Many personnel administrators engaged in recruitment and selection of managers believe that the trait approach has some validity. The traits usually considered are physical, personality, and intelligence, but comparing these traits in leaders has resulted in little agreement among researchers about which traits make the better leader. There are, of course, shortcomings in the methods of employing a trait approach, but if a man is confident, independent, and intelligent, he has a higher probability of succeeding.

First, the trait theory of leadership ignores the followers. The followers have a significant effect on the job accomplished by the leader. Second, trait theorists do not specify the relative importance of various traits. Should an organization attempt to find administrators who are confident or those who act independently? Third, the research evidence is inconsistent. Finally, the list of traits continues to grow. This cumbersome list leads to confusion and disputes and provides little insight into organizational leadership.

Personal-behavioral theories
LEADERSHIP CONTINUUM

The personal-behavioral approach to the examination of organizational leadership contends that leaders may best be classified by personal qualities or styles or by behavioral patterns. A number of individuals have presented theories of leadership that fit the personal-behavioral category. The personal-behavioral theories of leadership focus on an analysis of what the leader does in carrying out the administrative tasks. Tannenbaum and Schmidt (1958) postulated that the administrator in an organization often has difficulty in deciding what type of leadership action is most appropriate for handling a particular problem. The administrator may not be sure whether to make the decision personally or to delegate the decision-making authority to a colleague. To provide insight into the meaning of leadership behavior with regard to decision making, Tannenbaum and Schmidt suggested a continuum of leadership.

BENEVOLENT AUTOCRACY

McMurry (1958) felt that the cold realities of organizational life doomed what

is referred to as democratic leadership. The democratic and the autocratic leader must set objectives and guide personnel. Democratic leaders encourage two-way communication between themselves and members of their staffs. The benevolent autocrat is interpreted to be a powerful prestigious administrator who can be communicated with but who does not necessarily communicate with personnel. This type of administrator is perceived as being able to take prompt remedial action for activities within personal jurisdiction.

To support the benevolent autocrat theory, McMurry offered the following reasons for the demise of democratic leadership: (1) The climate within organizations is unfavorable. The "captains" of industry have worked hard to attain their positions in the administrative hierarchy. Thus, they are likely to be hard driving and would like to control the destiny of their organizations. These individuals are not likely to favor delegation of decision-making power. (2) Since most organizations must make rapid and difficult decisions, it is in their best interest to maintain the control of operations in a centralized group of managers. Thus, freedom of action is constrained by the need to make rapid decisions, and democratic leadership is not feasible because it encourages freedom of action. (3) Democratic leadership concepts are relatively new and unproven. The historical folklore of successful organizations (for example, profits) has followed traditional bureaucratic principles. These bureaucratic principles are generally compatible with autocratic and not with democratic leadership. Once an organization has begun to follow bureaucratic guidelines and develop autocratic leaders, these leaders begin to perpetuate themselves.

These three reasons, among others, are the evidence offered by McMurry to justify his claim that the benevolent autocrat is the most effective leader. This type of leader structures subordinates' work activities, makes the policy decisions affecting them, and enforces discipline. The benevolent autocrat may encourage participation in the planning of a course of action but is the "chief" in executing a decision. Briefly, the benevolent autocrat is concerned about subordinates' feelings, attitudes, and productivity; but despite these humanistic feelings, this individual runs the operation by using rules, regulations, and specified policies.

More than a decade has passed since McMurry first stated his leadership approach. What has occurred recently in society seems to indicate that the climate, centralization, and folklore arguments have weakened the number of organizations willing to attempt leadership approaches that are more humanistic and less benevolently autocratic and seems to be growing.

JOB-CENTERED AND EMPLOYEE-CENTERED LEADERS

Since 1947, Likert and his associates have studied leaders in industry, hospitals, and government, obtaining data from thousands of employees.

After extensive analysis of the studies, the leaders were classified as job-centered or employee-centered leaders. The job-centered administrator structures the jobs of personnel, supervises closely to see that designated tasks are performed, uses incentives to spur service, and determines satisfactory rates of production based on procedures such as time study.

The employee-centered manager focuses attention on the human aspects of personnel's problems and on building effective work groups with high performance goals. The employee-centered manager specifies objectives, communicates them to personnel, and gives personnel considerable freedom to accomplish their job tasks and goals.

Based on his extensive research, Likert (1967) suggested that data show that the type of leadership style used significantly influences various end result variables. Such variables as productivity, service, absenteeism, attitudes, turnover, and defective units were found to be more favorable from an organizational standpoint when employee-centered or general supervision was utilized. His recommendation was to develop employee-centered managers whenever possible.

TWO-DIMENSIONAL THEORY

A much publicized Ohio State University leadership study isolated two dimensions of leadership behavior identified through statistical analysis as *consideration* and *initiating structure* (Fleishman, Harris, and Burt 1955).

These two dimensions were used to describe leadership behavior characteristics in organizational settings. They assessed how supervisors think they should behave in their leadership role. A second questionnaire attempted to ascertain subordinate perceptions of supervisory behavior. Analysis of responses to these questionnaires allowed the Ohio State researchers to score a leader on consideration and initiating structure.

A leader who scored high on the consideration dimension reflected that he had developed a work atmosphere of mutual trust, respect for subordinates' ideas, and consideration of subordinates' feelings. Such a leader encourages good superior-subordinate rapport and two-way communication. A low consideration score indicates that the leader is more impersonal in dealings with subordinates.

A high initiating structure score indicates that personal roles and those of subordinates are structured toward the attainment of goals by the leader. This leader is actively involved in planning work activities, communicating pertinent information, and scheduling work.

MANAGERIAL GRID THEORY

Blake and Monton (1964) proposed that leadership styles can be plotted on a two-

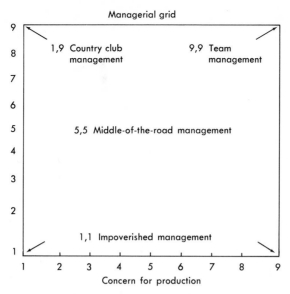

Fig. 12-1. Managerial grid theory.

dimensional grid. Five specific leadership styles are indicated in Fig. 12-1. These five leadership styles are only a few of the many that can be and are utilized.

Coordinates	Leadership style
1, 1	impoverished: a minimum effort to accomplish the work is exerted.
9, 1	task: the leader concentrates on task efficiency but shows little regard for human resources.
1, 9	country club: the leader focuses on being supportive and considerate of employees, but task efficiency is not a primary concern in this easygoing atmosphere.
5, 5	middle-of-the-road: adequate task efficiency and satisfactory morale are the goals of this style.
9, 9	team: the leader facilitates production and morale by coordinating and integrating work-related activities.

Ideally, the leader who is a 9, 9 individual would be the most efficient in an organization. Defining a 9, 9 leader for every type of job is an impossibility, but Blake and Monton implied that a managerial development program can move leaders toward a 9, 9 classification. They recommended the following management development phases:

Phase 1: laboratory seminar groups. Conferences are used to introduce the leaders to the grid approach and philosophy. A key part of the phase is to analyze and assess one's own leadership style.

Phase 2: teamwork. Each department works out and specifies its own 9, 9 description. This phase is an extension of phase 1, which included leaders from different departments in the conference groups. Thus, in the second phase, managers from the same department are brought together.

Phase 3: intergroup interaction. This phase involves intergroup discussion and analysis of 9, 9 specifications. Situations are created whereby tensions and conflicts that exist between groups are analyzed by group members.

Phase 4: goal setting. The leaders in the program discuss and analyze setting of goals.

The managerial grid approach relates task effectiveness and human satisfaction to a formal managerial development program. This program is unique in that (1) line managers, not academicians or consultants, run the program; (2) a conceptual framework of management, the grid, is utilized; and (3) the entire managerial hierarchy of the firm undergoes development, not just on a group level (for example, supervisors).

It is assumed that the development experience aids the manager in acquiring a more thorough concern for fellow employees and equips the manager with more expertise to accomplish task objectives, such as service and quality.

An examination of the various personal-behavioral theories indicates that similar concepts are discussed, but different labels are utilized. For example, the continuum, the benevolent-autocrat proposition, Likert, the Ohio State researchers, and the managerial grid approach all utilize two broadly defined concepts summarized in Table 8.

Each of the five approaches focuses on two concepts; however, some differences should be emphasized. First, the leadership continuum is based primarily on personal opinions. Although the opinions of the originators are respected, they must be supported with research evidence before more faith can be placed in each particular theory. Second, Likert implied that the most successful leadership style is employee-centeredness. He suggested that there is no need to look further to find the best leadership style. The critical question concerns whether the employee-centered style works in all situations.

Table 8. Personal-behavioral approach

Original source	Two concepts and derivation
Leadership continuum	Boss-centered and subordinate-centered; opinions of Tannenbaum and Schmidt (1958)
Benevolent autocrat	Benevolent autocrat and democrat; opinion of McMurry (1958)
Supportive	Job-centered and employee-centered; research at University of Michigan (Likert 1967)
Two-dimensional	Consideration and initiating structure; research at Ohio State University (Fleishman, Harris, and Burt 1955)
Managerial grid	Concern for people and concern for production; research of Blake and Monton (1971)

Instead of reporting studies and opinions that dispute Likert's claim, the Ohio State researchers found that from a production viewpoint the leader with a high initiation structure score was preferred by company executives. Thus, Likert's claim, or any other claim, that one best leadership approach has been discovered, is subject to debate.

The Ohio State theory and the managerial grid approach can be integrated into an *overlay theory* of leadership with overlay meaning that they are merged into one (Hensey and Blanchard 1969). Perhaps more integrated work along the lines of overlay would provide a better understanding of the personal-behavioral theories of leadership. An ultimate theory of leadership has not been discovered, but the endless list of styles causes semantic difficulties by referring to the same basic leadership behavior with different terminology.

Donnelly, Gibson, and Ivancevich (1971) summarized the five approaches discussed previously, as shown in Table 8.

Situational theory: leadership factors

An increasing number of behavior scientists have begun to focus their attention on an adaptive theory of leadership, that is, a leadership approach flexible enough to adapt to different situations. Included in this effort is a belief that the best leader is one who is able to adjust individual style to a particular group at a specific point in time to handle a given situation. The primary ingredients of a situational theory are the leader, the group, and the situation. The situation variable is of major importance since it affects what a leader can accomplish.

The situational theory advocates propose that the ideal leader is a person who is able to adapt personal style to cope with the situation at hand and with the personality of personnel. The work of Fiedler (1967) focused on adaptive leadership dimensions and assumed them to be situational factors that influence the leader's effectiveness. The dimensions identified are (1) leader-member relations: the degree of confidence the personnel have for the leader, the loyalty shown, and attractiveness of the leader, (2) task structure: the degree to which the followers' jobs are routine versus being ill-structured and undefined, and (3) position power: the power inherent in the leadership position. It includes the rewards and punishments that are typically associated with the position, the leader's official authority, based on ranking in managerial hierarchy, and the support that the leader receives from superiors and the overall organization.

By utilizing the three-dimensional model and empirical findings, Fiedler specified the type of leadership style that is most appropriate in different situations. He assembled data that relates leadership style to the three-dimensional measures of conditions favorable or unfavorable to the leader. The measure of leadership style adopted is one that distinguishes between leaders who tend to be permissive, considerate, and foster good interpersonal relations among group members (permissive) and leaders who tend to be directive, controlling, and more oriented toward task than toward people (directive). For example, considerate and permissive leaders obtain optimal group performance in situations in which the task is structured, but the leader is disliked and must be diplomatic. This type of leadership style is also effective in situations in which the leader is liked, but the group is faced with an ambiguous and unstructured task. When the situation is ambiguous and the task is structured, directive leadership is more effective.

The Fiedler model suggested that leaders who are directive can function best in certain types of situations, whereas leaders who are permissive function best in other types of situations. Instead of expecting a leader to adopt a set style, Fiedler identified the type of leader that functions best in the situation at issue. If a leader is to be effective in most situations, Fiedler suggested that flexibility is appropriate. The leader must examine the situation and decide whether to provide structured or unstructured instructions concerning the problem or goal.

Fiedler has presented a theory of leadership that takes into account the leader's personality as well as such situational variables as the task to be completed and the behavioral characteristics of the group of employees that the leader must influence. It is apparent that more research is needed before the theory gains widespread acceptance or even partial agreement among those studying leadership, but Fiedler has provided an excellent starting point for thinking in the 1970s.

It is evident that the "one best way" of leadership is not only elusive but has led to confusion. There is no one best way to lead people. In practice, leaders are seldom totally autocratic or totally democratic. The matter of leadership style is a complicated web of factors. Such items as the past experience of the leader, the organizational climate, and the personality of the leader are often mentioned in management literature as being most important in influencing leadership behavior.

LEADERSHIP FACTORS FOR EFFECTIVE BEHAVIOR

We have isolated some relevant factors in the leader network. In the context of the leadership framework, the effective leader is an individual who influences followers in such a manner as to achieve high-quality service, high group morale, low absenteeism, low turnover, and the development of followers. Fig. 12-2 specifies only four personal qualities that contribute significantly to a leader's ability to influence others. This is not intended to be a complete list of relevant factors in the leadership network. The four qualities selected, however, are suited for most leadership styles and are especially compatible with the situational theory of lead-

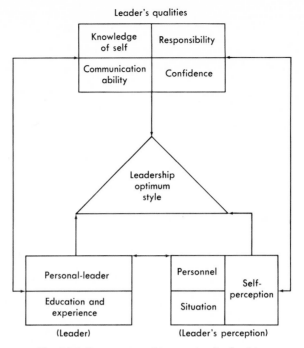

Fig. 12-2. Perspective of integrative leadership.

ership. They are also related, as shown by the solid line, to the perception factors identified.

Knowledge of self. One of the most important factors in the situation approach to leadership centers around leadership self-awareness. Leaders of people should be aware of their impact on those whom they lead. We are not assuming that they can predict accurately how their leadership style will affect followers in every situation. We are suggesting, however, that leaders should attempt to learn more about their influence on others.

Many of us maintain and develop inaccurate images of our personalities and interaction styles. For example, a leader may perceive herself as being a soft-spoken and easygoing individual, whereas her subordinates consider her a sharp-tongued and ill-tempered person. This type of counter evaluation or perception of the leader often reduces a group's effectiveness. It causes ineffectiveness because the leader continues to assume that she is one person and the group views her as the complete opposite. The result is often conflict, misunderstanding, and low morale.

Confidence. Leaders differ significantly in the personal confidence they have in their ability to lead others. The leader that lacks confidence would have difficulty in diagnosing different situations and adapting personal style to cope adequately with the situation. These difficulties result in the leader failing to perform certain functions that could lead to desirable results. For example, a leader with little confidence in herself will often assume that followers cannot adequately perform their job tasks. This may lead to the leader exercising close supervision over her subordinates. The closeness of supervision may prove disruptive because of the type of job being completed, the personality and type of personnel in the work group, and the large size of the work group.

A lack of confidence could also result in the leader making decisions that are not adequate or are viewed as being harmful by the group members. In effect, the confidence of a leader is related to some extent to the risk-taking aversions of the leader. The leader that lacks confidence makes decisions in many instances that compromise her follower's morale, rewards, and status in other groups.

Ability to communicate. Every leader in an organizational setting must be able to communicate her objectives to followers. The autocratic, service-oriented, people-oriented, and every other leader type must communicate expectations to followers. The leader who fails to communicate with followers may become incommunicative as an influence to others. This results because failing to communicate leads to chaos in general and to an inability to coordinate necessary follower activities in particular.

Responsibility. Leaders differ from other people in their willingness to assume responsibility, to take the initiative, to plan and carry through the tasks that are needed, and to take the credit or the blame, whichever the case may be.

The willingness to accept responsibility is a key attribute in effective leadership. The world is full of people who are afraid of responsibility and who are made anxious by the merest possibility that responsibility may be theirs. The acceptance of responsibility means acceptance of the possibility of blame for failure. Merely to think of these things causes anxiety for most of us. The acceptance of responsibility also means changing oneself and one's life. Accepting responsibility means some loss of freedom, and it means that one can no longer do what one wants, because it is necessary to do what the job at hand demands.

Our emphasis is on the leader's ability to diagnose herself and her total leadership environment. Perhaps what we are suggesting is that leadership training programs should stress diagnostic and adaptability skill learning. It should not be concluded that administrators can be easily educated to accurately diagnose work situations and

to adopt the appropriate leadership style.

If leaders are to become diagnostically skilled and flexible to the degree of changing their leadership style, depending on the circumstances at hand, patience is essential. The organization must be willing to plan, develop, and fund development programs; this is a time-consuming task.

LEADERSHIP IN THE NURSING SERVICE ORGANIZATION

To be an effective leader, the nursing service administrator must be knowledgeable of the range of leadership behavior available, the priority responsibilities of her role, and the nature of the forces influencing her actions. The responsibility of the leader is not primarily to provide directives but to maintain the evocative situation. Though she may be relatively inconspicuous, her role is crucial in keeping the goal in sight, creating a warm and permissive atmosphere for participation, recognizing consensus, and helping persons find their parts in cooperative effort.

Nursing service administrators attempting to introduce their patient care programs into health care systems are likely to find the following statements familiar:

1. My biggest adjustment has been to adapt myself to be a less authoritarian administrator, to get nurses to answer their own questions, and to let them make the decisions.
2. I thought we had free discussion in our nursing service, but we don't if nurses are still doing what they think I want them to do.
3. I'm secure in the decisions I'm making; I don't want to involve my nurses.
4. There was a time when I would have taken personal offense at their comments. Now I take their suggestions without feeling personally hurt.
5. Letting nurses learn from their own mistakes has taken longer than I had hoped, but now I feel strongly that it has been worthwhile.
6. We have lots of dialogue all right, but sometimes I wonder if we're producing, if it's leading anywhere.

These statements represent personal disclosures of feelings and ideas about what happens to an administrator when she provides leadership for introducing her patient care program or wishes to make alterations. Some of the comments imply growth and improvement, whereas others suggest frustration and resistance. Yet one common theme of the testimony is the leadership behavior of the nursing service administrator as she relates to her staff of nurses. The modern nursing service administrator is concerned about her leadership behavior, and this concern generates many questions relevant to the dynamics of leadership.

What leadership behavior is appropriate: autocratic or democratic?

Today many nurses consider the nursing service administrator to be in a salient leadership position for influencing the adoption of innovations. The complex problem of how the leader can be effective in bringing about new delivery programs in health care is receiving increased attention by nursing and other scholars (Bennis, Benne, and Chin 1962). Strategies for fostering change now emphasize the importance of personnel involvement in decision making, and this theory challenges the rationality of highly directive leadership (McGregor 1960). The administrator

of nursing service who successfully fosters innovations in the nursing service is not a lone leader impressing her decisions on her staff, but rather she provides nurses with opportunities for leadership by involving them in the decision-making process of the health care system. The need for including the nursing staff in decision-making to promote patient care programs and change does not mean, however, that an administrator's behavior must always approach permissiveness. Before a nursing service administrator acts, she should consider the total range of leadership behavior available.

The continuum or range of possible leadership behavior is illustrated graphically by Tannenbaum and Schmidt (1958). Each type of behavior is related to the degree of authority used by the administrator and to the amount of freedom available to her nurses in making decisions. The behaviors shown on the extreme left of Fig. 12-3 characterize the administrator who maintains a high degree of control, whereas those on the extreme right characterize the administrator who provides freedom for the nursing staff.

The continuum describes a number of alternative ways in which a nursing service administrator can relate to the staff she is leading. At the extreme left, the ad-

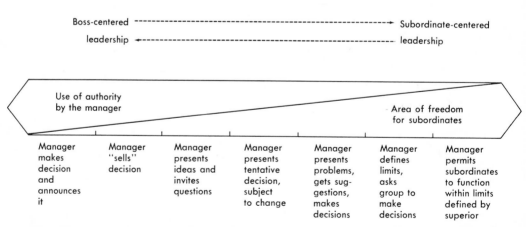

Fig. 12-3. Continuum of leadership behavior. (Adapted from Tannenbaum, R., and Schmidt, W.: Harvard Business Review 36:95-101, March-April 1958.)

ministrator's thoughts and perceptions determine decision making. Moving toward the right, one can see that decision making is increasingly determined by the nurse's thoughts and perceptions. Leadership should not be stereotyped as either forceful or permissive. Rather, leadership should be viewed as a process consisting of a range of possible alternative behaviors. The effective administrator chooses a behavioral alternative appropriate to the demands of each task she encounters.

It is difficult for a nursing service administrator to determine the degree to which leadership should be centered on herself or on her nurses. She may think that the nurses should help make decisions. At the same time, she may feel that she understands a problem better than do the nurses and that the decision should be her responsibility. Also, there are times when she may want to hear all points of view before making a decision, but she thinks it would be inefficient to spend all the time this would require. An administrator who finds herself in such a dilemma may be pushed in different directions of leadership without having sound reasons for her actions. She can, however, gain insight into her behavior choice by understanding the nature of the leadership responsibilities she has when guiding a group of nurses toward innovations in direct patient care and other nursing responsibilities.

What description of leadership is relevant for innovative behavior?

Leadership involves not only the immediate relationship of the administrator and her nurses, but also includes all aspects of group life and group management. One cannot talk about leadership without describing the group being led and the situation encountered.

Leadership for the forward-looking administrator is a process of stimulating and aiding groups of nurses to determine common objectives and to voluntarily design means for moving toward their achievement. The leader, in other words, provides facts and ideas and makes decisions that help the group to intelligently define and reach objectives. The various leadership acts involved in this process help nurses realize their innovative capacities and stimulate the productive use of their energies.

Although leadership behavior is in part dependent on the uniqueness of the group situation, there are fundamental aspects of leadership to which a nursing service administrator must be sensitive. The administrator needs to become familiar with the potentialities and characteristics of the individuals being led. She must perceive problems that face the nurses and determine whether a solution falls within group capabilities or outside its range. Group members look to the nursing service administrator for recognition and treatment according to their individual needs, and it is the nursing service administrator's responsibility to mold the group into a unit that can accomplish established ends and satisfy individual desires at the same time.

Nursing service administrators can simplify or complicate group operations. Sometimes they make group operations uncomfortable by their permissiveness, and at other times, they arouse animosity by their dictatorial nature. How the administrator is perceived by group members is very important. Often it is the individual nurse who, on the basis of personal perceptions, accepts or rejects leadership. The nursing service administrator is more likely to be effective if she is perceived as symbolizing the values and purposes of the nurses she leads. There must be a clear identity between group members and the nursing service administrator. If nurses perceive the nursing service administrator as being too different from themselves, they may think that they will not be represented properly or that communication with the leader will be threatening or difficult. This does not imply that a nursing service administrator and nurses must be identical in character and capabilities. It suggests, rather, that differences must be of a degree and kind that are acceptable to the group.

The future of the nursing group is a vital concern for the nursing service administrator. She must be sensitive to the long-range perspective of how the group will continue to meet the members' needs and how members will overcome future difficulties that might interfere with the group's purposes. In short, the nursing service administrator must anticipate problems and alternative solutions. She should be able to take steps to overcome forces that threaten the security or the success of the group or possibly even to use these forces to the advantage of the total group endeavor. Seeing a situation in broad perspective makes it possible for the nursing service administrator to initiate actions that encourage others and involve them more deeply in the group's work. The nursing service administrator should also realize that as nurses become more deeply involved in group activities, it is necessary to share her authority with them. She cannot permit her personal needs for control to block delegation of authority or relinquishment of decision-making power.

The nursing service administrator must consider numerous other aspects of leadership behavior. She must be willing to assume responsibility, take initiative, and plan and carry through tasks that need to be accomplished. This means that she has to accept the possibility of failure as well as success. She must be able to tolerate a high degree of tension. Organizational pressures often result in group frustration and hostility, and the nursing service administrator's degree of commitment and rationality may be severely tested. The same is true for her tolerance of isolation. As individual nurses step out to lead, they become distinct from the rest of the group, more vulnerable, and lonely.

Finally, communication skills are meshed with effective leadership. The objectives of the group must be stated so members will see in which direction the group must move. The means to achieve the goals must be spelled out so that unity of action can occur. This is the responsibility of the nursing service administrator.

This description of leadership behavior includes the major aspects of the role of the creative administrator. The nursing service administrator who is knowledgeable of her role gains insight into leadership dilemmas because she is better able to determine the degree to which she should control decisions. Determining appropriate leadership behavior is extremely complex, and it demands sensitivity to more than the leadership role. The nursing service administrator interested in maintaining appropriate behavior must also be aware of the forces that influence her actions. If she can understand what makes her prefer to act in a particular way, she may use this understanding to make herself a more effective leader.

What are some of the forces that affect leadership behavior?
HEALTH CARE ORGANIZATION

Among the more important forces contributing to behavior of the nursing service administrator are the health care organization scheme and the administrator's personality. Health care facilities, such as hospitals, public health agencies, and outpatient departments, have set patterns or norms that influence the behavior of the nursing service administrator. These norms exist because they contribute successfully to the organization's present operations. Particular types of behavior are accepted in the health care facility; if the nursing service administrator deviates from the norms, she usually meets with resistance. In some cases she is influenced by the expected behavior to such an extent that she loses her personal identity. The health care facility creates a network of determinants that causes the administrator's behavior to be inconsistent with her preferred personal strategy for action. There is often a marked discrepancy between what the nursing service administrator believes to be right and desirable and what is required by the institution.

The creative nursing service administrator in particular is often in a position in which institutional determinants and her own particular ideas or strategies for actions are conflicting. For example, will she subscribe to the institution's conventions on interdepartmental competition, efficiency, traditional procedures and tasks, and one-person decision making; or will she encourage cooperative involvement, airing of all points of view, and bring about participative decision making and shared responsibility? Stogdill (1956) suggested that when faced with conflicting pressures the leader may either conform to one or the other set of expectations and prepare to take the consequences or, as is more likely, take a compromise position and attempt to reconcile conflicts. Either alternative reduces the nursing service administrator's capacity to exercise a high degree of imagination, ingenuity, and creativity in leadership. Under such conditions, the potentialities of nursing service administrators are only partly utilized.

As the organizational complexity of health care facilities increases, the pressures generated become more restrictive. Even the strongest-willed nursing service administrator may find herself unable to exercise her unique nursing service abilities. Institutional pressures, Jennings (1960) explained, can force the leader to place a high priority on subtle and inoffensive social engineering. Human relations principles become a means by which the nursing service administrator seeks to meet the needs and expectations of the nursing staff and to cope with the determinants of the organization. As the nursing service administrator becomes politically skillful in gaining support, popularity, and rapport she moves away from substantive involvement and the initiation of new programs.

She becomes interested in her own survival completely separated from her leadership resources as a unique individual. Under the image of *human relations practitioner,* many nursing service administrators sacrifice their commitment to critical thought and independent behavior.

NURSING SERVICE ADMINISTRATOR'S PERSONALITY

Although an administrator of nursing service functions as a specialized part of the health care facility, she also has personal needs. While working with the human materials around her, she must work with the human materials in herself. Zalesnik (1963) and Porter (1973) suggested that the many dilemmas leaders face in choosing appropriate behavior are the result of their own inner conflicts. Competition and status are common types of internal personality conflicts.

The nursing service administrator operates in a competitive environment, and her behavior is often affected by inner conflicts resulting from competition. Zalesnik (1963:52-53) further suggested that if a leader does not resolve her concern with competing, she will develop a fear of failure. Setting unrealistic standards of performance or competing internally for unreachable goals can cause a nursing service administrator to feel that whatever she undertakes is destined to fail. Instead of risking failure, the nursing service administrator is likely to assume anonymity, a behavior that communicates resignation and noncommitment.

Competitive conflicts also are associated with success, and the result may be the same behavior that is associated with failure. The nursing service administrator's initial success in introducing a new program results in increased exposure. As she takes a position on controversial issues or supports a stand she becomes a target for criticism from nurses, patients, and fellow department heads. A nursing service administrator, foreseeing that her actions will result in criticism, may hesitate to make decisions that have far-reaching implications. To avoid criticism, the nursing service administrator may move from problem to problem without reaching solutions, again resulting in a behavior of noncommitment.

A nursing service administrator may also feel that her success is achieved through the displacement of someone else. The idea of success is associated with feelings of guilt and the urge to reverse the behavior that made it possible. When the nursing service administrator is about to reach a goal, she will deliberately prevent its fulfillment to avoid the success that may generate feelings of guilt.

Status conflict, which may also generate guilt, may arise when an administrator realizes that she is exercising power over nurses who are more capable than she is or when she realizes that differences in status make it impossible to treat her nurses as equals. Followers find it easier to take directions from a leader whom they consider superior. Yet, a nursing service administrator is forced to maintain a psychological distance that permits acceptance of leadership without resentment.

As soon as the nursing service administrator begins to achieve success and recognition, she is ripe for status conflict. She becomes torn between the responsibilities of acquired authority and the strong need to be liked. The nursing service administrators who formerly served as models now view her as a contender. At the same time, she no longer enjoys the open friendship of her previous peers or nurses. The following announcement from an individual rapidly becoming a recognized creative person serves as an example of status conflict.

The many activities we presently have under way seem to be more demanding than was anticipated. I am asking you to make an appointment with my secretary if you have to see me. Please do not construe this as the beginning of a closed-door policy. You must feel free to see me about anything when necessary. The appointment system is, I hope, an attempt to assure you that I will be able to spend some time with you without interruption.

How does status conflict affect leadership behavior? Sometimes nursing service administrators try to discard all symbols of status and authority, playing up their likeability. As they remove social distance in the interests of likeability they not only reduce work effectiveness, but also often lose the original intention of their behavior. Nurses, instead of meeting the nursing service administrator's need to be liked, gradually come to harbor feelings of resentment and anger toward her because the nursing service administrator's behavior inadvertently supplies a negative picture of what they perceive the leadership role should be.

Competition and status serve as examples to show that the nursing service administrator's inner force are determinants of leadership behavior. It is extremely difficult to separate inner forces from those residing in the realities of the institution. The creative nursing service administrator, however, must seek insight into herself and the values and traditions at work in the health care setting.

Nursing service administrators are concerned about leadership. They are sensitive to the complexity of the leadership behavior necessary for initiating innovative programs. To be an effective leader, the nursing service administrator must be knowledgeable of the range of leadership behavior available, the priority responsibilities of her role, and the nature of the forces influencing her actions. The better the nursing service administrator understands these factors, the more accurately she can determine appropriate leadership behavior that will enable her nurses to act more creatively and productively in the accomplishment of nursing service programs.

The effectiveness of the leader then is measured, not in terms of the leadership the nursing service administrator exercises, but in terms of the leadership she evokes; not in terms of her power over others, but in terms of the power she releases in others; not in terms of the goals she sets up and the directions she gives, but in terms of the goals and plans of action persons work out for themselves with her help; not in terms alone of service and projects completed, but in terms of growth in competence, sense of responsibility, and personal satisfactions among many participants.

Under this kind of leadership, it is not always clear at any given moment just who is leading, nor is this very important. What is important is that many may learn how to grasp a problem, to apply their minds to it, and to work together on it.

Leadership of this kind gets more done— more thinking, more action, more final products, and of even greater importance, more enhancement of human values.

REFERENCES

Applewhite, P. B.: Organizational behavior, Englewood Cliffs, N. J.: 1965, Prentice-Hall, Inc.

Bennis, W. G.: Leadership theory and administrative behavior, Admin. Science Q. **4**:259-301, 1959.

Bennis, W. G., Benne, K., and Chin, R.: The planning of change, New York, 1962, Holt, Rinehart & Winston, Inc.

Blake, R. R., and Monton, J. S.: The managerial grid, Houston, Tex., 1964, Gulf Publishing Co.

Cattell, R. B.: New concept for measuring leadership in terms of group syntality, Hum. Relations **4**:161-184, 1951.

Donnelly, J. H., Jr., Gibson, J. L., and Ivancevich, J. M.: Fundamentals of management, Dallas, Tex., 1971, Business Publications, Inc.

Fiedler, F. E.: A theory of leadership effectiveness, New York, 1967, McGraw-Hill Book Co.

Fleishman, E. A., Harris, E. F., and Burt, H. E.: Leadership and supervision in industry, Columbus, Ohio, 1955, Bureau of Educational Research, Ohio State University.

French, J. R. P., and Raven, B.: The basis of social power. In Cartwright, D., and Lander, A., editors: Group dynamics, Evanston, Ill., 1960, Row, Peterson & Co.

Hensey, P., and Blanchard, K. H.: Management of organizational behavior: utilizing human resources, New York, 1969, Prentice-Hall, Inc.

Jennings, E.: An anatomy of leadership: princess, heroes and superman, New York, 1960, Harper & Brothers, pp. 32-39.

Katz, D., and Kahn, R. L.: The social psychology of organizations, New York, 1966, John Wiley & Sons, Inc.

Likert, R.: The human organization, New York, 1967, McGraw-Hill Book Co.

Maslow, A. H.: Eupsychian management, Homewood, Ill., 1965, Richard D. Irwin, Inc. and The Dorsey Press.

McGregor, D.: The human side of enterprise, New York, 1960, McGraw-Hill Book Co.

McMurry, R. N.: The case for benevolent autocracy, Harvard Bus. Rev. **36**:82-90, Jan.-Feb. 1958.

Porter, E.: Strength-deployment-inventory, Pacific Palisades, Calif. 1973, Personal Strength Assessment Service.

Richards, M. D., and Greenlaw, P. S.: Management decision making, Homewood, Ill., 1966, Richard D. Irwin, Inc., p. 135.

Stogdill, R. M.: Leadership, membership and organization, Psychol. Bull. **47**:1-14, 1950.

Stogdill, R. M.: Patterns of administrative performance, Columbus, Ohio, 1956, Bureau of Business Research, Ohio State University Press.

Student, K. R.: Supervisory influence and work group performance, J. Applied Psychol. **52**:188-194, June 1968.

Tannenbaum, R., and Massarik, F.: Leadership: a frame of reference, Management Science **4**: 1-19, 1957.

Tannenbaum, R., and Schmidt, W. H.: How to choose a leadership pattern, Harvard Bus. Rev. **36**:95-101, March-April 1958.

Zalesnik, A.: The human dilemmas of leadership, Harvard Bus. Rev. **41**(4):50, 1963.

ADDITIONAL READINGS

American Management Association, Inc.: Efficient communication on the job: a guide for supervisors and executives, New York, 1963, The Association.

Likert, R.: New patterns of management, New York, 1961, McGraw-Hill Book Co.

Reddin, W. J.: Managerial effectiveness, New York, 1970, McGraw-Hill Book Co.

Chapter 13

A LOOK INTO THE FUTURE

It is relatively easy to look back; one can gather the facts and point out mistakes and show how a different action would have been better. Looking forward or forecasting with various degrees of uncertainty can be quite hazardous. Given such an obvious generalization, there are facts pointing to the occurrence of certain events in the next decade. Predictions have a purpose; ours is to collect some of the trends we have observed to be affecting organizational behavior.

In the past, external and internal environmental forces of great complexity rather than a planned program or master plan have shaped the development of nursing service administration to a high level of professional achievement. The pressures at work, requiring new responses in administrative functioning, have made the study and acquisition of knowledge in nursing service administration a requisite for effective performance.

A number of significant forces already operating are changing the nature of nursing practice and nursing service by requiring new leadership roles and subtly molding the character and style of tomorrow's nursing service administration. Intelligent action by the nursing profession will be needed to forecast changes occurring in the health field and affecting the future of nursing. Within this context we will enumerate broad changes bearing on nursing practice and nursing service and affecting medical and nursing staff relationships.

Health care as a basic human right and a national goal is now well established

(Stull 1969). It rests on the principle of equal access of health services for all people, regardless of their ability to pay and, to some degree, of their place of residence. In fact, this philosophy needs no longer be debated; it is a question of means, not ends. The acceptance of this principle establishes the motivation for the response of nursing service, namely, maximum service to meet people's expectations.

A goal set by the professional nursing organizations and the community (American Nurses' Association and National League for Nursing) in the 1960s concerned the patient's right to expect quality of care, quality of personnel, and quality of nursing service. These expectations will move closer to reality when nursing service accepts more comprehensive planning, feedback control from the environment, and accountability, promoting quality through evaluating the process of patient care. These pressures and expectations for quality have been rising much faster, especially of late, than the organizational capabilities and effectiveness level of the system in its present condition.

A force often discussed is the development of scientific knowledge and technology, with new horizons opening up constantly. This force has created, and will continue to create, great and new expectations from patients and the general public. These expectations must be understood and met by applying new knowledge to the solution of health problems in a manner that will benefit all people to a degree commensurate with costs. This must be accomplished in an environment that is not only constantly changing in its characteristics, but is also replete with conflicts concerning the purposes and values of health services, the differences of opinion about which services are most important, urgent, or most worthwhile, and the question of which services can be done most effectively and most economically. In the center of the turbulence is the nursing service administrator, her conceptual and physical acts are challenged to understand and cope with these divergent social, scientific, technological, and economic aspects of health care and their consequences.

Specialization, which accompanies scientific and technological advances, creates more complexity, interdependence, and the need for the development of a more formal system of integrative working arrangements (Arndt and Laeger 1970b). Therefore, the nursing service administrator faces an additional dilemma or challenge. Interdisciplinary coordination among high-level specialists requires that she cultivate much greater understanding and confidence and an awareness of the new thinking when she is planning, organizing, directing, and controlling her department and when she is applying the dynamic techniques of administration, that is, when changes are made in the structural, behavioral, or technological areas of the organization. In addition, interdisciplinary coordination requires the development of a sensitivity and tolerance for the various disciplines that comprise the total health care force; the separate contributions of these disciplines to overall successes is of considerable importance and necessitates skillful communication and reestablishment of a climate conducive to the conceptual acts of planning and organizing and the physical acts of directing and controlling.

The effective delivery of health care is evolving as a cooperative and coordinative system, one that combines a large number of subsystems, such as, medical and nursing programs, supportive service programs, management programs, and educational programs. This development has generated the need for an overall structure of administration, defined as a hierarchy of professional autonomies. Nursing service administration is one of the professional autonomies. This means that nursing service administrators cannot administer their expanding complex of organizations and technologies unless they work together more effectively, requiring new forms of cooperation and interdisciplinary, interinstitutional, and interagency involvement. Therefore, innovation in the organization and administration of health services can no longer be an accidental or random occurrence but must be a planned activity, rooted in programs of research, special studies, experimentation, and development.

The environment in which administrative operations occur now includes business technology, automated equipment of rapidly rising sophistication, producing more and better information faster and accelerating communications. This necessarily creates the need for faster action, quicker decisions, and more precise communications. The practicing nurse administrator will have to cope with the advancing technology of tomorrow. However, she must recognize that these are only tools to enhance effectiveness. Dealing with people is a constant challenge; people rarely respond as prescribed by any scientific law or formula. It is important that the nursing service administrator understand the use of the scientific method and approach in solving administrative problems.

Public policy has emerged in the health field as a reflection of the aspirations and frustrations of the people in search of solutions to problems unsolved by voluntary efforts. People have turned to the government for assistance. Although the people have benefited, there is always a concomitant price: a mounting multiplicity of regulations. The lessons always come slowly. People fail to realize that if they are committed to the ideal of health under conditions of democracy they must accept the fact that a successful and acceptable solution for their problems will not come through government edict or legislation. Rather, what is needed is a compound of the energy, initiative, ability, and character of the people in a joint venture with government. This will take imaginative thinking and bold initiatives on the part of the leadership from among those who serve, those who need help, those who budget, and those who control.

In the fulfillment of her role and responsibility, the nursing service administrator is visible and under continuous observation by the administration, the medical staff, the nursing staff, and a host of other groups and agencies who are evaluating, regulating, and negotiating with the institution. In addition, through her many professional relationships with local, state, and regional nursing associations, councils, and committees, she is regularly exposed to her peers. A variety of potential checks and balances exists on her administrative performance, more so than exists in many other fields. To what degree do those groups influence standards of work, behavior, and performance? Experience would indicate this varies considerably at the present time.

There is another factor that contributes to the development and performance of nursing service administration and that adds immeasurably to professional improvement, namely, accreditation. The standards set by the American Nurses' Association for organized nursing services and the criteria set by the National League for Nursing for evaluating nursing service in hospitals and related institutions also help determine professional improvement. The Joint Commission for Hospital Accreditation, in cooperation with the National League for Nursing, also established criteria for evaluation of nursing services. The state boards of nurse examiners have criteria for approvals of programs by law.

In the future, the demand will be for even higher standards, better performance, and more administrative excellence.

Service to people has always been a characteristic of nurses in the field. Although health care institutions must operate as successful business enterprises to survive financially, the primary motivation for nursing service administrators today and in the future must be based on a commitment to serve patients and their families and communities. This is the criterion of social responsibility. If this is not most apparent, visible, and self-evident, there will be more regulation in an attempt to gain other institutional responses to the public's need and expectation for services.

One of nursing service's administrative functions is to contribute to the control process for the successful conduct of operations for overall institutional goal achievement; consequently, motivation at the administrative levels must be consistent with hospital purposes, which are now defined by public policy. These functions must include acceptance of social responsibility and accountability.

The nursing profession is under pressure to become politically more active to (1) improve the care of all people and extend that care to comprehensive coverage, (2) become more recognized with other professions in the health services as a strong social force, and (3) share with other professions and groups the privilege of recognition, equal rights under the law, compensations for work well done, protection of individual rights, and the right to bargain collectively, whether staff nurse, supervisor, or administrator. The strength of the association is dependent on wealth, size of membership, degree of cohesiveness, and importance to the social system. Nurses are under pressure to join the American Nurses' Association; nurses should talk among themselves to build cohesiveness and to develop pride in their work. Nurses are under pressure to document their practices by recording the therapeutic and ecomonic value of their nursing services. This kind of data is helpful to legislative lobbyists for nursing. Every registered nurse who becomes actively involved in the political process becomes a lobbyist for the profession.

Social institutions such as hospitals, educational facilities, and religious institutions are molded by tradition, and, as such, they serve as the carriers of the culture and the keepers of the status quo. As a consequence, they actually precipitate some of the crises in today's society through their toleration of an imbalance between need, technology, and application. Admittedly, the transition from the old to the new is not easy, but whenever and wherever possible nursing service administrators must close the breach in the future.

Lambertson (1969) predicted that the occupation of nursing in the future will encompass two distinct groups: (1) practitioners of nursing developing innovative structures of patterns of practice and (2) practitioners of nursing practicing within the framework of existing structures or patterns of practice. We have added a third: practitioners of nursing capable of directly influencing the nursing structure in the open systems approach. In rendering comprehensive health care, no practitioner is completely independent. The nurses of the future are seen as the nucleus of the health team, with their practice as interdisciplinary and the patients as the focal point. The practitioners' responsibility and accountability have increased greatly. They are expected to be more autonomous and to take on more responsibility. Explicitness in their contribution to total patient care is becoming a must in nursing.

The pressure of cost alone may well move the profession toward more interdisciplinary education, a factor long overdue. The description of the forces at work in changing tomorrow's environment suggests the involvement and support of staffs from many fields and disciplines and in an operational structure conducive to effective performance. In tomorrow's and today's world of health affairs, effective organizational response to people's expectations requires collective effort and harmonious action from the community, boards of directors, medical and nursing profession administrators, and their representative associations. These groups and individuals are all involved, directly or indirectly, in planning, delivering, and financing health care.

What we are suggesting is that the resolution of our health care problems requires shared leadership, that is, a permanent alignment of all the forces involved in the provision of total health care, bonded together by a commonality of purpose and a singlemindedness that transcends the separate organizational professional and personal interests and motives of all who are involved in achieving it.

This brings about another nursing responsibility, that of recruiting, educating, and encouraging the kind of talent that is and will be required for the nurse to cope successfully with the complexity and number of the problems ahead. This also means that the rewards of a career in nursing and nursing service administration must be emphasized with more than money, status, and power. There must be an opportunity to satisfy psychological needs to fulfill the humanitarian goal of ministering to the health and welfare of those in need. Progress in the administration of the nation's health care institutions reveals the influence of professional nursing in achieving a higher standard and quality of administrative leadership. Today, the most potent factor the nursing profession can bequeath on the world of tomorrow is the nursing service administrator. We foresee that the care patients receive will only be as good as the nursing service administrator who directs that service; she will help shape the health care in the world of tomorrow.

Effective administrative practice is dependent on a synthesis of knowledge from the four schools of thought, which underlie our administrative theory and are applied to the purposes and problems of health care operations and to the broader areas of concern in the community health affairs. Effective administrative practice is also dependent on the knowledge base of the nurse practitioner, who must depend, likewise, on a broad spectrum of principles from a variety of disciplines in the solution of specific health problems and who is being encouraged to embrace greater understanding and appreciation of the social and economic consequences of the nursing care program administered to the individual patient.

That there is a body of knowledge that encompasses many fields and disciplines and is applicable to the specialized administration of health institutions has been recognized, established, and accepted by institutions of higher learning in the awarding of graduate degrees. Moreover, by agreement with voluntary agencies for accrediting, it has been possible for the major associations in the health field to create programs providing this knowledge.

Further support of the fact that progress has been achieved in this specialized education is evidenced by the success of the graduates and the respect their degrees receive from employing groups and agencies. In fact, the degree is accepted as a testimony of an interest in personal growth and development; the degree indicates a willingness to acquire more readily the values that professionalizes the responsibility.

Although there is some variation in the approach to graduate education and the curricula differ among schools, trends do indicate considerable unanimity of purpose. The nurses who will be nursing administrators five years from now already have their personalities well developed. These future nursing administrators will have already completed their formal education. Decisions that will affect tomorrow's administrative success must be made today on the basis of partial information.

For example, successful nursing administrators of the future will have a broad knowledge and appreciation of social values. They will be well aware of their organization's contribution to, or impact on, the local, regional, and even national health organization. They will develop ways and means to measure an organization's social values and contributions and in much more meaningful terms than nurses are capable of today.

In addition to having a broad knowledge of the social sciences, tomorrow's successful nursing service administrators will be relatively sophisticated in the field of the behavioral sciences and other combined disciplines. The knowledge the nursing administrator of the future has acquired will enable her to deal effectively with individuals and groups.

The future nursing service administrators will be competent in the quantitative sciences and in relating their technical competence to the world of action. Technology and computer simulations will reduce guesswork in the future; the quantitative sciences will take the place of this guesswork.

Another administrative qualification of the future will be an open systems perspective of health on national, international, or world level rather than the closed organizational views and regionalism of today.

A qualification for tomorrow's nursing service administrators will be understanding and willingness to accept the need for continuous education. In a period of rapid scientific and technological advancement, existing knowledge becomes obsolete in a matter of a few years. New thinking has to be applied; new administrative tools must be mastered as they become available. As the development of new knowledge accelerates, one can no longer afford the time-consuming, trial-and-error method of learning. Obsolescence will quickly overtake the administrators who hesitate to learn continuously.

Finally, the nursing administrators of tomorrow will have a strong sense of morality and humanity. In the 1960s administrators were concerned primarily with scientific management and with improving the standard of living. By 1980, nursing administrators, to be successful, will have to be concerned with improving the quality of life for patients and personnel.

These are broad predictions for successful administration in 1980. If these predictions are valid to a small degree, they point up some true contributions that the new nursing administrator can make to any organization of the future.

Some predictions from our model

1. The nursing administrator will see administration as a task of adjusting the variables of a social system.

2. In solving nursing problems, the nursing administrator will not be able to use a method that ignores the interdependence of variables.

3. The nursing administrator's use of single and supposedly linear relationships will oversimplify her work in problem solving.

4. None of the earlier approaches will have been proven incorrect; it will be shown that they merely tended to concentrate on structure, people, technology, or environment rather than see the whole system as a dynamic, continually changing entity. The result will be that many well-intended changes will have been negated in favor of other equally well-intended changes.

For example, instructors in continuing education consider individual needs and life aspirations. This often occurs at the very time that organizational structure and methods change, creating new sets of relationships; this is a time in which supervisors are introducing new technical systems and care requirements for patients are changing. The nursing administrator must learn to manage *total* systems, not separate components.

In very general terms, we see a future organization in which nurses will make many more decisions on their own, all objectives will be quantified, rewards will be increasingly nonmaterial, structure will be less defined for supervisory and middle and upper nursing service administrative levels, and schedules will be highly mechanized and programmed for the majority of members. We see an organization in which technical systems will change rapidly, demands from the environment will be seen as feedback on individual and organizational performance, and such feedback will be capable of radically influencing behavior within the system. We see an organization in which the full potential of the informal and interpersonal relationships will be developed and used in an attempt to reconcile people and organizations through involvement and commitment.

Finally, we see an organization in which nursing service administrators with expertise in the analysis of systems and in identifying intervariable relationships will make decisions with some knowledge of the ramifications of those decisions. They will also be conscious of their own administrative style, of the effect of the organizational variables, and of the behavior of the system as a whole. They will have more insights into the needs of their personnel, tension levels, and the realities of organizational life, that is, the objectives, tensions, communications, decisions, and actions within the social system.

But most important of all, the approach of administrators of total systems will be to integrate, that is, to see any one change as the predecesor to a series of changes within the system and possibly of the whole system. They will know that symptoms are rarely the problems and that to measure one performance criterion and ignore others will not measure the effectiveness of the system.

We began this book by noting that to understand a system we had to take it apart. The role of the administrator is to put it back together to operate on a total level. Every situation is different. Model building is one way of reducing this complex sociological phenomenon to manageable terms. But a framework of the parts does not constitute the whole; it can only provide a theoretical base for synthesis. Many large systems will become too complex for the individual to handle, even with the aid of models and data processors, and disintegration will occur. But in areas in which synthesis does occur in the struggle of organizational evolution, this synthesis will exist only as long as the system is managed and revitalized as a totality.

REFERENCES

Arndt, C., and Laeger, E.: Role strain in a diversified role set: the director of nursing service. I. Nurs. Res. 19(3):253-259, 1970*a*.

Arndt, C., and Laeger, E.: Role strain in a diversified role set: the director of nursing service. II. Sources of stress, Nurs. Res. 19(3):495-501, 1970*b*.

Lambertson, E. C.: The nurse in future health care delivery systems. Paper presented at United States Army, Baylor University, Program in Health Care Administration, April 1969.

Stull, R. J.: Management of the American hospital. In The American Hospital System, Pensacola, Fla., 1968, Hospital Research and Development Institute, Inc.

ADDITIONAL READINGS

American Nurses' Association: Commission on nursing services statement on the position: role and qualifications of the administrator of nursing service, New York, 1969, The Association.

American Nurses' Association: Standards for organized nursing services, New York, 1965, The Association.

American Hospital Association, Joint Commission on Accreditation of Hospitals: Accreditation manual for hospitals, Chicago, 1970, The Association.

American Nurses' Association: Section Regional Conferences for Professional Nurses: Improvement of nursing practice, New York, 1961, The Association.

American Nurses' Association: Statement on nursing staff requirements for in-patient health care services, New York, 1967, The Association.

Bennis, W. A.: Changing organizations, New York, 1966, McGraw-Hill Book Co.

Cleland, V.: The supervisor in collective bargaining, J. Nurs. Admin. 5:33-35, Sept.-Oct. 1974.

Committee For Economic Development: Union powers and union functions, New York, March 1964, Distribution Division.

Deutsch, M.: Conflict and its resolution. In Smith, E. G., editor: Conflict resolution: contributions of the behavioral sciences, Notre Dame, Ind., 1971, University of Notre Dame Press, pp. 36-57.

Goode, W.: Community within a community: the professions, Am. Sociol. Rev. 22:194-200, April 1957.

Kast, F. E., and Rosenzweig, J. E.: Organization and management, New York, 1970, McGraw-Hill Book Co., pp. 47-48.

Kerr, C.: Industrial conflict and its mediation, Am. J. Sociol. 60:230, 1954.

Leininger, M.: This I believe . . . about interdisciplinary health education for the future, Nurs. Outlook, 19(12):787-791, 1971.

Leininger, M.: The leadership crisis in nursing: a critical problem and challenge, J. Nurs. Admin. 4(2):28-30, 1974.

National Labor Relations Board: National labor relation act jurisdiction over health care institutions, Washington, D. C., 1974, The Board.

National League for Nursing: In pursuit of quality —hospital nursing services, New York, 1964, The League.

National League for Nursing: Nursing education accreditation: trends in accreditation, Report no. 3, New York, 1974, The League.

National League for Nursing: Quest for quality: a self-evaluation guide to patient care, New York, 1966, The League.

National League for Nursing: Self-evaluation guide for nursing services in hospitals and related institutions, New York, 1967, The League.

Nurse practitioner: what the future holds, editorial, Amer. Nurse, November 1974.

U. S. Department of Health, Education and Welfare Public Health Service: Toward quality in nursing: needs and goals, Report of the Surgeon General's Consultant Group on Nursing, Washington, D. C., 1963.

United States Army Medical Field Service School, Brooke Army Medical Center, Fort Sam Houston, Texas.

Yeo, R. D.: Reading the higher education tea leaves, Educ. Technol. 9(8):50-51, 1969.

Index